# Evidence-Based Pediatric NURSING

Sondae Stevens

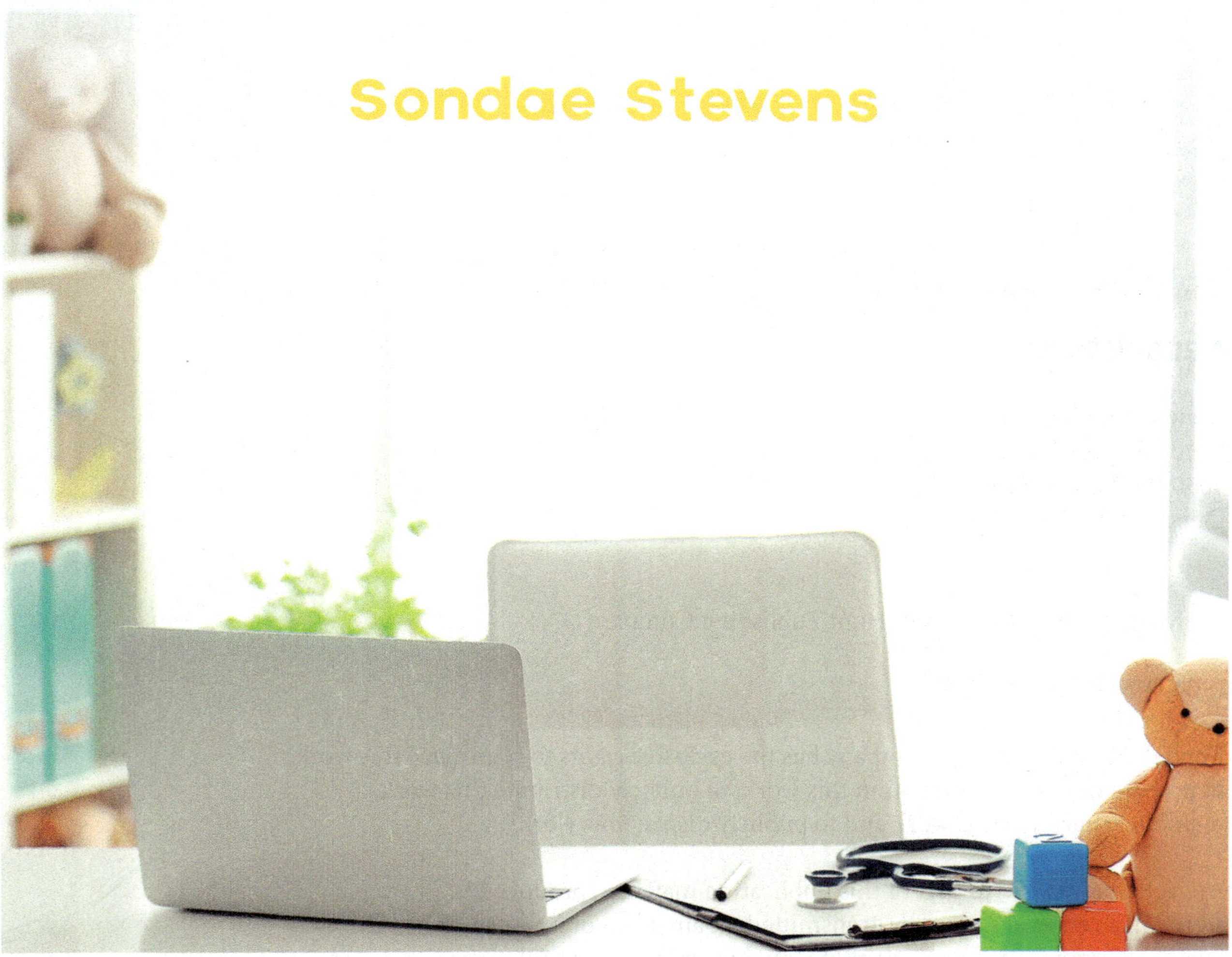

Kendall Hunt
publishing company

Cover image © Shutterstock.com

Kendall Hunt
publishing company

www.kendallhunt.com
Send all inquiries to:
4050 West mark Drive
Dubuque, IA 52004-1840



ISBN 978-1-5249-3552-8



Published in the United States of America

# BRIEF CONTENTS

# CONTENTS

# DEDICATION

My first book is dedicated to my family who supported my passion for writing, and my powerful, pediatric patients who inspired me to reach farther than I ever believed possible.

# ABOUT THE AUTHOR

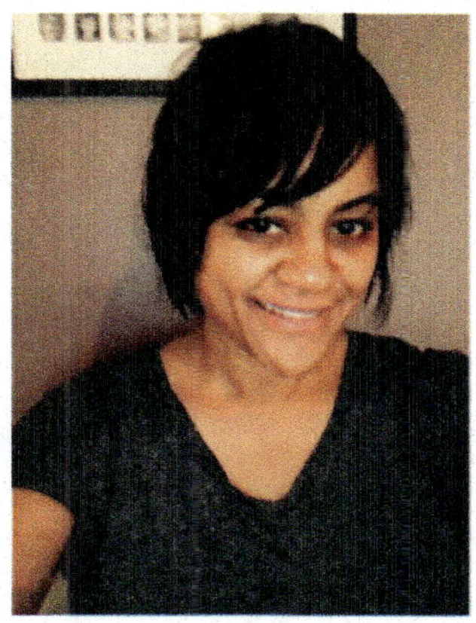

**Sondae Stevens** graduated from the University of California at Berkeley as an Integrative Biology major and Conservation Resource Studies minor. She enhanced her understanding of the relationship between the human body and the physical environment as a labor support doula, a postpartum doula, and a midwife assistant. She continued her education, went to DePaul University, and obtained her MS in Nursing. Nursing school afforded her the perfect environment to link her clinical experiences with the mother-baby continuum to evidence-based practice research while working on her Nursing degree.

As a nurse, she worked on the baby-side of the mother-baby continuum. She worked in General Pediatrics, Hematology-Oncology, and in Critical Care Home Health nursing. It was the experience of being a home health nurse that made her realize the importance of health promotion that keeps children with medical issues at home with their families.

Her passion for Pediatric patients led her to teach Pediatric clinical rotations as an adjunct professor at City Colleges of Chicago, and later become a tenured Assistant Professor and Certified Nurse Educator (CNE).

*Evidence-based Pediatric Nursing* came from a need to teach basic nursing care while incorporating research from an ever-changing health care system. This textbook attempted to bridge the gap between clinical practice, and evidence-based bedside nursing interventions. The strong focus on a preventative lifestyle for children on the illness-wellness continuum reminds nurses to be instrumental in the process of wellness. She hopes to complete another evidence-based textbook for her Obstetric nursing class.

# INTRODUCTION

*Evidence-based Pediatric Nursing* was created to address the contemporary changes in nursing education and bedside nursing using evidence-based practice. When nurses merge evidence-based best practices and bedside nursing, patients are the benefactors. However, cultural barriers in nursing and new norms in patient populations can make this a difficult process. The impact often places nursing research and nursing practice in opposite corners, and the patient stands alone in the middle. Nursing must keep in step, and be forward thinking to address the modern health-care system through the incorporation of evidence-based practice. To keep current, nurses need mechanisms to introduce new evidence-based practices systematically. These practices are an essential link that ensures consistency in nursing practice.

Nursing is particularly subject to cultural barriers because bedside nurses are most likely to ask a more senior bedside nurse for guidance (Estabrooks, Chong, Brigidear, & Profetto-McGrath 2005). It is not that the culture of communication between nurses is flawed; it is that the conversation can prompt a process to use best practices. Only a group effort can affect cultural change. Statements such as "that's the way we have always done that," or "that's the protocol" should require supporting evidence.

This text was designed to inspire the nurse to use a research framework that relies on evidence-based interventions for nursing practice. This framework benefits the novice student nurse as well as the seasoned bedside nurse. Nurses strive to use the best evidence from randomized, controlled trials. When not available, observational studies or case studies support nursing interventions in this book. The same process benefits nurses at the bedside to identify effective nursing interventions. The Cochrane Library, an online resource, contains the most up-to-date systematic reviews of randomized controlled trials. The Cochrane Library implements a formalized process that identifies all published and unpublished studies and evaluates them for quality. The Cochrane Library was used whenever possible, to guide the interventions in this book.

## RECURRING FEATURES

The Institute of Medicine (IOM) (2003) Quality and Safety Education for Nurses (QSEN) competencies, supported and gave context to the evidence-based interventions. Finally, the nursing process was used to identify quality nursing interventions to direct patient care. These competencies include Patient-centered care, Teamwork and Collaboration, Evidenced-based Practice, Quality Improvement, Safety, and Informatics. QSEN competencies connect to each chapter to help enrich the quality of the plan of care. Each chapter will also contain a clinical pearl for practice. Clinical pearls provide wellness tips, medical breakthroughs, and physiologic phenomenon for the bedside nurse. These recurring features support a holistic approach to caring for children.

Another recurring feature in this textbook, is the list of keywords. Unlike a traditional keyword list with a glossary, readers can find the meaning imbedded in the text. This is an active reading feature to promote student engagement. The list should act as a checklist that the reader understood the content. If not, the reader can return to the term embedded in the text.

Student nurses are a vital link for getting new evidence-based practices to the bedside. As they integrate experiences from texts, simulation, clinical sites, and skills labs, they ultimately need to practice in real life. The new graduate is too often thought of as a liability instead of an asset because they have not had the experience to be effective at the bedside. Evidence-based practice is a way to connect the new graduate to the health-care team and introduce responsibility for outcomes before they are proficient in nursing skills. Empowering a student nurse in this way promotes multidisciplinary communication and respect. This concise text provides a holistic model for pediatric nursing education and bedside nursing for all licensure levels, including new graduates and seasoned registered nurses.

CHAPTER 1

# PEDIATRIC CONSIDERATIONS

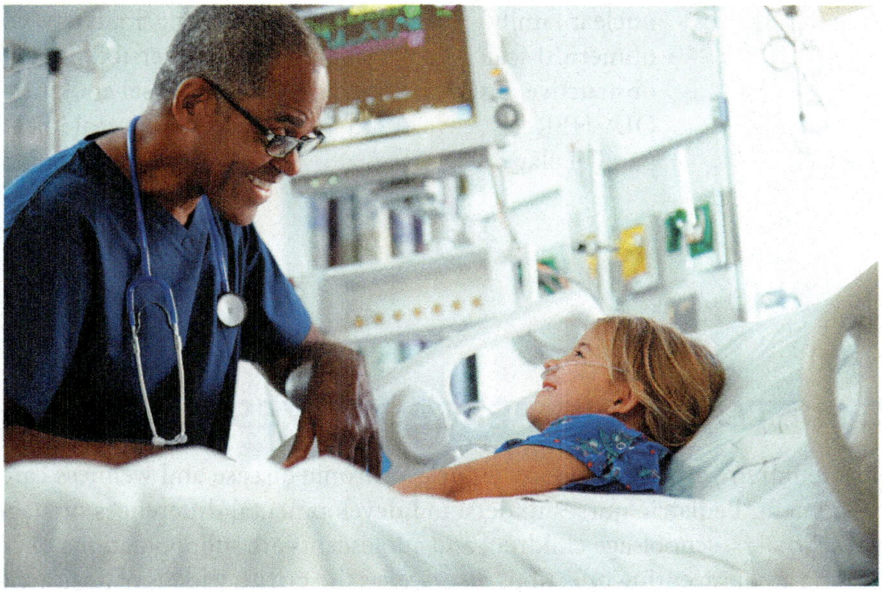

© Monkey Business Images/Shutterstock.com

## LEARNING OUTCOMES

1. Describe the history of pediatric legislation in America.
2. Recognize significant developmental features of families.
3. Synthesize data from physical assessment to create a focused assessment for families, playtime, emergencies, and end-of-life issues for infants through adolescents.
4. Utilize the nursing process to provide safe, comprehensive health care to pediatric patients.
5. Construct a comprehensive "family-centered" teaching plan for children from infants to adolescents.
6. Utilize therapeutic communication skills to accommodate children from infants to adolescents.
7. Identify situations specific to the child-bearing family that may cause ethical dilemmas and/or require legal actions.

## KEY TERMS

adoptive family
anticipatory grief
apnea monitor
asphyxiation
atraumatic care
associative play
authoritarian parents
authoritative parents
blended family
bolus
central venous access devices
complicated grief
cooperative play
cross-generational family
deltoid injection
democratic parenting
detachment
distraction
EMLA
electrocardiogram (ECG)
electroencephalogram (EEG)
FACES
family culture
family support system
family stressors
fentanyl
FLACC
foster family
guided imagery
helicopter parents
kangaroo care
lidocaine and prilocaine
magical thinking
noncommunicating children's pain checklist
nuclear family
numerical scale
obstructive lung conditions
OUCHER
parallel play
parental grief
patient-controlled analgesia (PCA)
peripheral venous access devices
permissive parents
relaxation
respiratory failure
respiratory insufficiency
restrictive lung disease
same-sex families
sense-pleasure skills
separation anxiety
sibling grief
single-parent families
social-affective skills
solitary play
stranger anxiety
submersion injury
universal choking sign
ventrogluteal injection
vulnerable population

## PEDIATRIC HISTORY AND PERSPECTIVES

Pediatric nurses treat children with acute disease, injuries, chronic disease and wellness care, through a lens of growth and development. Pediatric nurses understand developmental differences or stages of childhood. Infants, toddlers, preschoolers, school-age children, and adolescents are subpopulations of childhood.

Historically, treating and preventing infectious disease was the primary focus of health-care professionals. As vaccinations and better sanitation became available, the focus shifted to acute injuries and chronic disease. Infectious disease became less common than chronic disease. The goal then became to provide healthy children and their families with strategies for a healthy lifestyle. Children who accessed the health-care system had the opportunity to prevent infectious diseases.

In all situations, pediatric nurses support families through a special skill set that integrates the Society of Pediatric Nurses competencies, the nursing process, anatomy and pathophysiology, Quality and Safety Education for Nurses (QSEN) competencies and cultural competence.

Traditionally, pediatric nursing played a supportive role in pediatric medicine. Today pediatric nursing uses a holistic model that includes physical, emotional, intellectual, and spiritual assessments to deliver care to children and their families. The Society of Pediatric Nurses defines competencies for prelicensure, pediatric nurses. These include: applying anatomical and developmental differences in the neonatal, infant, toddler, children, and adolescent populations; providing children and families support for health promotion in context of the child's family; effective communication techniques that are culturally sensitive to the child, family, and health-care team; demonstration of safety techniques to prevent injuries or illnesses; an awareness of the economic, social, and political influences outside the family that act on the child's growth and development and family functioning; and the effects of the overlapping orbs of ethics, morality, and legislation (American Nurses Association, 2008).

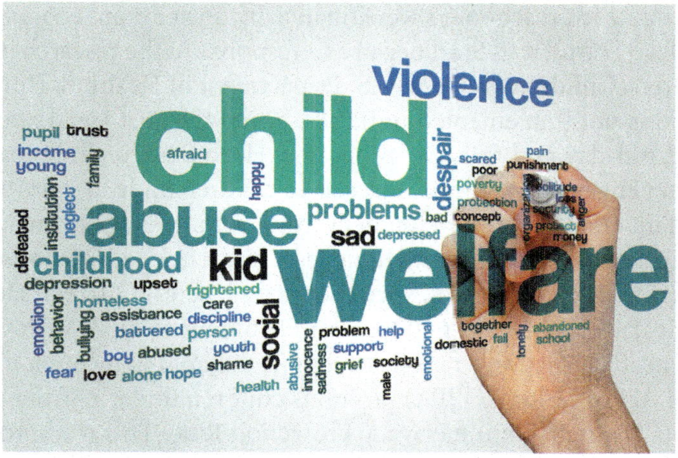

© ibreakstock/Shutterstock.com

Health care for every American has historically been challenging to implement. Government programs have struggled to support children since 1912 with the creation of the Children's Bureau of Child Welfare by President Taft (Sribnick, E. G. 2011). This was a grassroots effort that took 11 bills in Congress and 6 years to finally pass protection for children This was the first program to support children and families in America (Children's Bureau, U.S. Department of Health & Human Services n.d.). It took on issues such as infant mortality, birth rate, orphanages, juvenile reports, dangerous occupations, accidents and diseases, and child employment (Children's Bureau Timeline n.d.). President Lyndon B. Johnson rolled out several programs to help low-income families that included Medicaid. Medicaid became law in 1965 (Children's Bureau Timeline n.d.). Medicaid gave health-care insurance to low-income families (Children's Bureau Timeline n.d.). However, states were allowed to determine the level of coverage they would provide (Children's Bureau Timeline n.d.). This inconsistent coverage depended on where people lived, and subsequently, created disparities in lower income populations.

Inequitable health coverage is the fundamental flaw in the American health care system that is different from other developed countries. A system that ensures coverage for well-employed people leaves little protection for vulnerable populations like women, children and elderly citizens. The Affordable Care Act (ACA) extended Medicaid to cover almost all low-income people and decrease health care disparities. If the repeal of the ACA occurs, vulnerable, low-income families will not have access to high-quality preventative health care coverage, as Medicaid is the largest insurer in America. The CHIP (Children's Health Insurance Program) program was developed for children whose parents make too much money for Medicaid coverage, but cannot afford private insurance (Eligibility n.d.).

The CHIP program expired September 30, 2017, and remains expired until the US Congress passes new legislation. CHIP served 9 million children and covered check-ups, prescription drugs, immunizations, and dental care (Strauss 2017).

The Child Nutrition Act of 1966 was another program signed into law by President Johnson based on research that supported the link between nutrition, behavior, and learning (Children's Bureau Timeline n.d.) It was used to supplement breakfasts and lunches at school for children from low-income households (National School Lunch Program n.d.). This program was also subject to local government decisions about eligibility and did not use a national formula used in all states, and created health disparities (NSLP n.d.). However, it provided another option for food insecure households. Another popular program, the Special Supplemental Food Program for Women, Infants, and Children (WIC) was a part of the Child Nutrition Act and provided support for families at nutritional risk (Children's Bureau Timeline n.d.). This program has become a mainstay in the lives of families whose incomes are below 185% of the US Poverty Income guidelines (Women, Infants, and Children (WIC) n.d.). This benchmark equals an annual income of 45, 520 for a family of four in 2017 (Poverty Guidelines 2017).

President Johnson recognized preschoolers were financially, socially and economically disadvantaged and supported the program, Head Start. Head Start began as a response to the research link between breakfast and better test scores for children (Children's Bureau, U.S. Department of Health & Human Services n.d.).

However, Head Start was not implemented until 1995 when the first Head Start grants went into effect. In 1998, benefits included full-day and full year programs. Head Start includes early childhood education, health, nutrition, and parent engagement. Head Start serves children under 5 years of age. Head Start supports prenatal outcomes and infant and toddler development from birth. Head Start makes provisions for seasonal and migrant workers, indigenous Americans, and homeless children. Head Start works independently of local school districts and is usually accessed through social service agencies (Office of Head Start, n.d.).

Families in 2017 must earn less than $24,600 for a family of four to qualify (Poverty Guidelines 2017).

Children continue to need legislation to protect them in a changing technological world. The Children's Online Privacy Protection Act of 2000 (COPPA) prohibits children under 13 from posting identifiable information about themselves (Children's Online Privacy Protection Rule. This is to protect children from online predatory encounters. COPPA created a privacy policy, age restrictions, and required parental consent for websites to collect a child's personal information (COPPA 2015).

All of these programs help benefit children in need. Today, 15.6 million children live in food-insecure homes (United States Department of Agriculture 2015). The fight for better legislation for children must continue. Until all American children have food, access to health care, and high-quality early education, the funding of children's programs will remain at the mercy of partisan politics.

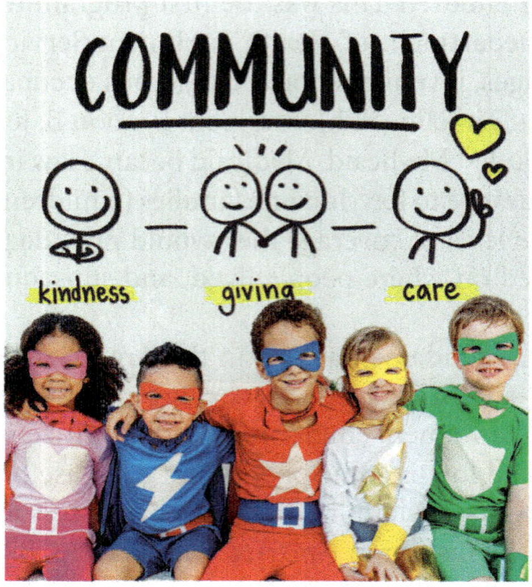


© Rawpixel.com/Shutterstock.com

Children are a **vulnerable population**, a disadvantaged subset or a population that requires specialized care. Special protections are essential because children are not able to adequately protect themselves and are subject to the choices and circumstances of their parents (Shivayogi, P. 2013).

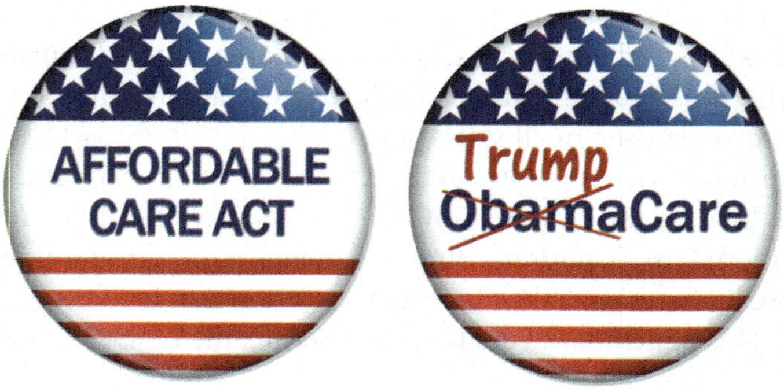


© Karen Roach/Shutterstock.com

According to the Kaiser Family Foundation (2017), by 2015, 28.5 million Americans still had no health-care coverage under the ACA, and 74% of uninsured people had at least one full-time worker in the household. The study notes most uninsured people come from low-income families and are people of color. People without insurance do not receive preventative medical care or care for chronic diseases. In 2015, 20% of people went without medical care because they could not afford it. These same people cannot access medical care until they are in need of emergency services that cost more than preventative care. As it stands now, the future of healthcare is experiencing dynamic change. Health-care professionals must participate in the process to ensure patients are getting what they need, as the health-care industry becomes more business driven. It has been fifty-two years since Medicaid began, and all low-income Americans do not have access to health insurance (Kaiser Family Foundation 2016).

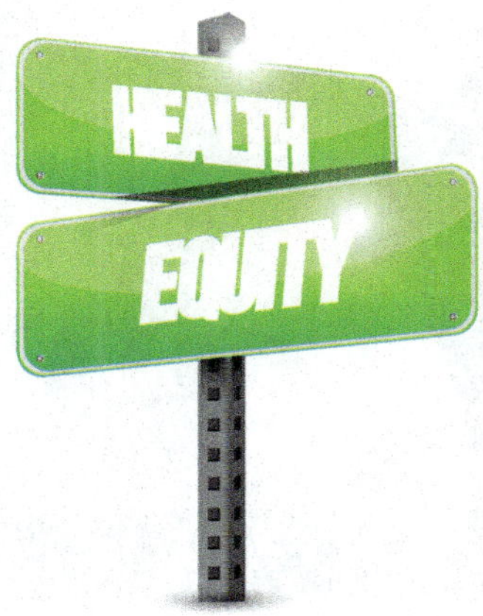

© alexmillos/Shutterstock.com

Healthy People, a federal government program run by the U.S. Health and Human Services, sets priorities for child health every 10 years. For the last 30 years, Healthy People created a report card to assess the health of the United States. The overarching goals are to improve the quality of American life through the decrease in disease, disability, injury and premature death, and health disparities. The goals also include health equity, improvement of social and physical environments to support healthy human development and lifestyle behaviors. One of the Healthy People 2020 objectives tracks the obesity rate for children and adolescents. The obesity rate for children and adolescents increased from the 2005–2008 rate of 16.1%. The goal was to decrease obesity to 14.5%. Unfortunately, 2011–2014 the rate was already 17%. More has to be done to support families with children at-risk for obesity. Healthy People identified a trend where obesity rates decreased with increasing income. Approximately 20% of children are obese who live at or just above the poverty line (Healthy People n.d.).

This relationship highlights the dependency between social issues and child health; both need to progress simultaneously. Pediatric nurses must gain sensitivity when talking with patients and families to these issues, so their nursing interventions and teaching approach realistic goals. Nurses need ongoing knowledge of social service supports and the changing political environment from administration to administration.

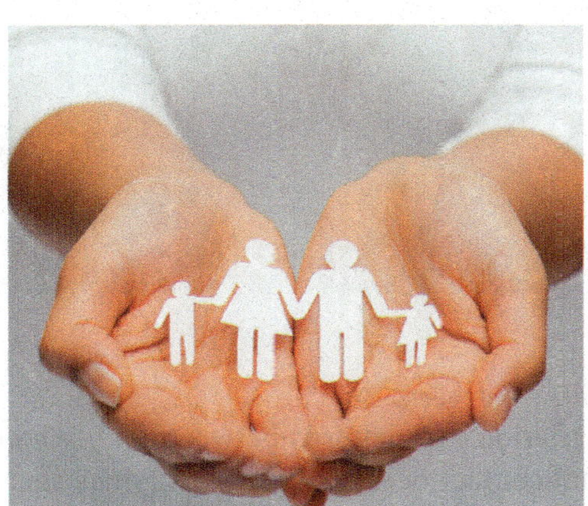
© Syda Productions/Shutterstock.com

## Family Structure

Families are all different and require different approaches. Families are complex systems, and each one has its own dynamic. Families have diverged from the media-driven images of the 1950s and 1960s into every conceivable permutation. However, all families have specific features that include familial roles, inherited patterns of behavior, and subtle, unspoken communications. The combination of these factors produces a family dynamic (Halpern-Manners, Warren., Raymo, & Nicholson 2015).

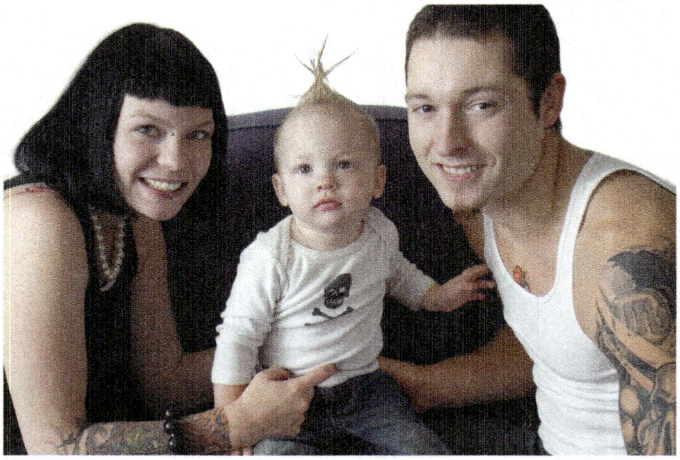

© Cindy Hughes/Shutterstock.com

Familial roles have shifted due to social pressures such as declining employment security, inequitable jobs, and frequent family transitions. Differentiation of gender roles and divorce also impact familial roles. These roles go beyond mother and father to breadwinner, the enabler, the problem child, or the responsible child. Family roles are created to fulfill family needs (Halpern-Manners, Warren, Raymo & Nicholas 2015).

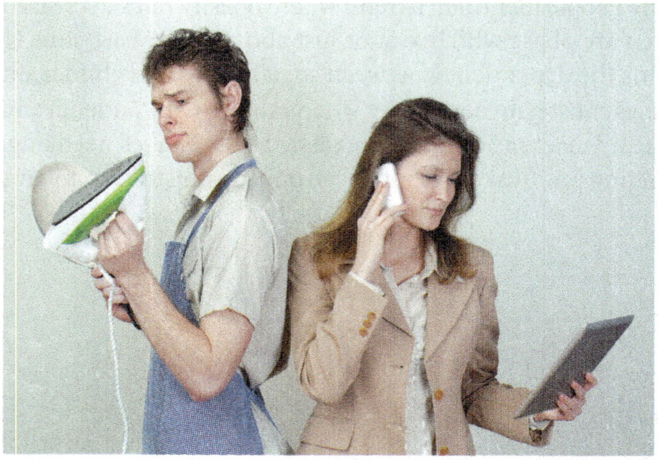

© Dmitri Ma/Shutterstock.com

Family dynamics include the relationship patterns between family members. Family dynamics impact future relationships even if minimal contact occurs. Family dynamics also impact self-concept, interaction with the world, and the psychological health of a child (Behere, A. P., Basnet, P., & Campbell, P. 2017).

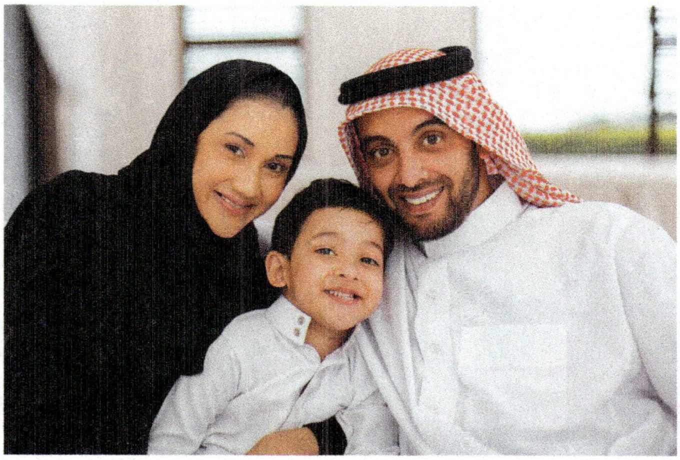

© michaeljung/Shutterstock.com

Families are usually not egalitarian. Parents chart the direction of the family and children play supportive roles in their family journey. Hierarchies set from previous generations can impact current and future generations. When caring for children and their respective families, understanding the roles and dynamics in the family can help a nurse deliver customized care.

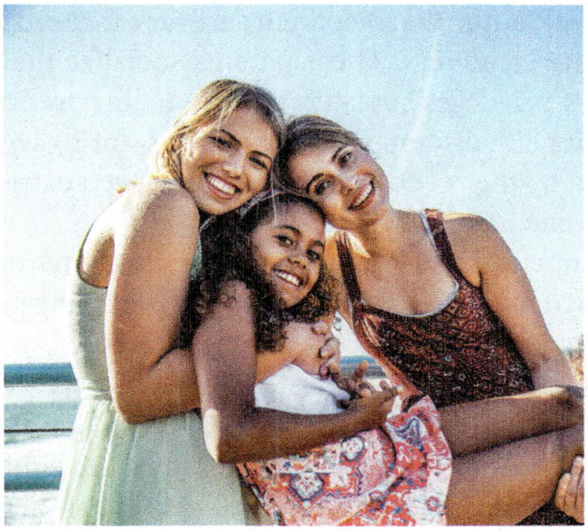

© oneinchpunch/Shutterstock.com

In healthcare, a family member can be anyone the family designates as the family. The composition of a family may fall into typical structures. According to Hampson & Beavers (2017), there are several family types a practitioner may encounter.

The American Academy of Pediatrics (2017) defines several family types. A **nuclear family** includes two opposite-sex parents and their children who can be biologic, step, adopted or foster children. The United States has an increasing number of **single-parent families** where there are one parent and one or more children living together. A **cross-generational family** has a family member, 65 years of age or older, living in the home. An **adoptive family** or **foster family** is a placement for a child or children who live in a regulated living environment without any members of the birth family, with one or two parents. A **never-married family** considers themselves a family without a legal marriage and has at least one child. A **blended family** or includes two parents and at least one stepparent, stepsibling, or half-sibling. **Same-sex families** include members of the Lesbian Gay Bisexual Transsexual Queer Intersex Asexual (LGBTQIA) community who have children. (AAP, 2017)

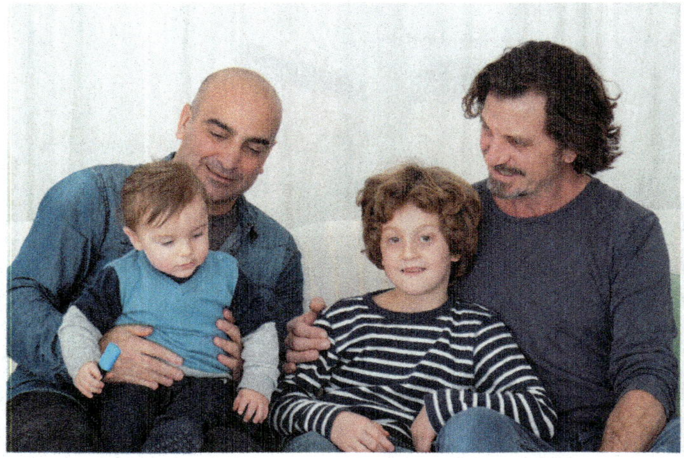

© Cineberg/Shutterstock.com

Parenting styles can differ from family to family. Pinquart (2016) defines parenting styles and finds no benefit to one structure over another on academic achievement of children. **Authoritarian parents** attempt to control the child's behaviors and attitudes through unquestioned rules and expectations. They believe children need parental control because of an inherent strong will that benefits from molding to societal influences. Authoritarian parents believe it is loving to teach the child to obey authority to ready them for school, work, and society. The rules are nonnegotiable. **Permissive parents** apply little to no control over the child's behaviors and consult the child when making family decisions. Parents have few demands of children and discipline is infrequent. **Authoritative parents** direct the child's behavior by setting rules and explaining the reason for each rule set. Unlike authoritarian parents, authoritative parents are task focused. Rules are open to interpretation for each task as opposed to resolute standards. These parents socialize their children to respect the family value system. Parents may take away privileges but later reinstate them based on new rules. **Passive parents** are uninvolved, indifferent, and emotionally distant. Passive parents want to avoid negative experiences. Passive parents are generally overwhelmed by the role of parent and may need extra support to comply with health-care interventions (Bettany & Kerrane, 2016; Pinquart 2016).

**Helicopter parents** try to compensate for the ultra-competitive environment most American children experience. These parents help, when helping is not necessary. The learning process inevitably involves failure, and this is something children have to learn because it is a reality in society. Protecting children from failure hinders their emotional development (Bettany & Kerrane 2016).

Socialization requires conflict, and children, even when they are infants must experience conflict to understand the natural strengths and weaknesses of an individual to manage conflict. Allowing children and parents the opportunity to experience conflict deepens the relationship between parent and child, and prepares parents and children to learn from experience instead of parental attempts to control experiences (Lewis & Weber 2015).

Nurses educate and reinforce parenting rules of American society that include realistic limits and expectations related to the developmental level of the child. Parents honor the child's feelings and provide role modeling and reinforcement for appropriate behavior. Most importantly, parents can consider the child's behavior, not the child. Children are not labeled "good" or "bad," they are praised for good behavior and disciplined over bad behavior. Children who are labeled good or bad may have a dysfunctional self-image within the family (Gray 2013).

Pediatric nurses complete a family assessment to identify the family's structure and function, to best support the child's development. An assessment identifies strengths and weaknesses in the family. Nurses perform comprehensive family assessments to identify strengths and weaknesses. Healthy families share similar characteristics such as effective communication techniques that include listening to one another, clear rules, responsiveness to emotional and social needs, affirmation and respect for all members, trust, shared responsibility, an adaptability to family stressors, shared values and rituals, and an ability to ask for help outside of the family (Cordova, Heinze, Mistry, Hsieh, Stoddard, Salas-Wright, & Zimmerman 2014). Parents contribute

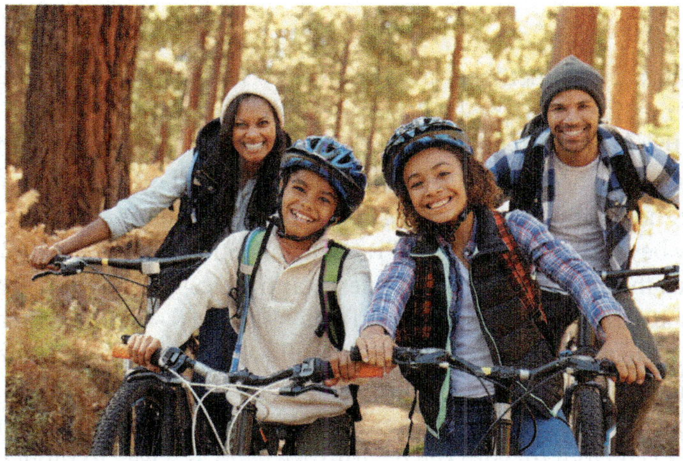

© Monkey Business Images/Shutterstock.com

to the assessment to create a complete the clinical picture. For example, if a parent believes a child isn't acting themselves, the nurse takes the parent's assessment of the child seriously and follows up with a set of vitals and an assessment. Some assessment signs are specific to a patient, using the assessment of the child's parents is an application of Family Centered Care. Likewise, the child's opinion must also be considered and incorporated into care when possible (Boztepe & Kerimoğlu Yıldız 2017).

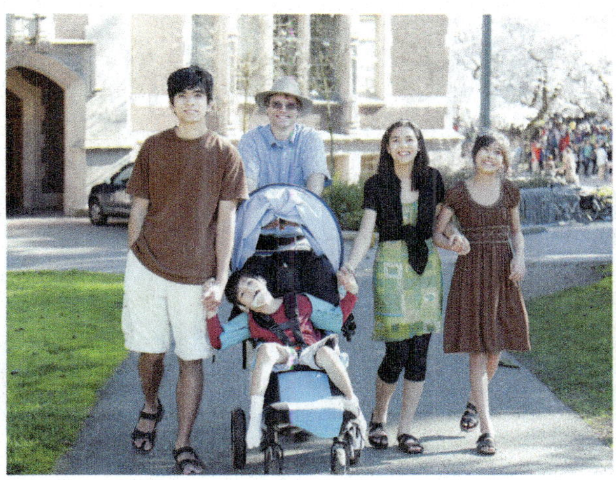

© Jared Jai Wicklund/Shutterstock.com

Nurses take a medical history of parents, siblings, and grandparents, and consult the family on the members of the family. Nurses identify developmental play the family can work on as the child grows, such as a preschool child learning to share toys and space. Nurses assess **family culture** that includes religion, behavior, attitudes, and values. A stressor is any interaction that causes a stress response. Stressors may consist of the number and age of children, parental workload, lack of support from one's spouse or other family members, and divorce (Clark, Michel, Early, & Baltes 2014).

Nurses must determine the family environment and if it is congruent with the child and their medical treatment. Nurses must determine the availability of and family interactions with community resources. Finally, nurses analyze the **family support system** for availability of extended relationships, that may include availability extended family, work, and peer relationships, social systems and community resources. These support systems can assist the family in meeting needs or adapting to a work or peer relationships (Wise 2017).

## Family Centered Care

Especially in adult populations, family members are considered visitors by the nurse when patients are partners in care. Historically, Pediatric medicine undervalued the role of the mother and family in a child's recovery. Often, parents were isolated from their children while doctors and nurses took care of all the medical needs of the child, but they could not replace the psychosocial benefits of being supported by family members (Harrison 2010).

Family-centered care benefits children regarding clinical care, parental satisfaction, and costs from birth to 12 years of age, and possibly beyond (Shields, Zhou, Pratt, Taylor, Hunter & Pascoe 2012). Nurses strive to engage family members to earn trust through listening and honest communication. Health-care professionals are experts in health care, but families are experts regarding their family members. Family-centered nursing care includes several aspects. Nurses must create a partnership with the child and all members of the family that present with the child (Kuo, Frick, & Minkovitz 2011). Family-centered care must incorporate cultural sensitivity and be flexible enough to incorporate all patients into the nurse–family relationship (Kuo, Frick & Minkovitz 2011).

The child and the family collaborate with the health-care team as a way to model teaching in the hospital. Families are trained to complete health care for their child family member. Nurses must also understand the availability of community resources to support families once they leave the hospital setting.

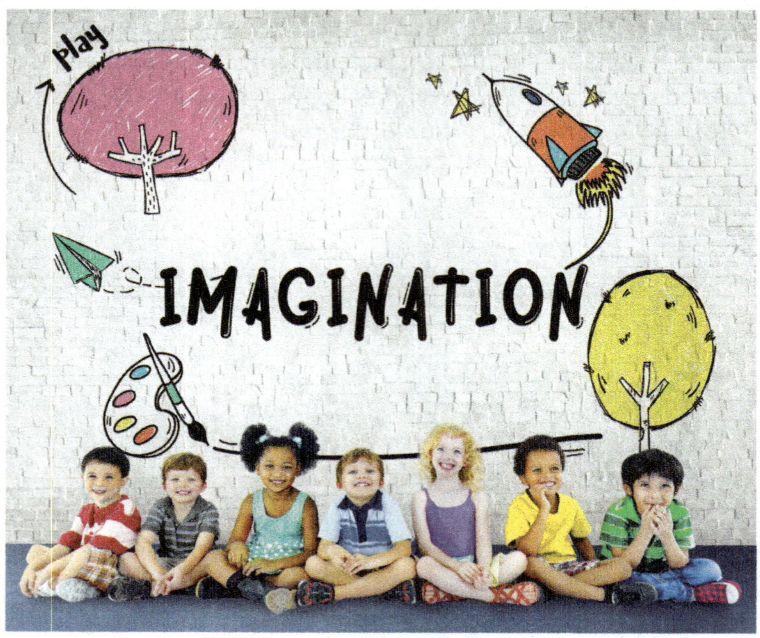




## Play

### QSEN Application

Evidence-based practice calls for nurses to "[i]ntegrate best current evidence with clinical expertise and patient/family preferences and values for delivery of optimal health care . . . knowledge of basic scientific methods and processes . . . and to include research evidence, clinical expertise, and patient/family values."

New research on the importance of play helps guide pediatric patient stays in the hospital. The nurse employs age-appropriate play to promote growth and development of the child.

From Quality and Safety Education for Nurses http://qsen.org/competencies/pre-licensure-ksas/#evidence-based_practice

According to the United Nations High Commission for Human Rights, play is a fundamental need for every child. However, for the last 50 years childhood play has decreased as adults utilize more control over children's activities (United Nations 2013).

There are consequences of this loss. The most dramatic decline has been in free play.
Free play is self-directed play created by the child and does not include organized play such as sports or crafting. Free play has two opposing forces working on it, parental fear and mainstream schooling. Parental fear originates with the responsibility to keep the child safe. There are many social pressures that exert forces on American children (Gray 2013).

Children in past decades played outside without parental involvement. However, concerns over violence and abduction trigger fear in parents. It is essential that if safe environments are not available in the child's neighborhood, parents must make environments away from the dangers and perceived dangers of risky environments. The benefits for children who have access to these free play environments build skills necessary to be effective members of society (Gray 2013).

When children engage in free play, they are experimenting with the world around them. According to Gray (2013), free play promotes self-understanding of interests, strengths, and weaknesses. Free play creates opportunities for problem-solving, decision-making, and self-control. Children become emotionally intelligent, by learning to manage emotions such as anger and fear. Children who engage with one another in free play learn to make friends and see other children as equals. However, the most important function of free play is happiness and autonomy. Children have a human drive to play opposed by the social demand for rigorous schooling at earlier and earlier ages. Since 1950, the suicide rate of children under 15 years of age has quadrupled, as the rates for 25–40-year-olds rose slightly. As politicians call for more schooling and more tests, children will need more opportunities to engage in free play (Gray 2013).

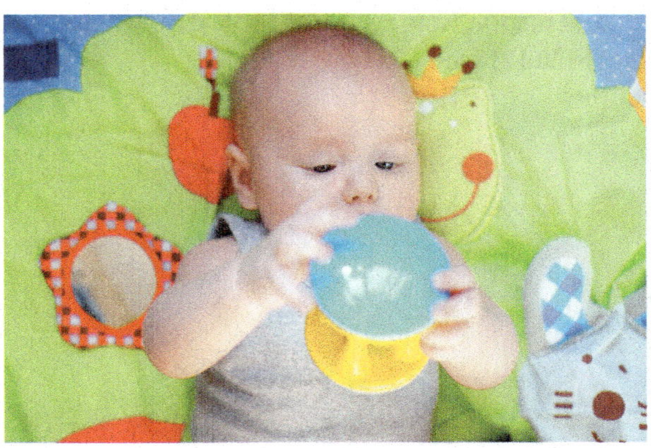

© Maria Sbytova/Shutterstock.com

**Fig 1-1** An infant engages in solitary play

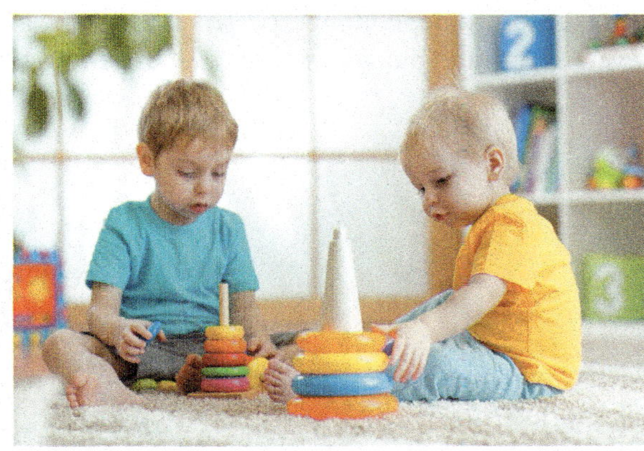

© Oksana Kuzmina/Shutterstock.com

**Fig 1-2** Toddlers participate in parallel play

Children engage in social play, exploratory play, and object play. Social play is any play that includes other children or adults. Mildred Parton (1932) defined four levels of play: solitary play, parallel play, associative play, and cooperative play (see Fig 1-1through 1-4). She found as these stages unfold from birth to school age, earlier stages could reappear. As a child develops skills to engage in cooperative play, they will still engage in solitary play. However, the solitary play develops and becomes more sophisticated. It is not immature to re-engage in earlier stages of play, the process may not be linear. It is developmentally beneficial to develop play throughout childhood, and expect variations from child to child (Parton 1932).

Children benefit from all types of play and need ample time to do so. Exploratory play may include art projects that express emotions or emotional situations. Children use the objects around them to create meaning. According to White (2012), this type of play leads to object play. Object play directly increases gross and fine motor skills and helps children understand the tools for living. These skills are the basis for higher order thinking in science, technology, engineering, and technology (STEM) (White 2012).

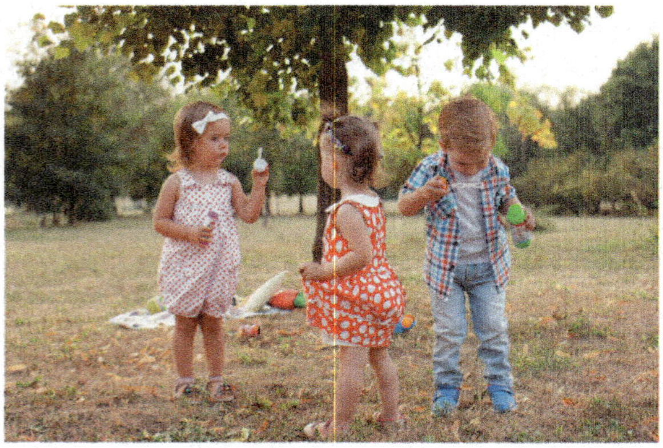


Fig 1-3 Preschoolers engage in associative play

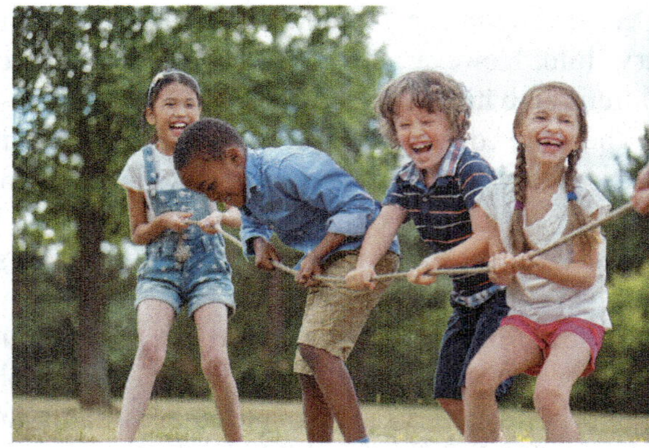


Fig 1-4 School-age kids cooperatively play

Children also spontaneously engage in pretend play. Pretend play creates a basis for creativity, language and literacy, and executive function (White, R. 2012). Pretend play promotes dynamic problem-solving because it uses divergent thinking or the identification of possible solutions to problems. This is a hallmark of a creative mind. Language and literacy increases with pretend play. Language consists of many symbols that represent ideas. Pretending necessitates the use of symbols and invokes empathy, formal computation, and counterfactual thinking or "what if" thinking. Children who understand the representation of symbols learn to read and comprehend that reading (White, R. 2012).

Executive functioning includes self-control of thought, action, and emotion (White, R. 2012). Executive function also translates to school readiness, development of memory, attention, intelligence, morality, and emotion regulation. Evidence of executive function by age four can predict long-term outcomes such as physical health, substance dependency, personal finances, and criminal behavior. Some studies indicate pretend play for even 10 minutes a day improves executive function (White, R. 2012) (see Fig 1-5).

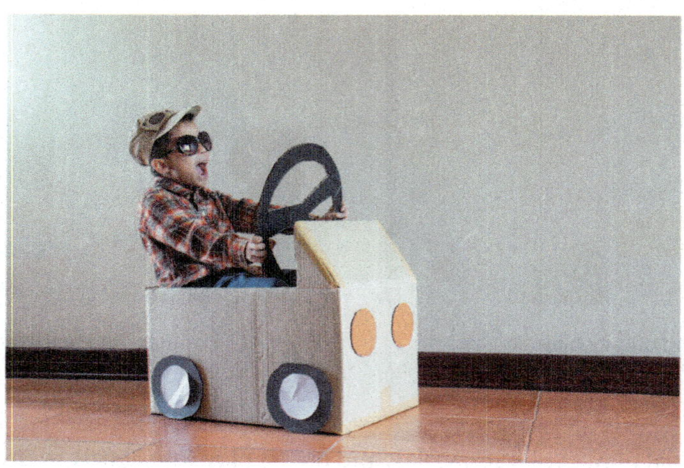


Fig 1-5 The development of the imagination is the work of childhood

Nursing can support children by incorporating a plan for age-appropriate medical play each day if their conditions permit. Play is a mechanism for the child to develop new abilities, modified in many creative ways based on the individual care plan. Parents are essential in the planning and implementation of play. It is an opportunity to teach parents about healthy, developmentally sound choices for their child based on their growth and development stage.

Play becomes the work of childhood that results in the development of several social skills including **social-affective skills** where children learn to take pleasure and fun in relationships. Play becomes the arena to exercise these skills, and these new abilities will improve with use (Jen, Wu & Gentry 2016).

## Play and Socialization

There are several roles children will adopt during play. The child who engages in **solitary play** engages in activity without stimulation from other people. Toddlers choose **parallel play** during free play. Toddlers play independently but among other children. Preschoolers engage in **associative play** where children play together without organization. School-age children engage in **cooperative play** where organized play happens in groups (Dyer, S., & Moneta, G. B. 2006).

For more examples, see Chapter 2 Growth and Development.

### Clinical Pearl

Parents need education about the impacts of media on young children's growth and development. Never before have children had the potential for 24 hours a day media exposure.

Excessive exposure to media has negative impacts on child physical, cognitive, social, and emotional well-being. Children cannot become reliant on media without parental facilitation. It is up to adults to protect the experience of childhood and encourage children to define their own lives without the pressure of unrealistic images portrayed in the media. (Jordan, A., and Romer, D. 2014).

Members of the pediatric health-care team use play to build a rapport and trust with a child. Nurses may count or sing a song to help a child through a procedure. The nurse may also incorporate play into wellness visits during the physical assessment.

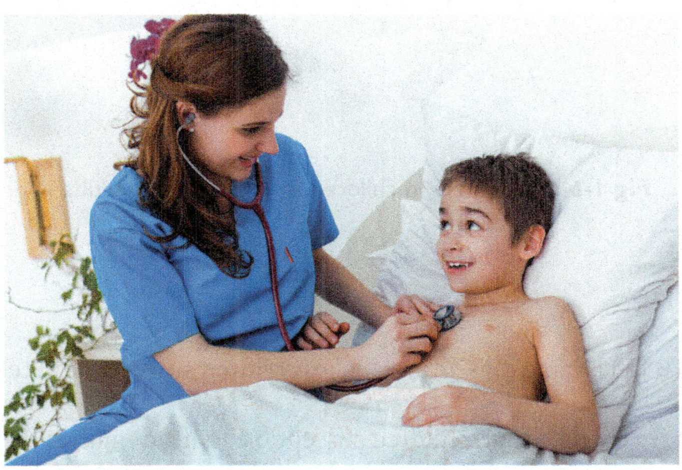

© Lighthunter/Shutterstock.com

### Physical Assessment

According to Caple (2016), a nursing assessment begins with vital signs and a good, physical exam. The physical exam generally proceeds through the steps inspection, percussion, palpation, and auscultation for each body system. The nurse begins the assessment with a warm and private room. The suggested examination occurs in a secure, comfortable position, and may occur on a parent's lap if desired. Make sure any intimidating equipment (needles or the otoscope), is stored away from the child's view. The nurse takes time for age-appropriate play and develops a rapport with the child prior to beginning an examination. The exam uses expected growth and development principles to obtain an accurate physical assessment. Once the child is at ease, and cooperative, the nurse proceeds with the assessment (Caple 2016).

**Atraumatic care** includes the use of interventions that minimize or eliminate physical and psychological distress in the child. Nurses explain each step of the exam, regardless of age, through the use of age-appropriate communication techniques and simple language. Nurses also use medical play. Children manipulate and handle medical equipment on the doll or draw a picture, and then translate that experience to their own care (Huff, Hamlin, Wolski, McClure, Eliades, Weaver & Shelestak 2009).

An assessment unfolds, for school-age children and adolescents, in a head to toe manner (Baid 2006). However, for infants and younger children, the assessment moves from least invasive to most invasive systems (Greydanus 2008). The heart and lung assessments begin the physical assessment, leaving the ears and throat for last (Greydanus 2008). The child and family are encouraged to ask questions during physical exams. A discussion, with time for questions about any findings, occurs after the examination.

Children are different from adults (see Fig 1-6). Their organs are immature and not always fully developed at birth. Familiarization with anatomical and physiological differences will help identify normal findings and abnormal findings, and guide the nursing process. Nurses begin with the prenatal history to determine the gestational age at birth. Preterm babies showed delayed growth and development related to gestational length (Greydanus 2008).

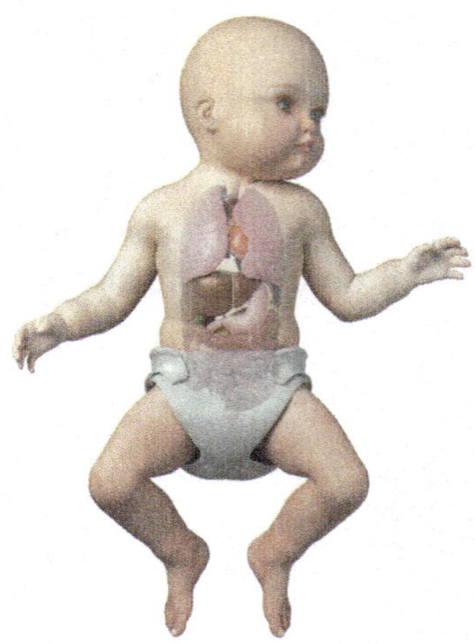

© Sebastian Kaulitzki/Shutterstock.com

**Fig 1-6** Differences in children as compared to adults

All from (Greydanus 2008)

- Body Surface Area (BSA) is large for size and makes children susceptible to temperature loss and dehydration (abdomen)
- Head is large with a weak and makes children susceptible to head injuries (head)
- Anterior fontanel closes between 12–18 months; posterior fontanel closes between 6–8 weeks (head)
- Brain cells myelinate 1 year of age (head)
- Tongue is large in the developing oral cavity and can obstruct the airway (mouth)
- Trachea is short and narrow and easy to occlude (throat)
- Cardiac output relates to rate, not preload and afterload, and makes heart rates fast (heart)
- Higher metabolic rate, increased oxygen demands, higher caloric input (Mouth)
- Ribs have a higher percentage of cartilage and makes the chest more flexible (lung)
- Alveoli are smaller and hold a smaller volume (lung)
- Diaphragmatic breathing releases more CO2 (lung)
- Protruding abdomen with weak abdominal muscles offer little protection from trauma (abdomen)
- Kidneys do not concentrate urine until 1–2 years of age making children susceptible to dehydration (above hipbone)

- Extracellular water is higher in infants and makes them susceptible to hypovolemia (arm)
- Bones have a higher percentage of cartilage and children are prone to fractures (leg)
- Muscle mass is small and underdeveloped (leg)

(Graydanus 2008).

Physical Assessment begins with a general inspection of the appearance of a child. The typical child presents as clean and appropriately dressed. Children make eye contact when they are comfortable. Children should have appropriate language, social, and physical skills (Greydanus 2008).

Vitals Sign Tree

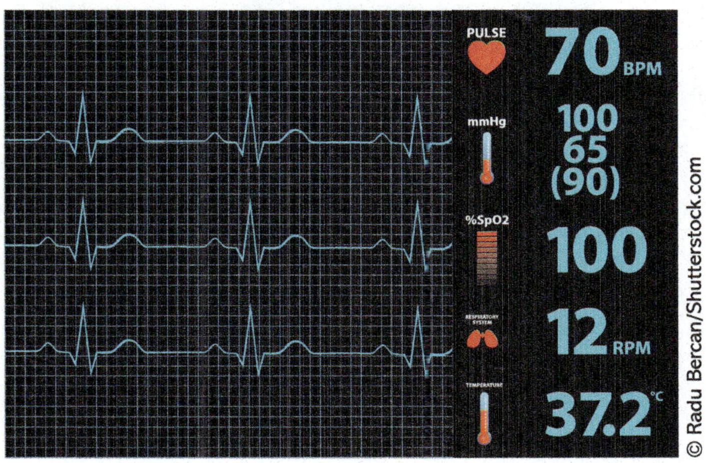


**Fig 1-7** Vitals begin the assessment

Head Assessment Tree (Greydanus 2008)

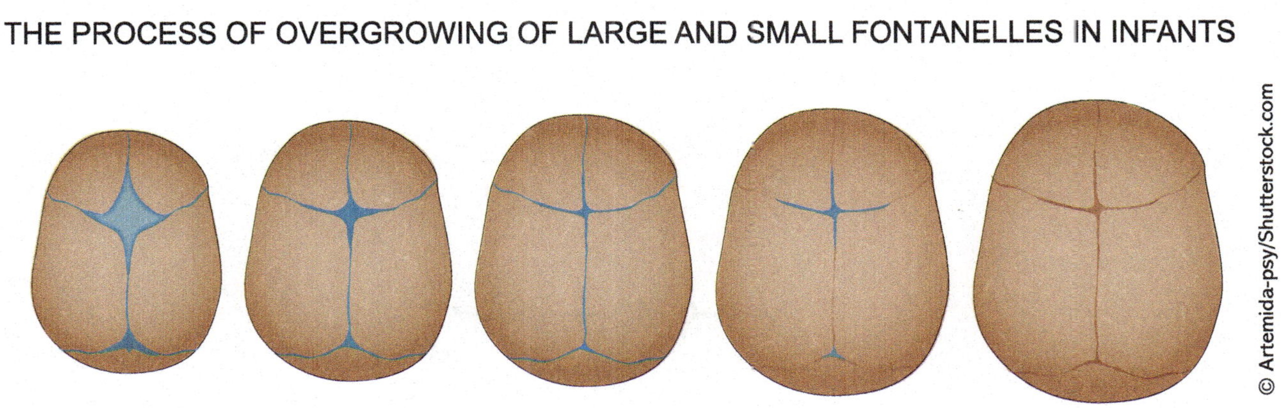


**Fig 1-8** The infant's head ossifies over time

Neurological Assessment (ATI Testing 2016)

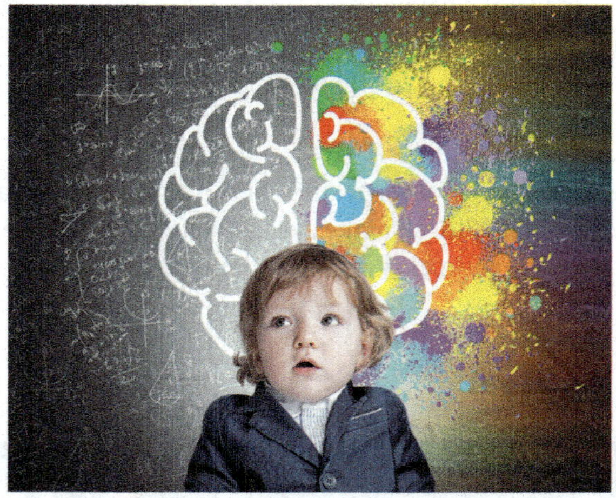



Chest Assessment Tree (Greydanus 2008)

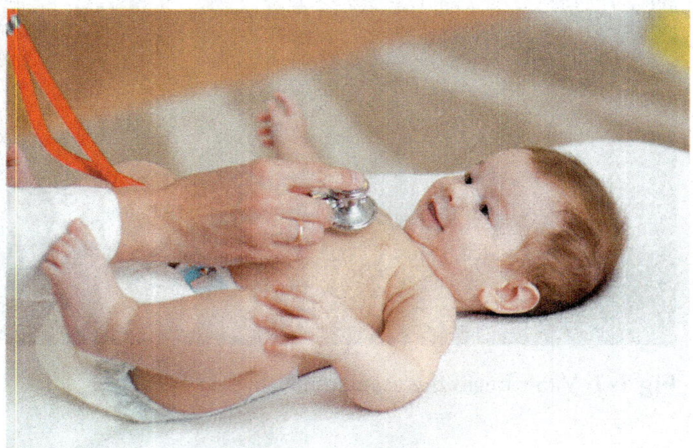



Circulatory Tree

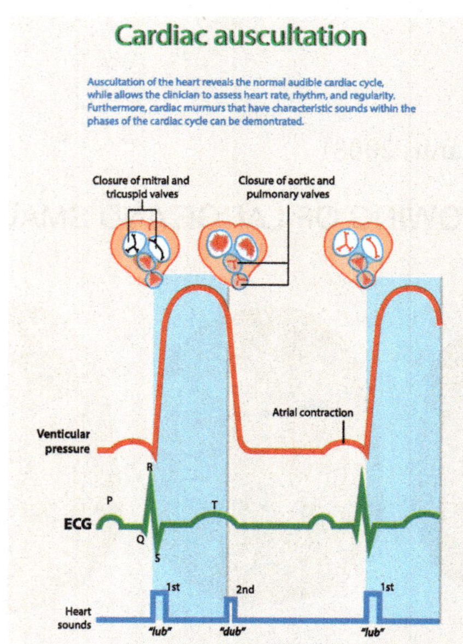




**Fig 1-9** Understand heart tones as a function of the valves opening and closing

Abdomen and Genitourinary System Tree (Greydanus 2008)

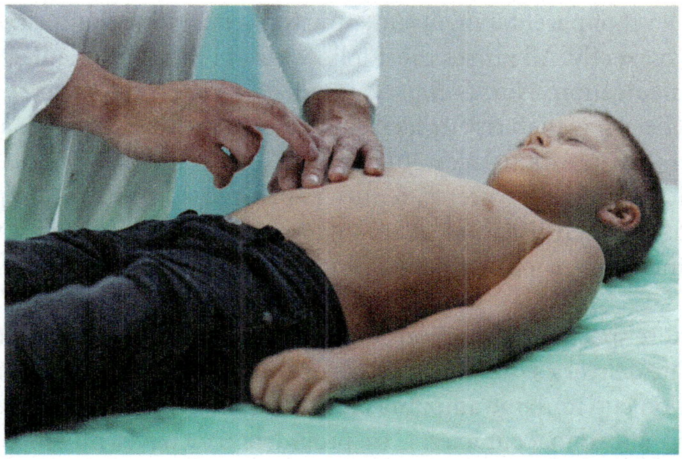



**Fig 1-10** The health-care provider percusses a child abdomen

Musculoskeletal Tree (Greydanus 2008)

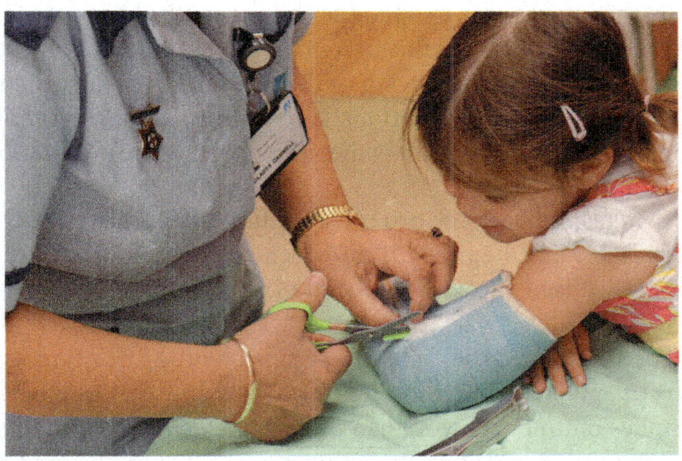

**Fig 1-11** Child in a fiberglass arm cast

Skin Tree (Greydanus 2008)

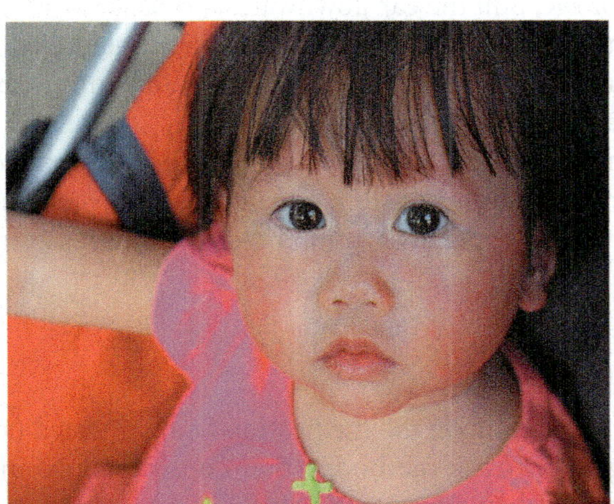



**Fig 1-12** Child with a skin rash on cheeks

## Medication Administration

The nurse determines the level of parental involvement with medication administration and teaches parents to administer medications correctly. All nurses must follow the Six Rights of Medication Administration, and calculate safe dosage for medication. Nurses must immediately report any discrepancies and get a revised order if necessary. Nurses check any high risk or facility-regulated medications with another Registered Nurse (Young, Cochran, Brehmer, Mei & Adkins-Bley 2015).

All children are verified using two patient identifiers prior to administration per the National Patient Safety Goals. Parents confirm identification of infants or nonverbal children. Two identifiers from the ID band must be confirmed: client name, date of birth, or hospital identification number (The Joint Commission 2017).

Many medications require specific nursing considerations. Nurses must consider the child's ability to swallow pills, and the appropriate delivery system. The nurse uses an oral medication syringe for small amounts of medication, and a medication cup for large amounts of medication. Nurses do not measure liquid medication in a teaspoon or tablespoon due to inaccuracies. Care providers may never mix medication with milk or formula because the infant might not swallow the entire feeding related to an altered taste of the milk or formula. The nurse can position the infant in a semi- reclining position similar to a feeding position, in an upright position, to prevent aspiration (Byington 1991).

Oral medications are placed into the side of the mouth in small amounts while the infant is upright. The nurse uses a gentle stroke on the infant's chin to open the child's mouth. The nurse teaches the parent and child not to crush tablets. The nurse may mix the medication in a small amount of nonessential food (such as applesauce). However, the nurse monitors the swallowing of the medication to ensure the dose was ingested. This technique is contraindicated for high-risk medications. A beverage of juice or water can follow administration to wash out the taste. A nipple may be used to allow the infant to suck the medication slowly, but medications are not given in a bottle (Byington 1991).

Children who are NPO take medications through a feeding tube. The nurse checks placement, through auscultation and a pH reading., and begins a liquid feed. The nurse does not add medications to the feeding bag; medications are infused through a special port. A water flush after the feeding is necessary (Miller 2015).

The nurse gives optic medications to the child in a supine or sitting position with an extended head. The nurse asks the child to look up, pulls the lower eye lid downward and applies medication in the pocket of the lower eyelid. The nurse applies ointments before nap or bedtime are best. If infants clench their eyes closed, then place the drops in the nasal corner. When the infant opens his eyes, the medication distributes over the eye. Follow with light pressure to the lacrimal duct for 3 minutes to prevent unpleasant taste (Farkouh, Frigo, & Czejka 2016).

The nurse gives otic medications to the child in a prone or supine position with the affected ear upward. If the child is under three years of age, pull the ear downward and back, to straighten out the ear canal. If the child is over three years of age the middle of the pinna is pulled back before administration of ear drops. The nurse warms refrigerated medications to room temperature prior to administration. The nurse massages the tragus for a few minutes following administration.

For nasal medications, the nurse administers drops with the head extended.by inserting the tip into the naris vertically, then angling it prior to administration. The nurse administers rectal medications beyond both rectal sphincters. It is important to for proper absorption holds the buttocks gently together for 5–10 minutes (Byington 1991).

## Injections

Injections come in several types depending on the medication being injected (see Fig 1-13). The nurse avoids tracking of medication by using the Z-track method. Other considerations include the child's age, weight, muscle development, the amount of subcutaneous fat over the site, the type and amount of the drug, and its absorption rate (Walsh 2017).

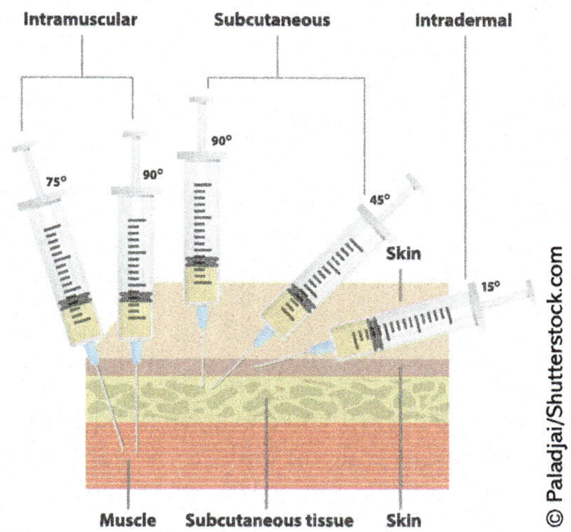


**Fig 1-13** Various angle for injections

The nurse gives intradermal medications on the inside surface of the forearm with a TB syringe with 25- to 27-gauge needle with an intradermal bevel. The needle inserts at a 15° angle, and never aspirates, and injects a small wheal (Caple & Balderrama 2017).

The nurse gives subcutaneous medications wherever there is adequate subcutaneous tissue. Common sites are the lateral aspect of the upper arm, abdomen, and anterior thigh. The nurse injects volumes of less than 0.5 mL in a 1 mL syringe with a 25- to 30-gauge needle. The typical insertion angle is 90°. Use a 45° angle for children who are thin (Pilgrim & Schub 2017).

The nurse uses a 22- to 25-gauge, 0.5- to 1-inch needle for intramuscular medications . The vastus lateralis is the recommended site for infants and small children in the supine, side-lying, or sitting positions (Byington 1991). A **ventrogluteal injection** requires the nurse to place the child in a supine, prone, or lateral position and inject 0.5–1 mL, depending on muscle size of the infant. The injection volume may be up to 2 mL in children (Byington 1991).

The nurse administers a **deltoid injection** with the child in a standing or sitting position. Injections can be up to 1 mL in volume. The nurse braces the child firmly to decrease movement of the needle while injecting and uses distraction before injection. Parents provide praise and comfort measures after the completion of the injection (Byington 1991).

The nurse may use a eutectic mixture of lidocaine and prilocaine (**EMLA**) applied to the site for 60 minutes prior to injection to ease the pain of injection. Therapeutic hugging can also help a child (Huff, Hamlin, Wolski, McClure, Eliades, Weaver & Shelestak 2009).

## Intravenous Medications

The nurse routinely assesses the venipuncture site per facility protocol for infection and infiltration prior to administration of medications. Terminologies such as a "little prick" or "a mosquito bite" are avoided. EMLA cream applied to the site for 60 minutes prior to the attempt may ease the pain. The nurse will introduce the child to the necessary medical equipment immediately before the procedure begins (Caple 2016; Byington 1991).

The nurse can use a **peripheral venous access device** with a 24- to 20-gauge catheter for IV medication administration. These devices support short-term IV therapy appropriate for administration at home with the assistance of a home health nurse (Cheung, Baerlocher, Asch & Myers 2009).

**Central venous access devices** can be short-term, non-tunneled catheter or peripherally inserted central catheters (PICC). Long-term catheters are tunneled or implanted infusion ports. A PICC is a good choice if multiple peripheral attempts are necessary (Uygun, Ibrahim, Okur, Mehmet Hanifi, Otcu, Selcuk, & Ozturk, Hayrettin 2011).

## Pain Management

Assessment of the pediatric patient depends on the child's cognitive, emotional, and physical development. Pediatric nurses manage pain through atraumatic, nonpharmacological, and pharmacological nursing interventions (Huff, Hamlin, Wolski, McClure, Eliades, Weaver & Shelestak 2009).

Pain is a psychosocial assessment that is prioritized after physiologic need tasks. Many factors impact the perception of pain. These include age, developmental stage, chronic or acute disease, prior experiences with pain, personality, family dynamics, culture, and socioeconomic status (McGrath 1994).

## Pain Assessment

Children experiencing pain produce a loud cry with an elevation in heart rate, blood pressure, and respiratory rate. Pediatric nurses use a self-reporting pain scale for children 4 years or older. Children under 4 are unable to report their pain accurately. However, multiple pain scales offer developmentally appropriate ways to assess all children's pain. A nurse chooses an appropriate pain tool to assess the child's pain and includes the parent or caregiver in rating the child's pain. The nurse assesses the location, quality, and severity of pain, and reassesses the child's pain level. Nurses use nonpharmacological, pharmacological, or both approaches to manage pain. However, pharmacological interventions are potentiated by nonpharmacological interventions and should be used together. Atraumatic measures include the use of a treatment room for painful procedures instead of "safe places," such as the hospital bed or the play room (Smith 2016).

## Pharmacological Nursing Interventions

The World Health Organization (WHO) (2012) recommends a two-step approach for pharmacological management of pain in children based on age. For children older than 3 months of age with mild pain, the first step is to administer a nonopioid, nonsteroidal anti-inflammatory drugs (NSAIDs) or acetaminophen (WHO 2012).

For children who have moderate or severe pain, the nurses administer a strong opioid. Morphine is the first-line treatment drug. An optimal dosage of medications controls pain without causing severe adverse effects. Nurses select the least traumatic route for medication administration. Medications are given routinely, not PRN (as needed), to manage pain that is expected to last for an extended period. Opioids relieve moderate to severe pain and may include morphine sulfate, hydromorphone, and fentanyl (WHO 2012).

The combination of a nonopioid and an opioid medication will potentiate the medications and effectively treat peripheral and central pain. This combination of medications creates an effective analgesic effect with fewer adverse effects than opiates alone (respiratory depression, constipation, and nausea) (WHO 2012).

## Pain Assessment Tool for Evaluation by Age

Young patients between 2 months and 7 years of age can use the **FLACC** (Face, Legs Activity, Cry, Consolability) scale. Children over 3 years of age can use the **FACES** scale (Fig 1-14) (WHO 2012).

The nurse uses the **Oucher** scale for children between 3 years of age and 13 years of age and measures pain response through the ranking of painful pictures. The **numerical scale** that ranges from 1 to 10 can be used by children 5 years of age and up (WHO 2012). **Noncommunicating Children's Pain Checklist** can be used with children 3 years of age and up (Smith 2016; Breau, McGrath, Camfield & Finley, G. A. 2002).

## Nursing Considerations for Giving Medications

The provider has several routes to choose from for medication orders. Each has benefits and risks. The oral route has benefits such as cost, convenience, and the ability to deliver medication over time. However, oral medications are ineffective for rapid relief of pain or pain that is fluctuating in nature (WHO 2012).

The topical or transdermal route can be used for **EMLA cream (lidocaine and prilocaine)** available in a cream or gel for any invasive procedure (IV insertion, biopsy) 60 minutes prior to a superficial puncture and 2.5 hours prior to a deep puncture. An occlusive dressing applied over the cream ensures contact with the

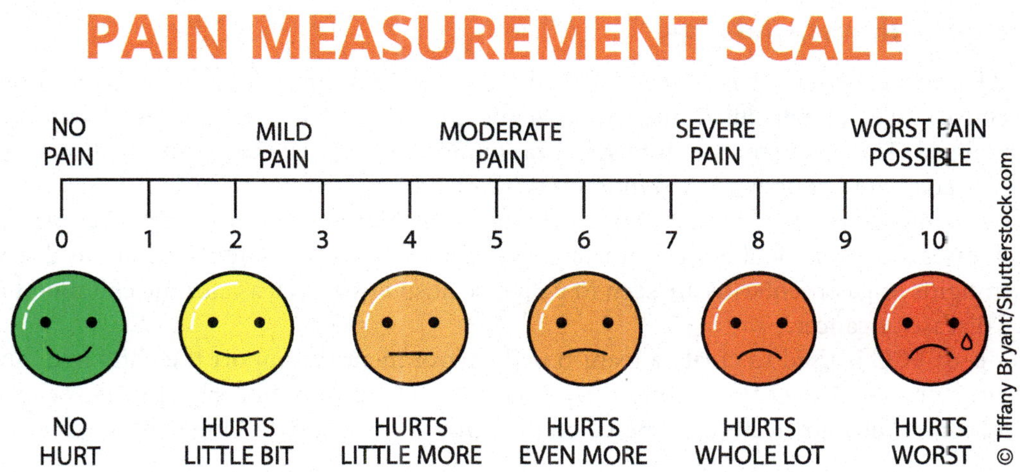


**Fig 1-14** The FACES scale

medication. Prior to the procedure, remove the dressing and clean the skin. However, the nurse needs a long window of time to complete this intervention (Stoltz & Manworren 2017).

Children over 12 years of age may use **fentanyl** is used to provide continuous pain control. The nurse gives fentanyl over 3-5 minutes to promote comfort and cmonitor for adverse effects. In case of respiratory depression, the nurse administers naloxone to reverse the effect of the opiate medication (WHO 2012).

Medications for the intravenous route can be ordered as a **bolus** and is given all at once for rapid pain control. Common opioid medications given in bolus doses include morphine and hydromorphone. A continuous schedule provides steady blood levels (WHO 2012)

The nurse monitors the use of **patient-controlled analgesia (PCA)** is used for self-administration of pain medication. The dose delivery has basal, bolus, or combination dose options. A PCA is a good option for children because there are lockouts after a maximum dose is delivered. The parent or caregiver manages the child's pain if the child cannot be responsible for the medication (WHO 2012).

## Nonpharmacological Interventions

Nonpharmacological interventions include **distraction** through the use of play, radio, a computer game, a movie, or a story to the child. When the sympathetic nervous system is inhibited, the sensation of **relaxation** occurs. Infants and young children relax when they are held and spoken to softly. Older children can assume a comfortable position and perform breathing techniques to induce relaxation. A nurse can use **guided imagery** to usher a child through an imaginary experience to help a child through a procedure (Wente 2013).

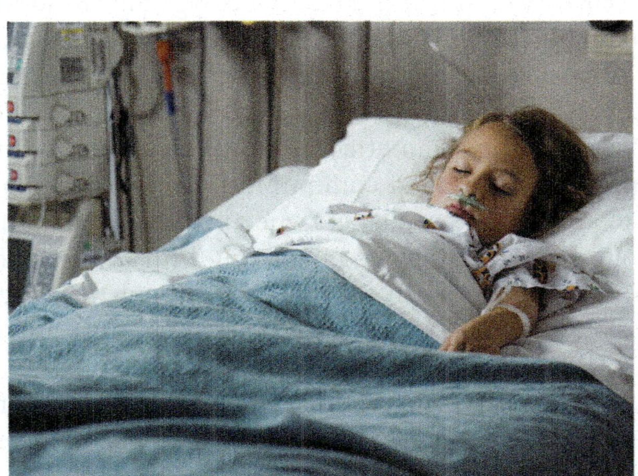

© Jos Temprano/Shutterstock.com

## Hospitalization, Illness, and Play

Children and families experience stress when hospitalized regardless of the reason for hospitalization. Children may have elective surgery, a scheduled surgery, or an unexpected traumatic event. Many factors affect a child who is hospitalized. The experience with hospitalization, illness severity, coping mechanisms, and parental responses are used to guide nursing interventions (Whelan 2007).

A nurse working in the hospital will encounter children with high acuity disease states because many minor childhood illnesses are cared for at home or through a pediatrician's office. Highly infectious diseases such as bacterial meningitis or gastroenteritis are seen in pediatric hospitals as well as chronic childhood illness such as sickle-cell disease or cancer.

The model of FCC is used to create a team-based environment to support the child and family during inpatient stays. Nurses can identify the child's response to hospitalization through a psychosocial assessment, in addition to, communication techniques based on the child's growth and development stage (Whelan, 2007).

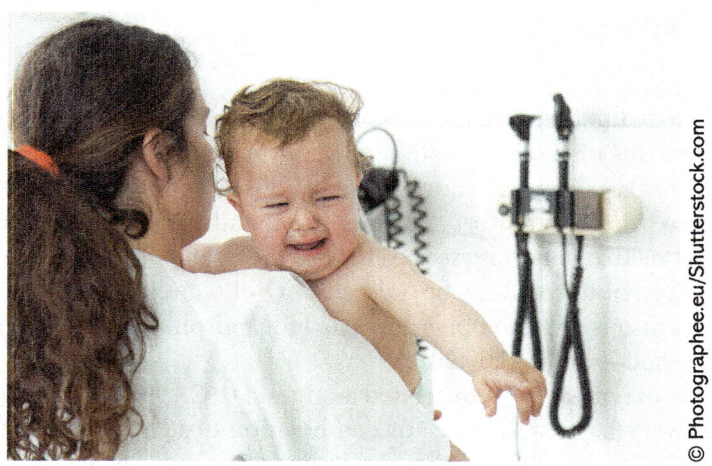


**Fig 1-15** It is normal for babies to cry upon separation from the primary caregiver

## Assessment

Infants experience **separation anxiety** around 9 months old (see Fig 1-15). Symptoms may manifest in different ways. An infant may protest or scream, cling to the parents, or use verbal and physical aggression toward strangers and the health-care team. Infants cannot describe their illness, follow directions, or understand the therapeutic value of procedures. Infants may have difficulty regulating emotional and behavioral responses, causing crying, the inability to be soothed, feeding problems, or dysfunctional sleep patterns. An infant can present as hypervigilant or extremely withdrawn and refuse feedings, and avoid engagement with their health care providers. Nurses must communicate with infants through nonverbal cues, and slowly introduce the child to the hospital environment. A calm demeanor from the healthcare team eases the transition for the child (Jordan, Franich-Ray, Anderson, Northam, Albert, Cochrane & Menahem 2013; Jovanovic 2011).

Toddlers may experience regression as an effect of hospitalization. A child may exhibit despair as withdrawal from others, depression, decreased communication, and developmental regression such as beginning to suck their thumb again or to use diapers when previously potty trained. Children from preschool and up may demonstrate **detachment** when interacting with strangers, forming new relationships, and may appear despondent. Preschoolers can communicate about the expression of their illness but cannot understand the causes of their illness. They can understand cause and effect experiences (Lehner 2015; Whelan 2007).

Preschoolers possess a quality called **magical thinking** where two events occur as cause and effect without any plausible evidence. For example, a preschooler could wish his or her younger brother would have never been born and feel guilty if the little brother gets hurt. This magical thinking can produce fears that are difficult to understand from an adult perspective. For example, child may believe their illness is a punishment for their bad behavior. Preschoolers typically show their reactions, rather than tell about their reactions (Boles & Roberts 2007; Whelan 2007).

School-age children can understand the way the body functions and can easily understand germs, infection, and multiple causes of illness. School-age children understand cause and effect. They understand the finality of death and no longer believe death is a sleep state. Nurses are honest with all pediatric patients, but by school-age, children sense if they are being misled. The greatest source of stress for these patients is the separation from their friends and their routine. Nurses can support these patients by reinforcing their medical knowledge as often as needed and making sure their home routine is incorporated into the plan of care as their medical condition allows (Boles & Roberts 2007).

Adolescents understand complexities and abstractions of the disease processes. However, they perceive illness severity based on its aesthetic impact on their body image. Adolescents seek to maintain control by appearing composed or detached. However, they will feel isolation from peers and worry about the impact on their school lives and social lives. Adolescents can be noncompliant in their medical regime because they want to be the same as their peers. Nurses can best support adolescents through referrals to support groups for adolescents. Adolescents find it easier to be compliant with support from their peers to maintain their medical regime (Canadian Paediatric Society 2008).

The family will also have a range of responses to hospitalization relative to the circumstances for bringing in the child. These emotions can range from anxiety from the unknown to fear and guilt from delaying the decision come to the hospital or frustration from not being able to care for the child adequately. The family also may have had negative experiences with the medical community. Nurses identify these issues and work with the family to adjust to the changing circumstances with their child. The hospitalization of the child may force family roles to shift based on financial concerns. There can also be stress incurred if finances are affected, especially for prolonged illnesses, or if there are other children who need care. Siblings may feel loneliness, guilt, jealousy, fear, or anger. The primary caregiver may experience role strain. The nurse will develop a plan of care to address these issues that arise (Lehner 2015).

## Psychosocial Assessment

The nurse determines the child's and family's understandings of the illness and the reason for hospitalization. Specific stressors such as family size, socioeconomic status, and health of the caregivers in the family affect the emotional well-being of the child and the family.

The nurse reviews past experiences with hospitalization and illness to help build a rapport with the child and family as well as assess the developmental needs of the child and family. An assessment of parenting roles and perceptions of changing roles provide important clues to identifying families who need additional resources and lack support systems (Lehner 2015).

## Nursing Interventions for All Children

The nurse gives explanations of treatments, procedures, and nursing care to the child, and provides anticipatory guidance for hospitalization. Family members are encouraged to stay overnight with the child during the hospital experience to reduce the child's stress. The nurse will attempt to integrate the child's routine into the plan of care as much as possible, promote autonomy, provide developmentally appropriate activities, and provide consistency in assigning caregivers (Lehner 2015).

## Infant Nursing Interventions

If parents are unavailable, and infants are not on isolation precautions, the nurse may bring the infant to the nurse's station to meet their psychosocial needs (Maguire, Webb, Passmore, Cline 2012).

## Toddler Nursing Interventions

The nurse encourages parents to provide routine care for the child, such as changing diapers and feeding as well as medications if the child will be receiving medications at home. The nurse promotes autonomy in the child by offering appropriate choices (Lehner 2015).

## Preschooler Nursing Interventions

The nurse explains any procedures using simple, clear language with the preschooler, as medical terms can be misinterpreted. As with the toddler, the nurse promotes autonomy through choices, allows ample time for the child to express feelings, and validates the child's fears and concerns. The nurse uses play and provides toys that allow for emotional expressions, such as a pounding board to release feelings of protest or crayons to draw symbols of what they are feeling. Children are less intimidated by medical equipment if they can handle the instruments, as is developmentally appropriate (McGrath & Huff 2001).

## School Age Child Nursing Interventions

The nurse offers concrete, factual information about any procedures or treatments, providing time for the child to express feelings and ask questions. The nurse creates routine for long hospitalizations, especially including time for school work, and promotes contact with friends if possible. The nurse encourages the parents to enlist peers to help bring homework, and help the child complete homework (Lehner 2015).

## Adolescent Nursing Interventions

Adolescents require direct, factual information. The nurse empowers the adolescent in the planning of care to foster independence and responsibility. Adolescents need a supportive peer group, especially those with the same medical diagnosis (Canadian Paediatric Society 2008).

## Child Life Specialists

Nurses engage children in play as time allows. However, there is a specific health-care professional called a Child Life specialist who specializes in age-appropriate play (see Fig 1-16). They create opportunities for normative play, medical play, and therapeutic play for children recovering in the hospital (Burns-Nader & Hernandez-Reif 2016; McGrath & Huff 2001). The American Academy of Pediatrics (AAP) designates child life specialists as essential to the health-care team (Smith, Desai, Sira & Engelke 2014).

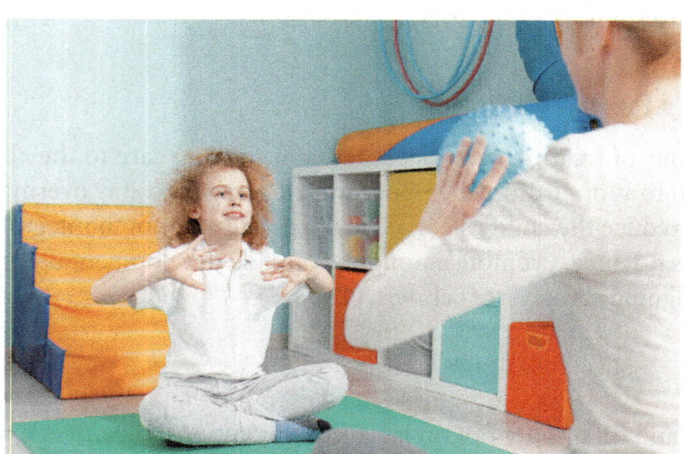



**Fig 1-16** Play is a therapeutic exercise

Child life specialists cater to the needs of children in the hospital. They study child development, counseling, and child psychology. Child life specialists help prepare children for treatments or procedures they will face as inpatients. Their primary function is to buffer the stress and anxiety inherent in the hospital experience. They also attempt to maintain a child's growth and development in spite of the hospitalization. Child Life Specialists can also help with other siblings that may be in the hospital setting. They also use the FCC model of carein pediatric hospital settings. As health-care delivery improves, Child Life Specialists should become a standard of care in all pediatric settings (Smith, Desai, Sira, & Engelke 2014).

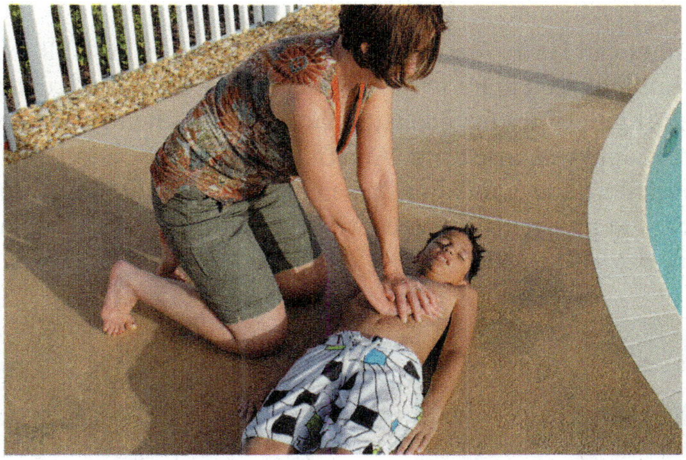
© Mike Focus/Shutterstock.com

## Pediatric Emergencies

Children must adjust to a constantly changing body and a dynamic skill set of physical activities. Nurses perform an assessment, implement emergency nursing interventions, and teach the caregivers child safety prevention.

Children can have a respiratory, drowning, apparent life-threatening event, SIDS, or poisoning emergency. Nurses must have the assessment skills to identify the differences and expedite effective interventions to manage these pediatric emergencies.

## Respiratory Emergencies

A respiratory emergency can originate from **respiratory failure** or the loss of the ability to exchange gas in the lung. Or respiratory distress can originate from inadequate ventilation, or **respiratory insufficiency**. Either condition can result in apnea or the cessation of respirations for more than 20 seconds. Apnea causes hypoxemia or bradycardia, and respiratory arrest or the complete absence of respirations. Apnea or respiratory failure can result from airway obstruction from aspiration of a foreign body (Gunning, K. E. 2003).

Toddlers are at risk for respiratory arrest from many events. Toddlers may develop primary inefficient gas exchange related to cerebral trauma, brain tumor, overdose, asphyxia, or CNS infection. They can experience **obstructive lung conditions** such as chronic bronchitis or asthma. Toddlers may also develop **restrictive lung disease** that impedes lung expansion such as respiratory distress syndrome, or pulmonary fibrosis (Caronia 2017; Robinson 2016).

## Assessment

Signs of early respiratory distress include restlessness, tachypnea, tachycardia, hypertension, diaphoresis, nasal flaring, retractions, a head bob during inspiration in infants, grunting, dyspnea, wheezing, and refusing to eat. Signs of advanced hypoxia include bradypnea, bradycardia, hypotension, cyanosis, decreased level of consciousness (LOC) and coma (Schub, E. B. 2016).

Signs of choking include the **universal choking sign** (see Fig 1-18; clutching neck with hands), an inability to speak, dyspnea, dysphonia, a weak cough, wheezing or no sound at all, and cyanosis (Janahi et. al. 2017).

## Diagnosis

Diagnosis follows directly from the assessment and confirmed through Arterial blood gases (ABGs) that reveal respiratory acidosis and chest x-rays to determine an obstruction or atelectasis (Janahi et. al. 2017).

## Interventions and Teaching

The nurse follows the American Heart Association (AHA) guidelines for CPR for respiratory and cardiac arrest if the child stops breathing (see Figure 1-17). The health care team uses current basic life support and advanced cardiac life support guidelines for neonates and pediatric clients. In a hospital setting, the nurse activates the protocol for the rapid response team (American Heart Association 2015).

The nurse's responsibilities include maintaining a patent airway (suctioning), monitoring vital signs, providing oxygen as necessary, and preparing for intubation should it become necessary. The nurse also gives medications and fluids (Engel 2015).

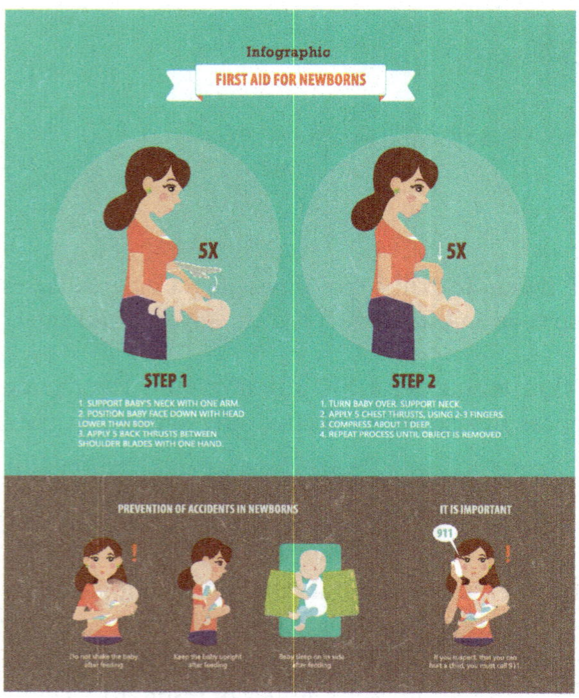


© twins_nika/Shutterstock.com

**Fig 1-17** Parent teaching for newborns

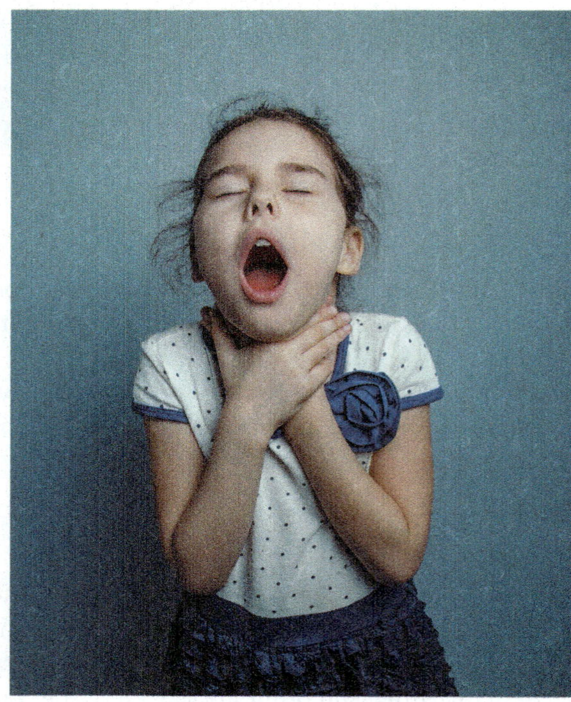

© maxim ibragimov/Shutterstock.com

**Fig 1-18** Universal choking sign

## Obstructed Airway

The nurse uses the AHA guidelines for a choking child that includes combination of back blows and chest thrusts for infant patients. Children and adolescents need abdominal thrusts to remove the obstruction. The nurse checks for the obstruction periodically but does not do a blind finger sweep as this can obstruct the airway again. The nurse places the breathing child into the recovery position (a side-lying position with legs bent at knees for stability) (American Heart Association 2015).

The nurse educates the child and family about the signs of choking and to "not treat" until the child stops coughing. Coughing is the body's natural response to choking, and parents are encouraged to work with this protective mechanism until it fails. The family needs current CPR training, and childproof techniques for the house, especially for young children (American Heart Association 2015).

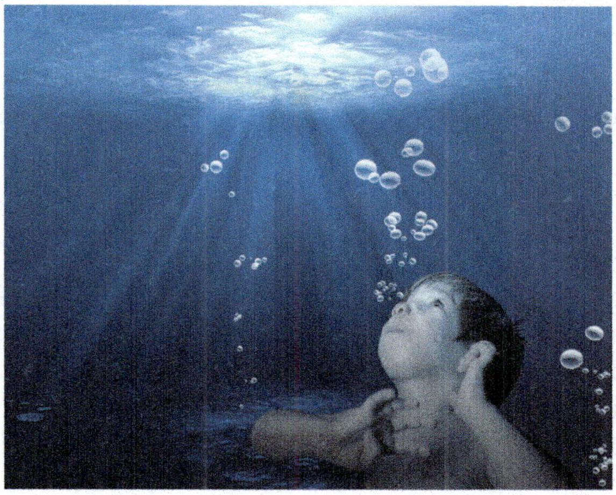


## Drowning

Drowning occurs while submerged in a fluid that is at least 1 inch deep. Common places for drowning include the bathtub, toilet, bucket, pool, pond, or the lake. **Submersion injury** (near-drowning) incidents are those in which children have survived for 24 hours after being submerged in fluid. Risk factors include children over 1 year of age and adolescents, unsupervised in bathtub or pool, diving, and child abuse (Carter & Sinclair 2011).

## Assessment

The nurse documents the history of the event that includes the location, time of submersion, type, and temperature of the fluid. The child may have hypothermia, with respiratory distress and wet breath sounds that include tachypnea, circulatory insufficiency. There can be a loss of consciousness and abdominal swelling from water ingestion. The child may have a spinal cord injury. The nurse monitors the child a Glasgow Coma score. The nurse watches for signs of respiratory distress and cerebral edema for 24 hours (Carter & Sinclair 2011).

## Diagnosis

Diagnosis is confirmed by symptoms and a chest x-ray for atelectasis or infiltration. Electrocardiogram (EKG), Arterial Blood Gas (ABG), and blood glucose monitoring indicates the severity of the injury. Interventions depend on the extent of cerebral hypoxia (Carter & Sinclair 2011).

## Interventions and Teaching

The nurse administers oxygen, fluids, medication and/or assists with intubation for mechanical ventilation. The nurse and respiratory perform chest physiotherapy to promote the clearance of the fluid from the lungs (Carter & Sinclair 2011).

The nurse uses therapeutic communication to keep the family informed of the child's status. The nurse teaches the child and family safety interventions for the home environment that include toilet locks, supervised baths and swimming, keeping pool areas locked, and using life jackets while boating or swimming in large bodies of water (Weiss 2010).

## Apparent Life-Threatening Event

An apparent life-threatening event occurs when an infant exhibits apnea, marked change in skin and muscle tone, gagging, and choking. Risk factors include gastroesophageal reflux (GER), respiratory infections, seizure, and urinary tract infection (UTI) (Choi, H. J., & Kim, Y. H. 2016)).

### Assessment

A detailed description of the event from an observer begins the assessment. The nurse documents the maternal history, and any family history of seizures. The infant present with apnea, hypotonia, choking, gagging, or coughing, and cyanosis (Choi, H. J., & Kim, Y. H. 2016).

### Diagnosis

Diagnosis identifies underlying causes such as GER, seizure disorder, sleep apnea, a cardiac condition, hypoglycemia, an electrolyte imbalance, an infection, or a non-accidental injury. An esophageal pH monitoring, electroencephalogram (EEG), Electrocardiogram, Echocardiography, blood glucose monitoring blood work, a urinalysis, and video surveillance provide evidence for an etiology and other indications as to the origin of the event. An **electrocardiogram (ECG)** identifies long QT syndrome or dysrhythmias related to an electrolyte imbalance. An **electroencephalogram (EEG)** detects abnormal brain function such as epilepsy (Choi, H. J., & Kim, Y. H. 2016).

### Interventions

Encourage the family to learn CPR and prepare the child and family for various diagnostic testing. The nurse explains the **apnea monitor** to parents of children with sleep apnea. The alarm sounds when the child stops breathing. The nurse encourages parents to use a safe sleep position (infant supine position with the face free in a comfortably heated room) and refrain from smoking in the home environment (Choi, H. J., & Kim, Y. H. 2016).

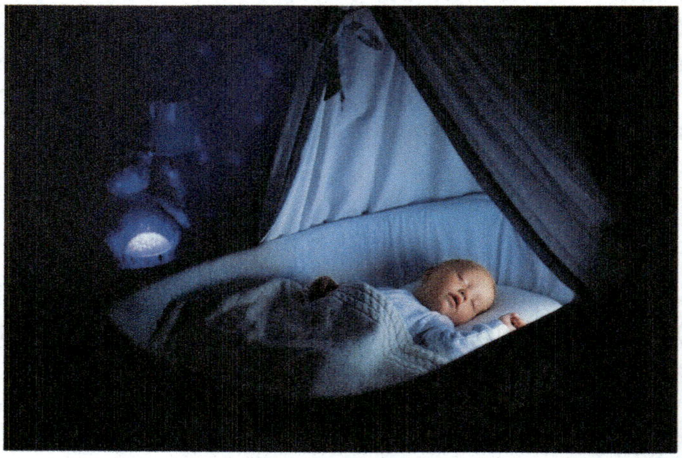

© FamVeld/Shutterstock.com

## Sudden Infant Death Syndrome

Sudden infant death syndrome (SIDS) is the unexpected, unpredictable death of an infant without an identified cause. The nurse teaches all families preventative measures. Risk factors include maternal smoking during pregnancy, secondhand smoke, co-sleeping with parent or adult, a nonstandard bed such as a sofa, soft bedding, water beds, pillows, prone or side-lying sleeping, a low-birth weight, prematurity, twin or multiple birth, low-Apgar scores, viral illness, family history of SIDS, and poverty (Smith, N. C., & Engelke, Z. M. 2017).

### Assessment

The nurse takes a history of events prior to the discovery of the infant, history of illnesses of pregnancy and birth history, and a presence of risk factors (Smith, N. C., & Engelke, Z. M. 2017).

### Interventions and Teaching

The nurse provides emotional support and encourages the family to express feelings. The nurse provides referrals to community resources when available. Preventative education includes placing the infant on the back for sleep, avoiding tobacco smoke, not over bundling the infant and causing overheating, keeping the face free, room sharing without bedsharing, and keeping loose bedding and soft objects out of the bed. The parents should check on infants under 1 years of age at night to make sure the child's face is free of blankets. Parents may offer a pacifier at naps and night if breastfeeding is well established (after 6 weeks of age). Breastfeeding and up-to-date immunizations decrease the risk of SIDS (Smith, N. C., & Engelke, Z. M. 2017).

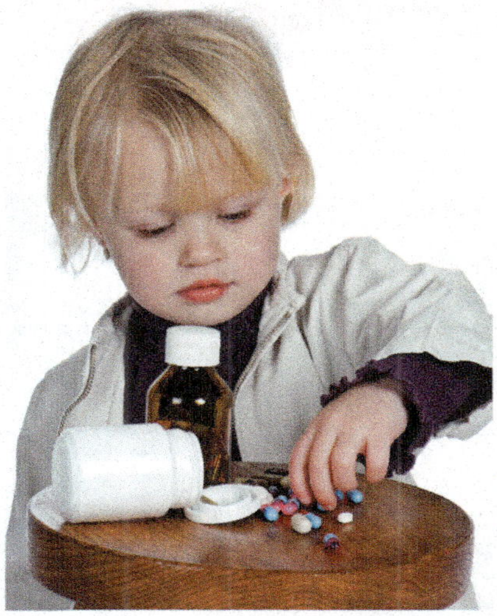

© Anneka/Shutterstock.com

## Poisoning

Poisoning includes the ingestion toxic substances. Poisoning is common in curious toddlers and adventurous adolescents. Nurses use prevention teaching to help make parents aware of the danger of common household items. Risk factors include children younger than 5 years of age, improperly stored medications and household chemicals, exposure to cosmetics, and lead ingestion from lead-based paint or soil (Engelke, Z. M., & Schub, T. B. 2016).

### General Assessment

The nurse obtains a history of the poisoning including the time of ingestions, the name of the poison, and the quantity of the poison ingested. The nurse looks for combination drugs such as acetaminophen and codeine or slow release medications to indicate severity of poisoning. The nurse determines the amount of left over medication to estimate the child's consumption. When in doubt, the nurse should assume the maximum amount was ingested. Interventions depend on the type of poison the child has ingested. The child who ingested poison may present with nausea and vomiting; sudden sleepiness, confusion or decreased alertness; and abdominal cramping (Crisp & Rainbow 2007).

## Acetaminophen

Acetaminophen is toxic at 140 mg/kg. A child who has ingested acetaminophen shows signs of nausea, vomiting, sweating, and pallor in the first 2–4 hours. In 24–36 hours, the child shows an improvement in symptoms. However, they can develop hepatic failure 36 hours–7 days evidenced by pain in upper-right quadrant, confusion, stupor, jaundice, and coagulation disturbances (Larsen & Fuller 1996).

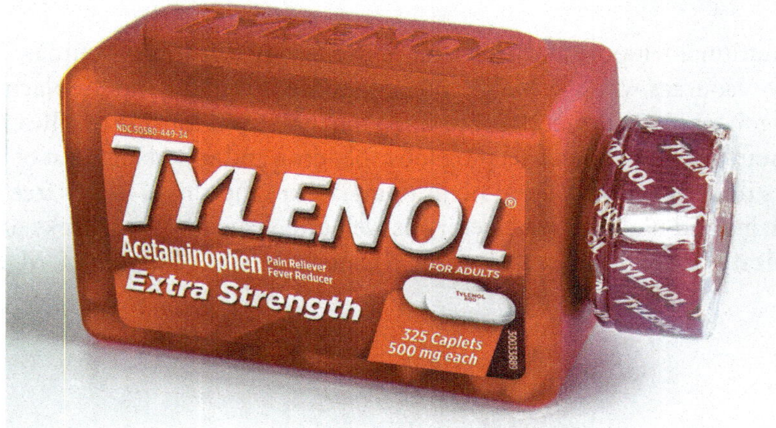




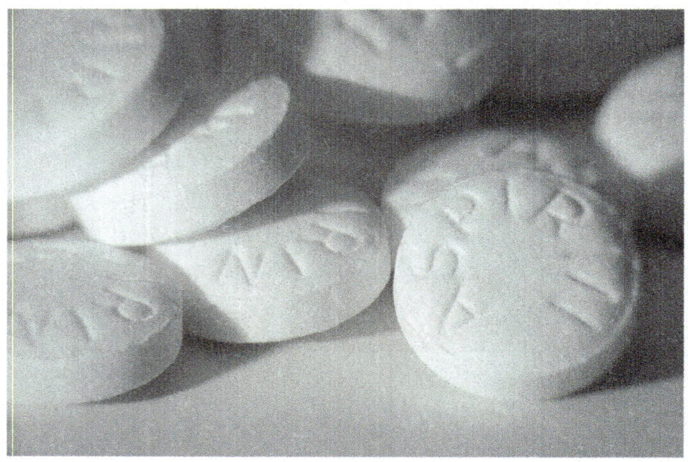



## Acetylsalicylic Acid (Aspirin)

Aspirin in doses above 150mg/kg is troubling. Early signs of toxicity include tachypnea, vomiting, agitation and confusion, diuresis, and hyperthermia. Older children may report tinnitus. The typical presentation of respiratory alkalosis leading to metabolic acidosis does not always correlate to children (Crisp & Rainbow 2007).

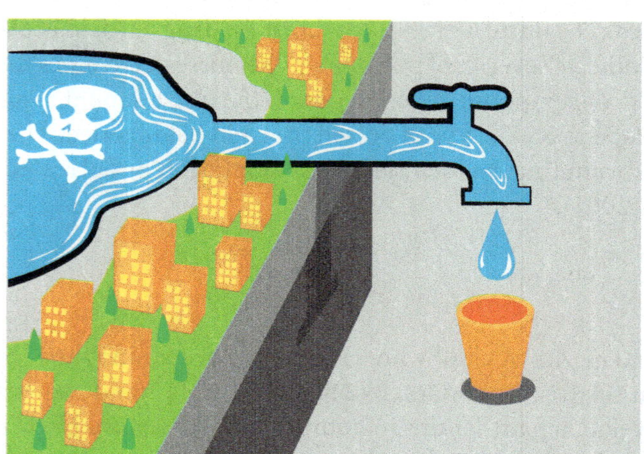

## Lead

Lead is a neurotoxin where children can develop clumsiness, hearing or growth impairment, speech regression, or deteriorate in their cognition or attention. The risk for lead toxicity is greater if the child has an iron deficiency (Crisp & Rainbow 2007). Children with a high lead level can develop encephalopathy, paralysis and coma (Lawrence, P. C., & Schub, T. B. 2017).

Chronic exposure causes lead storage in bones that continuously poisons the child. Lead impairs Vitamin D synthesis and may lead to rickets (Weidemann, Weaver & Fadrowski 2016).

Lead impairs the glomeruli and the renal tubules in the kidney. This impairs GFR, calcium function, and causes chronic kidney disease (CKD) (Weidemann, Weaver & Fadrowski 2016).

Elevated lead levels are a public health issue when children and families have known contamination in their drinking water. Nurses should support public health efforts so that all American children have potable water to drink.

## Supplemental Iron

The child's reaction to iron poisoning occurs in three phases. Acute symptoms begin 30 minutes to 6 hours after ingestion. The child presents with nausea, vomiting, diarrhea, gastric and symptoms may resolve. A latent period lasts up to 12 hours. The next phase includes fluid shifts can cause hypotension and increasing lethargy. The final phase includes liver failure 48–96 hours after consumption when toxic levels of ammonia produce neurological symptoms such as GI hemorrhage, renal and hepatic failure, and, coma, shock, and possible death (Crisp & Rainbow 2007).

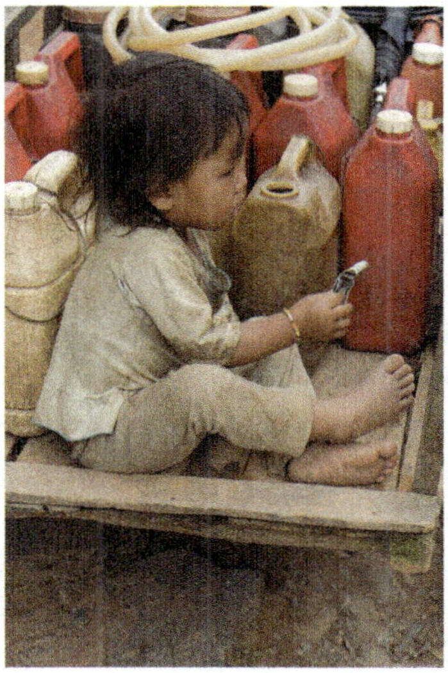



## Hydrocarbons and Corrosives

Hydrocarbons are derived from petroleum and include gasoline, propane, butane, paint thinner, and glue. Ingestion of hydrocarbons causes aspiration pneumonia (O'Malley, G. F. 2015). Children who ingest hydrocarbons present with burns to the mouth choking, coughing, nausea, and vomiting, lethargy, weakness, tachypnea, cyanosis, stridor, and abdominal pain (Lupa, Magne, Guarisco & Amedee 2009).

Corrosives refer to household cleaners, batteries, denture cleaners, and bleach. Children who ingest corrosives experience pain and burning in mouth, throat, and stomach. Child develop edema in the lips, tongue, and pharynx and have white mucous membranes. Children may have violent vomiting with hemoptysis, drooling, anxiety, and shock (Lupa, Magne, Guarisco & Amedee 2009).

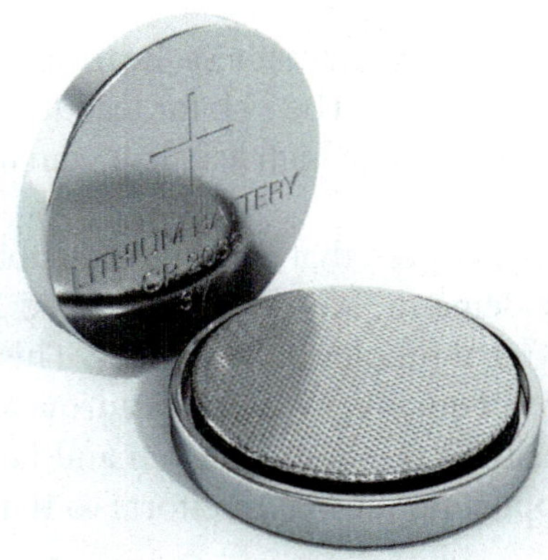


© cigdem/Shutterstock.com

## Interventions

Interventions for poisoning match the type of poison and the amount the child has ingested. First, caregivers remove the poison from the vicinity of the child, collects medication evidence, and initiates cardiopulmonary (CPR) support if necessary. Then a call to the local or regional poison control center provides specific instructions for care to the caregivers. Once admitted, the nurse monitors vital signs, administers IV fluids as prescribed, and uses chelation therapy for heavy exposures. Syrup of ipecac is contraindicated for routine poison control treatment (Crisp & Rainbow 2007).

The nurse keeps the family informed of the child's condition. The nurse also offers case management for children who have chronic signs of poisoning and makes referrals to a community nurse, teacher, or early intervention.

## Antidotes

There are known antidotes for some poisons. Student nurses who remember these antidotes can look for opportunities to apply this learning in the clinical setting.

Acetaminophen toxicity reverses with an oral dose of N-acetylcysteine.

Acetylsalicylic acid is absorbed using activated charcoal, gastric lavage, sodium bicarbonate to balance metabolic acidosis. The nurse monitors oxygen levels and providers adjust ventilation rates to manage acidosis, administers Vitamin K to increase clotting times, and support the hemodialysis procedure if necessary.

Supplemental iron poisoning in children requires emesis, lavage, or chelation therapy with deferoxamine mesylate for severe cases (Crisp & Rainbow 2007).

Children that ingest hydrocarbons need special treatment. The provider will not induce vomiting to prevent further tissue damage in the GI tract from hydrocarbons. The provider intubates the child, performs gastric decontamination, and treats the child for chemical pneumonia (O'Malley 2015).

Children that ingest corrosives (drain cleaners, toilet cleaners, batteries, and bleach) are similarly concerning because they destroy tissue and compromise the child's airway from burns. The child is kept NPO in such circumstances. It is undesirable for the child to vomit or receive treatments to neutralize the acid. (O'Malley 2015).

## Teaching

Teachings for children and families are focused on prevention. The nurse reminds parents to keep hazardous materials in a locked cabinet, out of reach of children. In addition, adults should not take medications in front of children, dispose of old medications, keep medications in locked cabinets, and never refer to medicine as candy (Engelke & Schub 2016).

Parents who take a child safety class prevent more accidental injuries than parents who do not (Kendrick et. al. 2013).

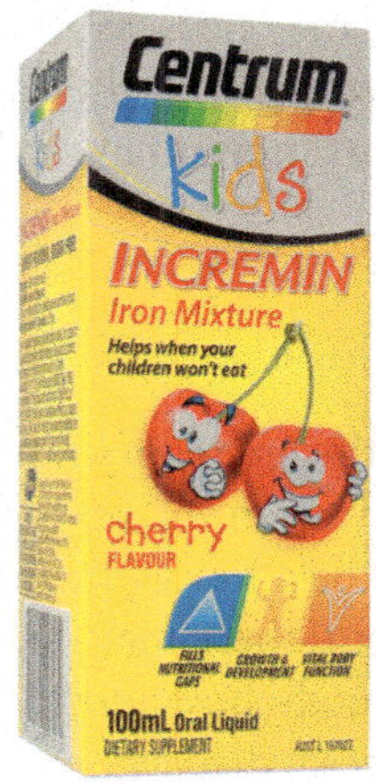


© CTR Photos/Shutterstock.com

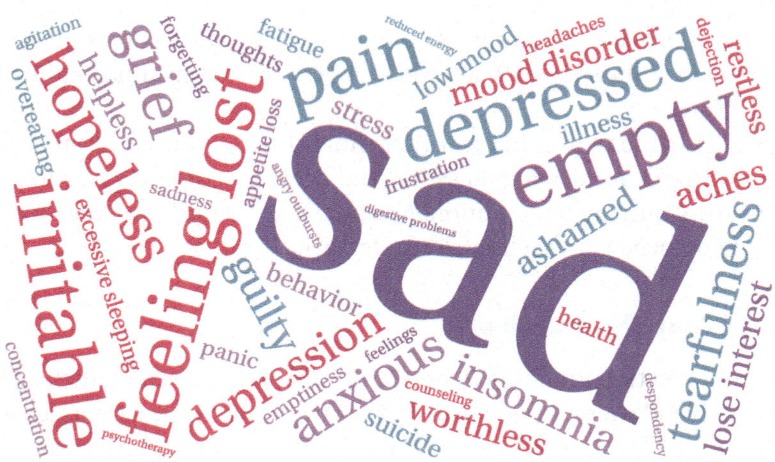


© arloo/Shutterstock.com

## End-of-Life Issues

The effect of losing a child has long-term and short-term effects. Families experience grief and mourning in different ways. **Anticipatory grief** occurs when death is expected. **Complicated grief** extends for more than 1 year following the loss. Complicated grief causes intense thoughts distressing yearning, feelings of loneliness, distressing emotions and feelings, and disturbances in personal activities, such as sleep. Complicated grief requires a referral to an expert in grief counseling (Schonfeld & Demaria 2016).

**Parental grief** is intense, long-lasting, and complex. There are secondary losses related to the death of the child, such as absence of hope and dreams, disruption of the family unit, loss of identity as a parent (Schonfeld & Demaria 2016).

Grief is unique to every family member. **Sibling grief** depends on age and developmental stage and will present differently than parental grief (Schonfeld & Demaria 2016).

Infants and toddlers from birth through 3 years of age do not understand death the way adults do. Toddlers display egocentric thinking that skews their comprehension of death. Toddlers show a range of strong emotions such as sadness, anger, depression, and anxiety. These emotions intensify when parents feel the same way. Preschool children from 3 to 6 years of age may interpret separation from parents as punishment for bad behavior or view dying as temporary. Preschoolers lack a concept of time and may think the dead person is sleeping (Schonfeld & Demaria 2016).

School-age children need logical or factual explanations. They develop an adult concept of death as inevitable, irreversible, or universal for the first time. They may also develop a fear of the disease process, death process, or the unknown, and sense a loss of control as a result. Fear is often displayed through uncooperative behavior. Adults may engage the school-age child to ask questions about funeral services and what happens to the body after death (Schonfeld & Demaria 2016).

Adolescents between 12 and 18 years of age may possess an adult-like concept of death but may have difficulty accepting death because they are discovering who they are, establishing an identity, and dealing with issues of puberty. Adolescents need peer support more than parental support to process the grieving process (Schonfeld & Demaria 2016).

### Nursing Assessment and Considerations

There is a progression of signs that let the health care team know the child is approaching death. Nurses may notice a sensation of heat on a child's skin even when the body feels cool. There may be decreased sensation and movement in lower extremities. There will be a loss of the senses of hearing as the last sense to diminish. The child's appetite will decrease as will thirst, and there may be swallowing issues. The child may be confused or lose consciousness. The child will develop metabolic acidosis, and will breathe with a Cheyne–Stokes respiration (fast, deep breathing, and periods of apnea), display bradycardia and hypotension, and lose bowel and bladder functions (Schonfeld & Demaria 2016).

The health care team can provide the family the opportunity for anticipatory grieving. The Nursing staff can provide privacy, a consistent nursing staff, and the opportunity for spiritual, cultural, or religious rituals (Schonfeld & Demaria 2016).

Palliative care aims to provide pain relief from terminal illnesses for children and families. The nurse consults with the client and family for desired measures and provides comfort measures, food, and hydration. Controlling pain is the priority nursing intervention. Nonpharmacological measures such as relaxation, imagery, and distraction help to manage pain (Schonfeld & Demaria 2016).

### Nursing Interventions for the Family

The nurse provides clear information to the client and family about the disease, medications, procedures, and expected events. Nurses teach and support parents to care for their loved one. Parents are encouraged to remain near the child as much as possible. Nurses promote the client's autonomy as developmentally and physically appropriate and prioritize the visitation of family and friends (Schonfeld & Demaria 2016).

Nurses support parents to understand the client's behaviors. Books, movies, art, music, and play therapy may provide an outlet for healing. The nurse delivers professional support and guidance from a trusted member of the health-care team that is neutral and accepting. The nurse encourages the celebration of special memories and people, reading of favorite books, providing favorite toys/objects, physical contact, sibling visits, and continued verbal communication, even if the client seems unconscious. The process is more important than the chosen activities (Schonfeld & Demaria 2016).

After death, give time to the family to stay with the body as long as they wish. The nurse removes any tubes and equipment with the help of a family member if they desire. The nurse provides the family emotional support (Schonfeld & Demaria 2016).

The nurse refers to the client by name and encourages all family members to share stories about the client's life (Schonfeld & Demaria 2016).

It is just as important that nurses practice self-care. Nurses who attempt to maintain good health, develop empathy, take time off of work, and develop well-rounded interests have longevity in the nursing profession. Nurses create professional and social support systems for themselves to support their nursing practice (Schonfeld & Demaria 2016).

## CHAPTER HIGHLIGHTS

- Pediatric patients are a vulnerable population who benefit from federal government programs to protect their health care.
- Families help to direct the nursing process in pediatric patients.
- Play must be incorporated into interactions with children as play is the work of childhood.

- Children have different anatomical and physiologic differences that direct their health care.
- Hospitalized children require interventions to keep them at the height of their growth and development potential.
- Child Life Specialists are a part of the health-care team to help children maintain their growth and development.
- Grieving families need support, privacy, and time to process the death of a child.

## REFERENCES


American Academy of Pediatrics (2017). Types of Families. Retrieved from https://www.healthychildren.org/English/family-life/family-dynamics/types-of-families/Pages/default.aspx

American Dental Association. (2012). Eruption charts. Retrieved from http://www.mouthhealthy.org/en/az-topics/e/eruption-charts

American Heart Association. (2015). Web-based Integrated Guidelines for Cardiopulmonary Resuscitation and Emergency Cardiovascular Care—Part 11: Pediatric Basic Life Support and Cardiopulmonary Resuscitation Quality. Retrieved from ECCguidelines.heart.org.

American Nurses Association. 2008. *Pediatric Nursing: Scope and Standards of Practice.* Silver Spring, MD: Nursebooks.org.

ATI Testing. 2016. Nursing Care of Children. Retrieved from http://www.atitesting.com/ati_next_gen/DisplayResources.aspx?Name=rm_rn_ncc_2016_ebook_20170417.pdf.

Baid, H. (2006). The process of conducting a physical assessment: a nursing perspective. *British Journal Of Nursing, 15*(13), 710.

Behere, A. P., Basnet, P., & Campbell, P. (2017). Effects of Family Structure on Mental Health of Children: A Preliminary Study. *Indian Journal Of Psychological Medicine, 39*(4), 457–463. doi:10.4103/0253-7176.211767

Best Practices, n.d. Retrieved June 21, 2017, from http://www.ipfcc.org/bestpractices/better-together.html.

Bettany, S. M., & Kerrane, B. (2016). The socio-materiality of parental style. *European Journal of Marketing, 50*(11), 2041–2066. Retrieved from https://search-proquest-com.chamberlainuniversity.idm.oclc.org/docview/1844593014?accountid=147674.

Bidell, T. R., & Shweder, R. A. (2009). *The Child : An Encyclopedic Companion.* Chicago: University of Chicago Press.

Boles, R. E., & Roberts, M. C. (2007). Children's perceptions of illness and death. In S. Ayers, A. Baum, C. McManus, & et. al. (Eds.), *Cambridge handbook of psychology, health and medicine* (2nd ed.). Cambridge, UK: Cambridge University Press. Retrieved from https://chamberlainuniversity.idm.oclc.org/login?url=http://search.credoreference.com/content/entry/cupphm/children_s_perceptions_of_illness_and_death/0?institutionId=8802.

Boztepe, H., & Kerimoğlu Yıldız, G. (2017). Nurses perceptions of barriers to implementing family-centered care in a pediatric setting: A qualitative study. *Journal For Specialists In Pediatric Nursing, 22*(2), n/a.

Breau, L. M., McGrath, P. J., Camfield, C. S., & Finley, G. A. (2002, September). Psychometric properties of the non-communicating children's pain checklist-revised. Retrieved November 12, 2017, from https://www.ncbi.nlm.nih.gov/pubmed/12237214.

Burns-Nader, S., and Hernandez-Reif, M. 2016. "Facilitating play for hospitalized children through child life services." *Children's Health Care,* 45(1), 1–21. doi:10.1080/02739615.2014.948161.

Byington, K. C. (1991). Your guide to pediatric drug administration. *Nursing, 21*(8), 82.

Canadian Paediatric Society (2008). Issues of care for hospitalized youth. *Paediatrics & Child Health, 13*(1), 61–64.

Caple, C. M. (2016). Physical Assessment in Children: Performing. *CINAHL Nursing Guide.*

Caple, C. M., & Balderrama, D. M. (2017). Administration of Medication: Intradermal Injection. *CINAHL Nursing Guide,*

Caple, C. M., & Walsh, K. C. (2016). Administration of Medication: Administering Medications via IV Bolus or IV Push. *CINAHL Nursing Guide.*

Caronia, J.R. (2017) Restrictive Lung Disease. Retrieved November 14, 2017, from https://emedicine.medscape.com/article/301760-overview.

Carter,E. & Sinclair,R. (2011). Drowning, *Continuing Education in Anaesthesia Critical Care & Pain,* 11(6). p210–213, https://doi.org/10.1093/bjaceaccp/mkr041

Cheung, E., Baerlocher, M. O., Asch, M., & Myers, A. (2009). Venous access: A practical review for 2009. *Canadian Family Physician, 55*(5), 494–496.

Children's Bureau Timeline. n.d. Retrieved June 17, 2017, from https://cb100.acf.hhs.gov/childrens-bureau-timeline.

Children's Bureau, U.S. Department of Health & Human Services (n.d.) Retrieved from https://cb100.acf.hhs.gov/sites/default/files/cb_ebook/cb_ebook.pdf

Children's Online Privacy Protection Rule ("COPPA"). 2015. Retrieved June 17, 2017, from https://www.ftc.gov/enforcement/rules/rulemaking-regulatory-reform-proceedings/childrens-online-privacy-protection-rule.

Choi, H. J., & Kim, Y. H. (2016). Apparent life-threatening event in infancy. *Korean Journal of Pediatrics, 59*(9), 347–354. http://doi.org/10.3345/kjp.2016.59.9.347

Clark, M., Michel, J., Early, R., & Baltes, B. (2014). Strategies for Coping with Work Stressors and Family Stressors: Scale Development and Validation. *Journal Of Business & Psychology, 29*(4), 617–638.

Cordova, D., Heinze, J., Mistry, R., Hsieh, H., Stoddard, S., Salas-Wright, C. P., & Zimmerman, M. A. (2014). Family Functioning and Parent Support Trajectories and Substance Use and Misuse among Minority Urban Adolescents: A Latent Class Growth Analysis. *Substance Use & Misuse, 49*(14), 1908–1919.

Crisp, S., & Rainbow, J. (Eds.). (2007). *Emergencies in paediatrics and neonatology.* Retrieved from https://ebookcentral-proquest-com.chamberlainuniversity.idm.oclc.org

Duncan, D. (2015). Candida and breastfeeding. *British Journal Of Midwifery, 23*(2), 98–100.

Dyer, S., & Moneta, G. B. (2006). FREQUENCY OF PARALLEL, ASSOCIATIVE, AND COOPERATIVE PLAY IN BRITISH CHILDREN OF DIFFERENT SOCIOECONOMIC STATUS. *Social Behavior & Personality: An International Journal, 34*(5), 587–592.

Eligibility. n.d. Retrieved June 17, 2017, from https://www.medicaid.gov/medicaid/eligibility/index.html.

Engel, S. C. (2015). Drowning episodes: Prevention and resuscitation tips. *Journal Of Family Practice, 64*(2), E1-E6.

Engelke, Z. M., & Schub, T. B. (2016). Parent Education: Teaching Parents about Preventing Accidental Poisoning in Children. *CINAHL Nursing Guide,*

Estabrooks, C. A., Chong, H., Brigidear, K., & Profetto-McGrath, J. (2005). Profiling Canadian nurses' preferred knowledge sources for clinical practice. *Can J Nurs Res 37*(2) p. 118–40.

Farkouh, A., Frigo, P., & Czejka, M. (2016). Systemic side effects of eye drops: a pharmacokinetic perspective. *Clinical Ophthalmology (Auckland, N.Z.), 10,* 2433–2441. http://doi.org/10.2147/OPTH.S118409

Gray, Peter. 2013. *Free to Learn.* New York, New York: Basic Books.

Greydanus, Donald E. The Pediatric Diagnostic Examination New York : McGraw-Hill Professional. 2008. eBook., Database: eBook Collection (EBSCOhost)

Gunning, K. E. (2003). Pathophysiology of Respiratory Failure and Indications for Respiratory Support. Retrieved from http://jpck.zju.edu.cn/jcyxjp/files/ge/04/MT/0453.pdf https://doi.org/10.1383/surg.21.3.72.14672

Halpern-Manners, A., Warren, J. R., Raymo, J. M., and Nicholson, D. A. 2015. "The Impact of Work and Family Life Histories on Economic Well-Being at Older Ages." *Social Forces, 93*(4), 1369–1396.

Hampson, R. B., & Beavers, W. R. (1996). FAMILY THERAPY AND OUTCOME: RELATIONSHIPS BETWEEN THERAPIST AND FAMILY STYLES. *Contemporary Family Therapy: An International Journal, 18*(3), 345–370.

Harrison, T. 2010. "Family-Centered Pediatric Nursing Care: State of the Science." *Journal of Pediatric Nursing-Nursing Care Of Children & Families, 25*(5), 335–343.

Healthy People 2020 Leading Health Indicators: Progress Update. n.d. Retrieved June 30, 2017, from https://www.healthypeople.gov/2020/leading-health-indicators/Healthy-People-2020-Leading-Health-Indicators%3A-Progress-Update.

Huff, L., Hamlin, A., Wolski, D., McClure, T., Eliades, A. B., Weaver, L., & Shelestak, D. (2009). Atraumatic Care: EMLA Cream and Application of Heat to Facilitate Peripheral Venous Cannulation in Children. *Issues In Comprehensive Pediatric Nursing, 32*(2), 65–76.

Institute of Medicine. (2003), Health professions education: A bridge to quality. *Washington DC: National Academies Press.*

Janahi, I. A., Khan, S., Chandra, P., Al-Marri, N., Saadoon, A., Al-Naimi, L., & . . . Greer, W. (2017). A new clinical algorithm scoring for management of suspected foreign body aspiration in children. *BMC Pulmonary Medicine, 17*(1), 61. doi:10.1186/s12890-017-0406-6

Jeffery Media Productions (2017). Normal Pediatric Vital Signs (PALS) Retrieved from https://acls-algorithms.com/wp-content/uploads/2017/03/PALS-Vital-Signs.pdf

Jen, E., Wu, J., & Gentry, M. (2016). Social and Affective Concerns High-Ability Adolescents Indicate They Would Like to Discuss With a Caring Adult. *Journal Of Advanced Academics, 27*(1), 39–59. doi:10.1177/1932202X15621904

Joint Commission (2017) National Patient Safety Goals. Retrieved from https://www.jointcommission.org/assets/1/6/2017_NPSG_HAP_ER.pdf

Jordan, A., and Romer, D., eds. 2014. *Media and the well-being of children and adolescents.* New York: Oxford University Press.

Jordan, B., Franich-Ray, C., Anderson, V., Northam, E., Albert, N., Cochrane, A., & Menahem, S. (2013). Maternal Report of Infant Emotional Well-Being Following Their Infant's Hospitalization for Neonatal Cardiac Surgery. *Infant Mental Health Journal, 34*(4), 259–266.

Jovanovic, J. 2011. "Saying Goodbye: An Investigation into Parent-Infant Separation Behaviours on Arrival in Childcare." *Child Care in Practice, 17*(3), 247–69.

Kaiser Family Foundation. (2016). Uninsured Rate Among the Nonelderly Population. Retrieved from https://www.kff.org/uninsured/fact-sheet/key-facts-about-the-uninsured-population/

Kendrick, D., Mulvaney, C. A., Ye, L., Stevens, T., Mytton, J. A., & Stewart-Brown, S. (2013). Parenting interventions for the prevention of unintentional injuries in childhood. *Cochrane Database of Systematic Reviews*, (Issue 3), CD006020. doi:10.1002/14651858.CD006020.pub3

Kiesler, J., & Ricer, R. (2003). The abnormal fontanel. *American Family Physician, 67*(12), 2547–2552.

Koren, Kuo, D. Z., Frick, K. D., & Minkovitz, C. S. (2011). Association of Family-Centered Care with Improved Anticipatory Guidance Delivery and Reduced Unmet Needs in Child Health Care. Maternal And Child Health Journal, 15(8), 1228–1237.

Larsen, L. C., & Fuller, S. H. (1996). Management of acetaminophen toxicity. *American Family Physician, 53*(1), 185

Lawrence, P. C., & Schub, T. B. (2017). Lead Poisoning (Plumbism). *CINAHL Nursing Guide*,

Lehner, D. C. (2015). Toddler Developmental Delays After Extensive Hospitalization: Primary Care Practitioner Guidelines. *Pediatric Nursing, 41*(5), 236–242.

Lewis, K. and Weber, S. 2015. Perspectives on Parent-and-Child Work in Waldorf Early Childhood Education. Spring Valley: New York. Waldorf Early Childhood Association of North America.

Maguire, D, Webb, M., Passmore, D., Cline,G. (2012). NICU Nurses' Lived Experience: Caring for Infants With Neonatal Abstinence Syndrome. *Advances in Neonatal Care. 12(5):281–285, October 2012.*

McGrath, P. A. (1994). Psychological aspects of pain perception. Retrieved November 12, 2017, from https://www.ncbi.nlm.nih.gov/pubmed/7702468

McGrath, P., & Huff, N. (2001). 'What is it?': findings on preschoolers' responses to play with medical equipment. *Child: Care, Health & Development, 27*(5), 451–462.

Office of Head Start. n.d. Retrieved June 17, 2017, from https://www.acf.hhs.gov/ohs/about.

O'Malley, G. F. (2015). *Hydrocarbon Poisoning.* http://www.merckmanuals.com/professional/injuries-poisoning/poisoning/hydrocarbon-poisoning

O'Malley, G. F. (2015). *Caustic Ingestion.* http://www.merckmanuals.com/professional/injuries-poisoning/poisoning/caustic-ingestion#v1118891

Lupa, M., Magne, J., Guarisco, J. L., & Amedee, R. (2009). Update on the Diagnosis and Treatment of Caustic Ingestion. *The Ochsner Journal, 9*(2), 54–59.

Miller, J. (2015). Verifying NG tube placement in children. *Nursing, 45*(10), 9.

National School Lunch Program (NSLP). n.d. Retrieved June 17, 2017, from https://www.fns.usda.gov/nslp/history_10#free.

Parten, M. B. (1932). Social participation among pre-school children. *The Journal of Abnormal and Social Psychology, 27*(3), 243–269. http://dx.doi.org/10.1037/h0074524

Pilgrim, J. M., & Schub, E. B. (2017). Administration of Medication in Children: Robinson, H. C. (2016). Respiratory Conditions Update: Restrictive Lung Disease. Retrieved from https://www.ncbi.nlm.nih.gov/pubmed/27576233 Subcutaneous Injection. *CINAHL Nursing Guide*,

Pinquart, M. (2016). Associations of Parenting Styles and Dimensions with Academic Achievement in Children and Adolescents: A Meta-Analysis. *Educational Psychology Review*, *28*(3), 475–493.

Poverty Guidelines. 2017. Retrieved June 17, 2017, from https://aspe.hhs.gov/poverty-guidelines.

QSEN Competencies. n.d. Retrieved June 30, 2017, from http://qsen.org/competencies/pre-licensure-ksas/.

Riley, M. & Bluhm, B. (2012). High Blood Pressure in Children and Adolescents *Am Fam Physician*. 2012 Apr 1;85(7):693–700.

Santrock, J. W. 2007. "*Parten's classic study of play.*" *A topical approach to life-span development* (3rd ed.). New York: McGraw-Hill. p. 573. ISBN0-07-313376-0.

Scheiman, M, Amos, C., Ciner, E., Marsh-Toole, W., Moore, B., Rouse, M. (2002) Pediatric Eye and Vision Assessment. Retrieved from https://www.aoa.org/documents/optometrists/CPG-2.pdf

Schonfeld, D. J. & Demaria, T. COMMITTEE ON PSYCHOSOCIAL ASPECTS OF CHILD AND FAMILY HEALTH, DISASTER PREPAREDNESS ADVISORY COUNCIL. (2016). Supporting the Grieving Child and Family. Pediatrics 138 (3) p Retrieved November 19, 2017, from http://pediatrics.aappublications.org.chamberlainuniversity.idm.oclc.org/content/138/3/e20162147Schub, E. B. (2016). Oxygen Therapy by Face Mask: Providing for the Pediatric Patient. *CINAHL Nursing Guide*,

Shields L, Zhou H, Pratt J, Taylor M, Hunter J, and Pascoe E. 2012. Family-centered care for hospitalised children aged 0–12 years. *Cochrane Database of Systematic Reviews 2012*, Issue 10. Art. No.: CD004811. DOI: 10.1002/14651858.CD004811.pub3.

Shivayogi, P. 2013. Vulnerable population and methods for their safeguard. Retrieved June 17, 2017, from https://www.ncbi.nlm.nih.gov/pmc/articles/PMC3601707/.

Smith, J. G., Desai, P. P., Sira, N., and Engelke, S. C. 2014. "Family-Centered Developmentally Supportive Care in the Neonatal Intensive Care Unit: Exploring the Role and Training of Child Life Specialists." *Children's Health Care*, *43*(4), 345–368. doi:10.1080/02739615.2014.880917.

Smith, N. C., & Hurst, A. M. (2016). Physical Assessment Performing in the Newborn. *CINAHL Nursing Guide*,

Smith, N. C. (2016). Pain Assessment in Children: Performing. *CINAHL Nursing Guide*,

Smith, N. C., & Engelke, Z. M. (2017). Parent Teaching: Prevention of Sudden Infant Death Syndrome. *CINAHL Nursing Guide*,

Stoltz, P & Manworren, R (2017). Comparison of Children's Venipuncture Fear and Pain: Randomized Controlled Trial of EMLA® and J-Tip Needleless Injection System *Journal of Pediatric Nursing: Nursing Care of Children and Families* (37) p. 91–96

Strauss, V. (2017, Oct). 9 million kids get health insurance under CHIP. Congress just let it expire. *The Washington Post*. https://www.washingtonpost.com/news/answer-sheet/wp/2017/10/01/9-million-kids-get-health-insurance-under-chip-congress-just-let-it-expire/?utm_term=.62c1d48ad3ff.

Thiadens, A. J., Hoyng, C. B., Polling, J. R., Bernaerts-Biskop, R., van den Born, L. I., & Klaver, C. W. (2013). Accuracy of Four Commonly Used Color Vision Tests in the Identification of Cone Disorders. *Ophthalmic Epidemiology*, *20*(2), 114–122. doi:10.3109/09286586.2012.759596

Toruner, E. K., & Uysal, G. (2012). Causes, reporting, and prevention of medication errors from a pediatric nurse perspective. *Australian Journal Of Advanced Nursing*, *29*(4), 28–35.

United Nations (2013). General comment No. 17 (2013) on the right of the child to rest, leisure, play, recreational activities, cultural life and the arts (art. 31). Retrieved June 30, 2017, from http://ipaworld.org/childs-right-to-play/article-31/

United States Department of Agriculture (2015). "Household Food Security in the United States in 2014" Retrieved from https://www.ers.usda.gov/webdocs/publications/84973/err237_summary.pdf?v=42979

Uygun, Ibrahim, Okur, Mehmet Hanifi, Otcu, Selcuk, & Ozturk, Hayrettin. (2011). Peripherally inserted central catheters in the neonatal period. *Acta Cirurgica Brasileira*, *26*(5), 404–411. https://dx.doi.org/10.1590/S0102-86502011000500014

Weidemann, D., Weaver, V., & Fadrowski, J. (2016). Toxic environmental exposures and kidney health in children. *Pediatric Nephrology, 31*(11), 2043–2054. doi:10.1007/s00467-015-3222-

Weiss, J. (2010, July 01). Prevention of Drowning. Retrieved November 14, 2017, from http://pediatrics.aappublications.org/content/126/1/178

Wente, Sarah J.K. (2013). Nonpharmacologic Pediatric Pain Management in Emergency Departments: A Systematic Review of the Literature.Retrieved from http://ovidsp.tx.ovid.com.chamberlainuniversity.idm.oclc.org/sp-3.27.1a/ovidweb.cgi?&S=NIJGFPBGAFDDHPMLNCFKMFFBBKCNAA00&Abstract=S.sh.62%7c1%7c1

Whelan, T. (2007). Hospitalization in children. In S. Ayers, A. Baum, C. McManus, & et. al. (Eds.), *Cambridge handbook of psychology, health and medicine* (2nd ed.). Cambridge, UK: Cambridge University Press. Retrieved from https://chamberlainuniversity.idm.oclc.org/login?url=http://search.credoreference.com/content/entry/cupphm/hospitalization_in_children/0?institutionId=8802

White, Rachel. 2012. Power of Play. Retrieved from https://mcm.org/wp-content/uploads/2015/09/MCMResearchSummary1.pdf.

Wise, S. (2017). Family structure, child outcomes and environmental mediators. Retrieved November 10, 2017, from https://aifs.gov.au/publications/family-structure-child-outcomes-and-environmental-mediators/export

Women, Infants and Children (WIC). n.d. Retrieved June 15, 2017, from https://www.fns.usda.gov/wic/wic-income-eligibility-guidelines.

World Health Organization (WHO) (2012). Retrieved from http://apps.who.int/iris/bitstream/10665/44540/1/9789241548120_Guidelines.pdf

Young, K., Cochran (Brehmer), K., Mei, M., & Adkins-Bley, K. (2015). Ensuring Safe Medication Administration through Direct Observation. *Quality In Primary Care, 23*(3), 167–173.

CHAPTER 2

# GROWTH AND DEVELOPMENT

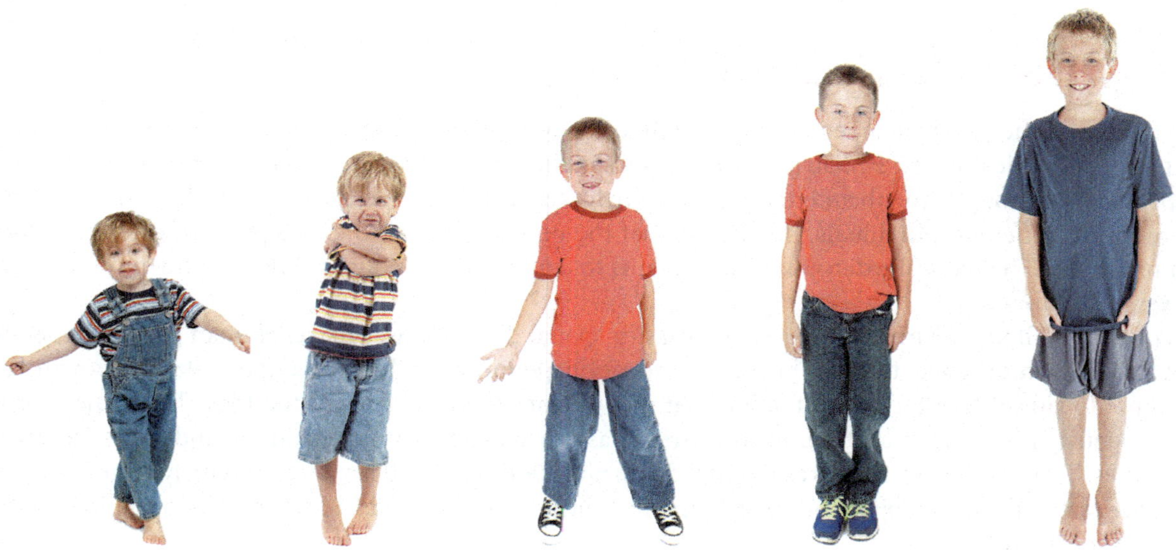

© Suzanne Tucker/Shutterstock.com

## LEARNING OUTCOMES

1. Describe the developmental theories of Erickson and Piaget.
2. Utilize the nursing process to provide safe, comprehensive health care to developing infants, toddlers, preschoolers, school-age children, and adolescents.
3. Recognize significant developmental milestones in infants, toddlers, preschoolers, school-age children, and adolescents.
4. Synthesize data from theories, physical assessment and developmental milestones to create a focused assessment.
5. Plan nursing interventions and evaluate outcomes that are developmentally appropriate for infants, toddlers, preschoolers, school-age children, and adolescents.
6. Teaching/learning principles in providing anticipatory guidance in the prevention of disease across childhood.

7. Construct a comprehensive "family-centered" teaching plan for children and their families.
8. Provide anticipatory guidance in the delivery of family-centered women's health care through client teaching to promote and maintain wellness.

## KEY TERMS

Animism
Anticipatory guidance
Associative play
Attachment
Autonomy
Bonding
Centration
Cephalocaudal
Competitive play
Cooperative play
Conservation
Egocentrism
Holophrases
Intersectionality
Magical thinking
Negativism
Object permanence
Parallel play
Physiologic anorexia
Pretend play
Proximodistal
Ritualism
Separation anxiety
Solitary play

## Principles of Growth and Development

Understanding the predictable, emerging growth and development patterns in children are essential to the practice of pediatric nursing. Pediatric nurses use these principles to deliver customized care across the pediatric spectrum. Although growth and development are linked; they are processes that unfold in time and space, differently, in different individuals. It is the goal of the pediatric nurse to create plans of care that promote both processes. The natural extension of this goal is to support the family as children undergo the dynamic process of childhood.

Growth in all organisms refers to an increase in spatial dimensions, or size. Human growth depends on many factors including genetics, sex, hormones, nutrition, pollution, and socioeconomic status. Growth occurs in a **cephalocaudal** (see Fig 2-1) direction that moves from the head toward the toes. The growth process simultaneously proceeds in a **proximodistal** trend, as it originates from the midline and moves toward the extremities. The fetal head emerges as the first discernible body part and remains extremely large in comparison to the rest of the developing body. Fetal growth continues as the head and trunk develop, before the arms and legs (Fowler 2016).

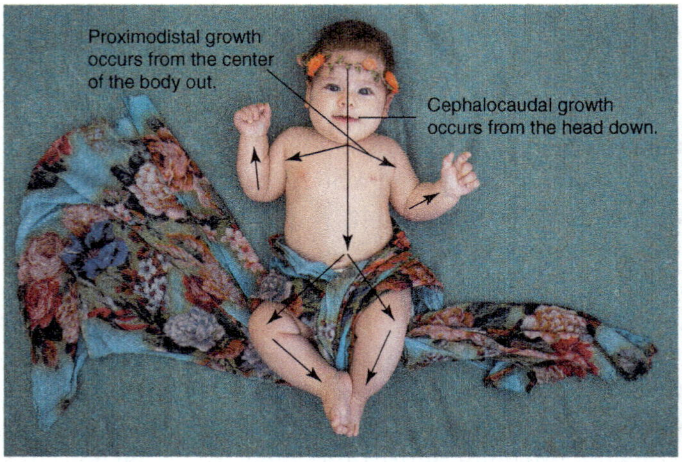


Modified from © Zoltan Gabor/Shutterstock.com

**Fig 2-1** Growth occurs from a cephalocaudal and proximodistal directions

Human beings possess a large skull that protects the developing brain. A child's genetic code creates a blueprint for the nascent brain. However, according to Harvard University Center for the Developing Child, the "architecture" of the human brain, or the potential of the human mind develops between the child and the environment. This interaction reinforces neural connections in the brain that are difficult to change later in development. Growth and development interact in dynamic ways to produce a mature adult (Center on the Developing Child at Harvard University 2017).

The development process yields an increase in complexity and maturation in the brain. Neurons sequentially connect to process information more complexly. Muscles progressively build to increase strength, endurance, flexibility, and coordination. Kidneys mature to increase the concentration and filtration of urine, the digestive system expands as levels of enzymes necessary for digestion increase, and the endocrine system releases hormones within weeks of conception and peaks during puberty (Fowler 2016).

Child development consists of an individualized, continuous process shaped by many factors such as genetics, sex, hormones, nutrition, psychosocial environment, pollution, socioeconomic status, and culture (National Research Council (US); Institute of Medicine (US), 2004). Children develop as they acquire skills through interaction with their environment. The rate of development is variable, but the sequence is not. Pediatric patients require additional assessments of chronological and developmental age to yield a holistic clinical picture.

The most important application of growth and development principles for the pediatric nurse is to offer **anticipatory guidance** about upcoming physical challenges. Physical growth will determine particular environmental modifications parents will need to enforce, and children will have to navigate. Anticipatory guidance allows parents time to understand the next stage and provides ample time for questions as a proactive technique that promotes child safety (DeSafey 2012).

Nurses use developmental concepts to direct patient care. A developmental approach makes a child feel comfortable and facilitates his or her cooperation. An age-appropriate toy acts to calm, distract, and teach a child while the pediatric nurse obtains an assessment. Clear, honest, and developmentally appropriate communication makes the child, the nurse, and the family feel like a team against medical challenges (Fowler 2016).

Nurses further support a child's growth and development by monitoring, implementing, and teaching about optimal nutrition and rest. The holistic theory of nursing equally encourages exposure to opportunity, cognitive and psychosocial stimulation, and caring guidance. The developmental theories of Erikson and Piaget help assess the psychological, cognitive, and moral dimensions of children and guide the nurse to better help patients during health and disease (Fowler 2016).

Nurses must use critical thinking to understand the junction of growth and development of the pediatric client. Early identification of developmental delay and whether that delay is related to hospitalization helps guide interventions for the child.

## QSEN Application

Patient-centered care calls for nurses to "recognize the patient or designee as the source of control and full partner in providing compassionate and coordinated care based on respect for patient's preferences, values, and needs." Nurses need knowledge of patient preferences; coordination and integration of care with other providers to provide transitions and continuity, physical and emotional support, the availability of friends and family for support, and the effect of cultural, ethnic, and social identifications. Nurses need the skills to draw out patient values, provide them an environment that is respectful to those values, and communicate those values to other members of the health-care team. Patient-centered care is important in assessing growth and development to gain a valid conclusion as to how the process is unfolding".

When a nurse understands the developmental and chronological age of the child, the nurse can design customized care for the child.

From Quality and Safety Education for Nurses http://qsen.org/competencies/pre-licensure-ksas/

# Developmental Theorists

## Erickson

The psychosocial theory of Erik Erikson (1968), and the cognitive theory of Jean Piaget (1950) assist nurses in making assessments and interpreting the patient response (Fowler 2016). These assessments allow nurses to create plans of care that serve the child intellectually, emotionally, and physically.

Erik Erikson, a German psychoanalyst with a background in Montessori education, studied the psychosocial development of human beings. Erikson excelled to Professor of Human Relations at Yale University. Erikson's ideas changed the role of children in modern society. He took a giant step away from the contemporary Freudian psychosexual model of children, toward a developmental conflict model. In this theory, the human relationship is the interface that explains human development. Each stage reflects a conflict that needs resolution before moving to the next stage. Erikson represents development in eight stages from birth to death. Each quantitative stage highlights a conflict necessary to assimilate to increase development and a healthy personality. Each conflict integrates knowledge and builds toward the next stage. Incomplete stages leave psychological remnants of the conflict and remain in the personality. The Erikson stages from birth to adolescence apply to pediatric populations. (Erikson 2013).

**Table 2-1** Erikson Stages

| Age | Psychosocial Crisis |
|---|---|
| Infant<br>0-1 | Trust vs Mistrust |
| Toddler<br>1-3 | Autonomy vs Shame |
| Preschooler<br>3-6 | Initiative vs Guilt |
| School Age<br>6-12 | Industry vs Isolation |
| Adolescent<br>12-18 | Identity vs Role Confusion |

Information sources from Erickson 2013. Table courtesy of Sondae Stevens.


Erikson's theory directs nursing interventions to increase health promotion and health maintenance. This approach supports parents around common concerns from potty training and temper tantrums to adolescent experimentation and limit testing. The nurse reconciles some child–parent tensions by teaching parents to understand the developmental perspective of the child. The impact of hospitalization causes a disruption of **bonding** and **attachment** processes for children and their families upon admission. Nursing must seek to identify and support families who encounter this phenomenon (ATI Testing 2016).

Bonding occurs in the first Erikson stage of trust vs. mistrust and refers to a feeling of connectedness from the adult to the child (ATI Testing 2016). The fit of personalities between mother or caregiver and child begins the parenting journey. Sensitivity to this fit encourages nursing interventions to increase bonding. Nurses use therapeutic frameworks to support mother-baby dyads. Many things can disrupt this new relationship including medical treatments, prematurity, and messages from the media. Simple bonding problems from labor medications or cesarean birth benefit from consistent support from the Obstetric nurse. These issues resolve quickly, especially when mothers decide to breastfeed their baby and have familial support. More complex bonding problems require a referral for social services or psychological issues. Nursing time spent on bonding and subsequent attachment may prevent issues of care later in the relationship (ATI Testing 2016).

Attachment supports an emotional and spiritual connection between child and caregiver. Attachment is a measure of connectedness from child to adult. Children display attachment when they seek the attachment figure out when they are scared or hurt. Adults exhibit a secure attachment when they respond to this relationship. The nurse consciously works with parents to promote the appropriate development of the child and family, especially during hospitalization (ATI Testing 2016).

## Piaget

Jean Piaget, a Swiss psychologist, known for his groundbreaking work in child development, also changed the perception of childhood. He served as Director of the International Bureau of Education to help educate the children of the world. Unlike Erikson, Piaget focused on the qualitative features of knowledge acquisition (Smith, d.)

Piaget believed children grow and develop their reasoning processes as a result of their interactions with the environment. Therefore, children need to explore and interact with outside stimuli to develop more advanced reasoning processes. (Chambers 2013).

Piaget believed children are not smaller, sillier, cuter versions of adults. Younger children think in a subjectively different way from older children and adults. Children in the same Piaget stage, apply a similar logic to their reasoning (Chambers 2013).

According to Piaget, children direct cognitive development. Children actively participate in life and do not passively wait for cues from adults to learn. Children play to learn about the world around them. Children explore their physical environment and construct their understanding of objects and events (Chambers 2013).

Piaget's theory includes four stages or periods of cognitive development. Cognitive development increases information processing and language development. Piaget explained the thinking that characterizes each of these stages through childhood (Chambers 2013).

Piaget defines four stages: sensorimotor, preoperational, concrete operational, and formal operational. The sensorimotor period develops the infant's senses to interpret the world. The development of cognitive skills includes **object permanence**, separation, and mental representation (ATI Testing, 2016). Object-permanence refers to the understanding that an object, or person, exist even when out of sight (Chambers 2013).

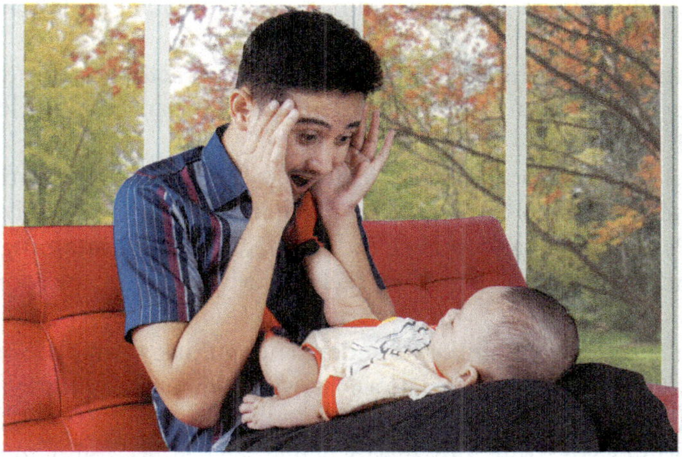

© Creativa Images/Shutterstock.com

**Fig 2-2** A baby begins to learn about object permanence

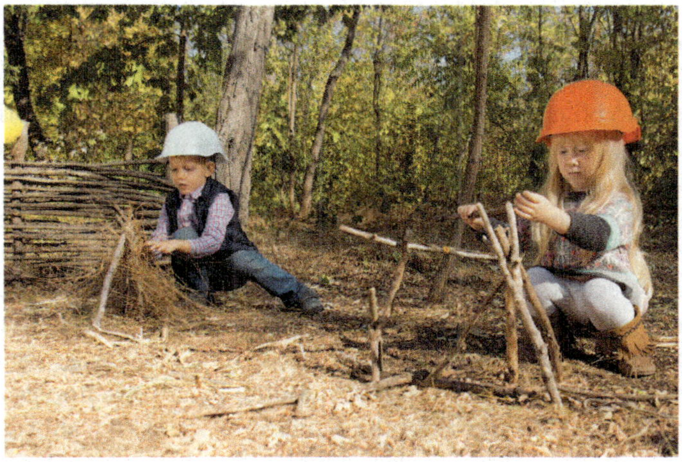

© Viacheslav Nikolaenko/Shutterstock.com

**Fig 2-3** Children learn through their environment

**Table 2-2** Infant Language Development

| Age | Stage |
|---|---|
| 3 weeks | Crying 1-1 1/2 hours per day |
| 6 weeks | Crying 2-4 hours per day |
| 2 months | Single vowel sounds |
| 3-4 months | Cooing; turns head to sounds and makes consonant sounds |
| 9-10 months | Understands "no"; 2 word to 3 word phrases |
| 1 year | 3-5 words |



The game "peek-a-boo" serves as the classic example to teach infants this concept. This phenomenon occurs at approximately 9 to 10 months of age. Separation challenges infants and parents, especially the first time. The bonding and attachment periods build trust, and separation strengthens that bond. Infants build separation skills from their parents and/or caregivers so they can experience more of the world. The baby learns to play in safe spaces that are adjacent to and in view of the caregiver. Eventually, the infant learns to trust that they are not alone and can tolerate longer time periods without requiring direct contact with parents (ATI Testing 2016).

Handover techniques such as saying goodbye and using a ritual ease the anxiety for both mother and child (Jovanovic 2011). In homes where there are other siblings, or children are in day care centers this is accomplished rather quickly.

Separation anxiety emerges as a normal stage in development. It acts as a reflex when the infant is in perceived danger. It draws the mother or caregiver back to the child. The anxiety lasts longer in the mother after separation (Jovanovic 2011).

Both mother and child should practice this process to develop their relationship. It is important for children to understand separation can happen, and that the primary caregiver returns soon after. It creates a sense of trust. Parents must also realize the importance of maintaining trust with their infant. Parents should refrain from breaking the handover technique by sneaking away or tricking the child (ATI Testing 2016).

Mental representation is the infant's ability to understand and use symbols. Some infants may use sign language to communicate. The infant may associate a coat, with someone leaving. Symbols become a new way to communicate (ATI Testing 2016).

The preoperational period spans from 2 to 7 years of age. The child's ability to use symbols to represent language emerges. Their ability to use logic does not. Children display **egocentrism** and **animism** in the preoperational period. Egocentrism makes children unable to represent a perspective different from their own. Adults should model empathy, but children's behavior will not reflect this at this time. When children play hide-and-seek, adults see their egocentrism. Piaget (1929) believed egocentrism caused children to project their feelings and thoughts onto other objects (Chambers 2013). Often children partially hide from the adult, yet they feel completely hidden. Preoperational children display animism or the belief that inanimate objects possess emotions and thoughts (ATI Testing 2016).

The concrete operational period spans from approximately 7–11 years of age. Children use logical thought to understand the physical world, which is a significant milestone. Children understand rules and limitations of physical objects. Concrete operational thinkers now understand the concept of **conservation**. Conservation refers to certain inherent physical properties of objects that do not change when a superficial change is made to their appearance (Chambers 2013). The classic example uses two different sized containers using the same amount of water. Undoubtedly, a preschooler claims that the amount of water in a tall, slender glass was greater than the amount of water in a short, wide glass. This occurs even when children see the amounts of water were equal before being transferred into these containers (Fowler, 2016).

# Assessment

## Communication with the Infant

Infants begin to communicate immediately through crying, body language, and eye contact. Nurses communicate with infants when they hold them for feedings, talk and even sing to them when they are in quiet alert, and comfort and swaddle them, if they are upset. Creating a calm, comfortable environment soothes the infant and builds on the rapport between infant, nurse, and family (ATI Testing 2016).

Nurses who create a comfortable, warm environment and take a slow approach to physical contact with an infant get better assessments. Nurses who take time to play with the infant will find a readiness of the infant to participate in the assessment. Creating a rapport with an infant may be intimidating. However, nursing is part of a team effort. Pay attention to the ways the family speaks to the child. If done successfully the nurse will have a place on the team and possibly in the family's heart (ATI Testing 2016).

## Cultural Influences

The dynamic, multicultural nature of health care demands nursing deliver care to an ever-diversifying patient population. By 2030, 40% of Americans will identify as a minority (Siantz, M. L. 2008). The desire to eliminate health disparities depends on future nurses who reflect the diversification of the patient population and those willing to be advocates of diversity. Current nurses need cultural awareness, cultural knowledge, cultural skill, and cultural encounters to become culturally competent (Ferguson, S. L., and Campinha-Bacote, J. 1997). The term culture includes race, gender, sexuality, and class.

All cultures have norms around parenting and meeting developmental milestones. Nurses must account for this in their growth and development assessment. Racial stereotypes have detrimental effects on the growth and development of both the marginalized children and those that benefit from the marginalization. Race and class both impact access to health care. According to the Center for Disease Control, the infant mortality rate was double for black women as white women in 2005 and 2008 (CDC Health Disparities & Inequalities Report (CHDIR) 2015).

Nurses must utilize the concept of **intersectionality** to understand the ways racism, sexism, sexuality, and ableness overlap, and subsequently impact children. By reducing an experience to one effect, only one perspective emerges. The problem of seeing discrimination from one view oversimplifies and ignores other aspects of the discrimination. The impact must be viewed through multiple lenses and synthesized to create a holistic picture of the family and the children (Crenshaw, K. 1991).

## Premature Infants

Premature infants who are born before 37 weeks are considered premature. Babies are categorized as late preterm (34–36 weeks gestation), moderately preterm (32–34 weeks), very preterm (less than 32 weeks), and

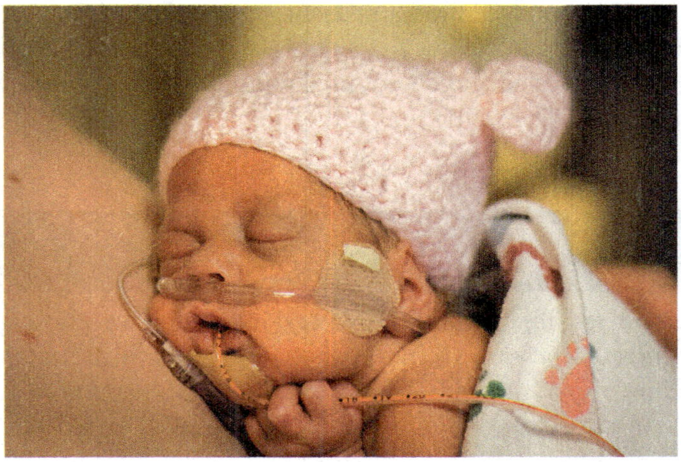

Maesse Photography/Shutterstock.com

**Fig 2-4** A premie on oxygen with an orogastric tube

extremely preterm (before 28 weeks). Premature babies are challenged to begin life without developed organ systems (Loftin, R. W., Habli, M., Snyder, C. C., Cormier, C. M., Lewis, D. F., & DeFranco, E. A. 2010).

Premies have not developed a fully functioning respiratory, hepatic, genitourinary, or immune system. Premies lack brown fat and subcutaneous fat making them prone to heat loss, tachypnea, and hypoglycemia. Premature babies may have feeding problems related to poor suck and swallow reflexes. They start life in the lowest percentiles on the growth chart and need extra time to catch up to the milestones of typical infants (Greydanus 2008).

## Infants

An infant's developing brain can make more than one million neural connections every second. This effect continues in the first few years of life. These connections provide the framework for brain architecture that will direct future learning, behavior, and health. Genetics create beginning brain structure, and interaction reinforces these connections through repeated use. It appears that the major factor in brain development is a "serve and return" between parents and children, and children and their community. Serve and return develops as a result of the bonding and attachment process. An infant may develop social behavior through smiling. An adult response reinforces the neural circuit. If this process does not occur, infant brains can flood with stress hormones and hinder normal brain development (Center on the Developing Child at Harvard University 2017).

### Physical Assessment

The typical newborn will have head circumference averages between 33 and 35 cm (13 and 14 in). A typical infant's head circumference grows 2 cm (0.75 in) per month during the first 3 months, 1 cm (0.4 in) per month from 4 to 6 months of age, and 0.5 cm (0.2 in) per month during the second 6 months (ATI Testing 2016).

The crown to rump length is 31–35 cm (12.5–14 in), approximately equal to head circumference. The head to heel length averages 48–53 cm (19–21 in). Newborn weight averages 2,700–4,000 g (6–9 lb.). Newborns typically lose up to 10% of their birth weight by 3 to 4 days of age. Typical fluid shifts, loss of meconium, and limited but adequate intake, especially in infants who breastfeed, indicates weight will fluctuate. Babies regain their birth weight by the tenth to the fourteenth day of life, depending on the feeding method used (ATI Testing 2016).

Infants gain weight at a rate of 680 g (1.5 lb.) per month during the first 5 months of life. A typical 6-month-old baby weighs 7.26 kg (16 lb.). Birth weight doubles by the age of 5 months, and triples by the age of 12 months. Babies average 9.75 kg (21.5 lb.) at 1 year of age. Infants height increase approximately 2.5 cm (1 in) per month until the child is 6 months of age. The child's birth length increases by 50% by the age of 12 months (ATI Testing 2016).

An accurate birth weight is an important parameter to assess infant growth and breastfeeding efficacy. However, birth weights can artificially inflate due to IV fluid administration. The most accurate birth weights occur in mothers who are orally hydrated and do not use IV fluids in labor (Noel-Weiss, J., Woodend, K. A., Peterson, W. E., Gibb, W., and Groll, D. L. 2011).

#### Clinical Pearl

Labor interventions often call for fluid administration and increase newborn weights. Fluid administration to the mother can artificially increase a baby's birth weight, and artificially decrease the baby's weight at the first two-week wellness appointment. Doctors and nurses should consider this if an exclusively breastfed infant has lost more than 10% of their weight (Noel-Weiss, J., Woodend, K. A., Peterson, W. E., Gibb, W., and Groll, D. L. 2011).

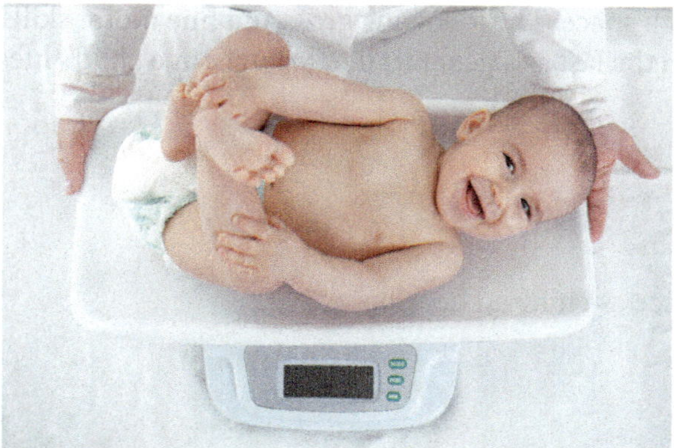

© didesign021/Shutterstock.com

**Fig 2-5** An infant on an infant scale

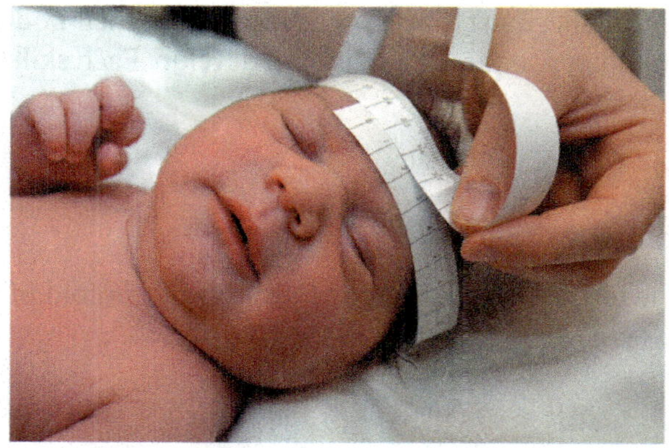

© ChameleonsEye/Shutterstock.com

**Fig 2-6** Infant head is measured around the widest circumference

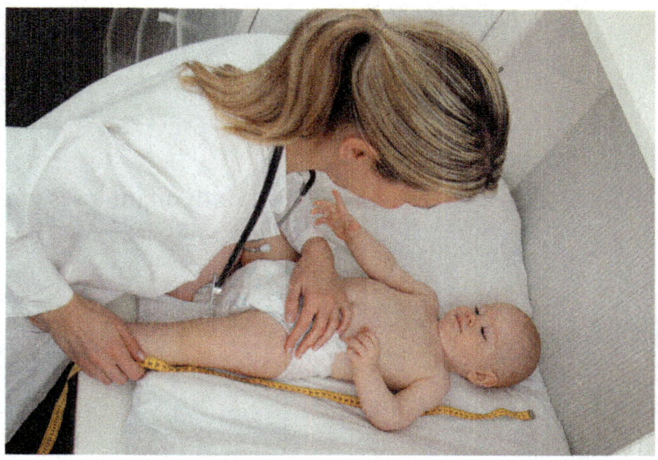

© riopatuca/Shutterstock.com

**Fig 2-7** Length is measured from the top of the head to the heel

Growth results in an increase in physical parameters of height, weight, and bone growth. Growth charts are created by the Center for Disease Control and are used as a standard to measure the pediatric client's growth over time (ATI Testing 2016).

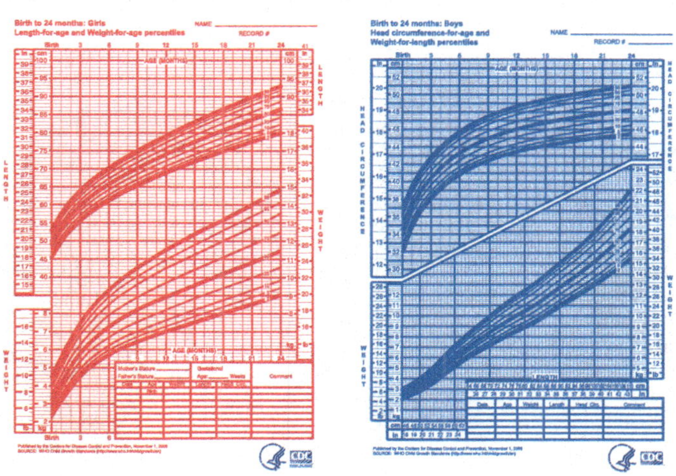

**Fig 2-8** Infants are plotted on the growth chart as a percentile

Infants must learn how to manipulate their bodies through space. The following gross and fine motor skills unfold in a sequence as children develop. Each skill builds on the last as a general rule throughout a child's life.

## Milestones

### Infant Milestones

The following gross and fine motor skills unfold in a sequence as children develop.

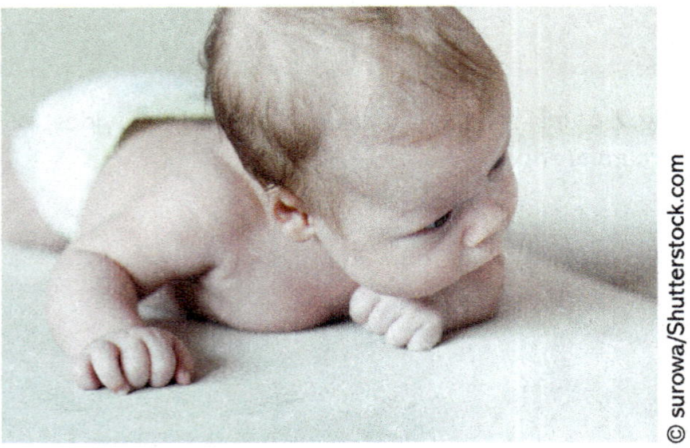


2-month infant lifts head

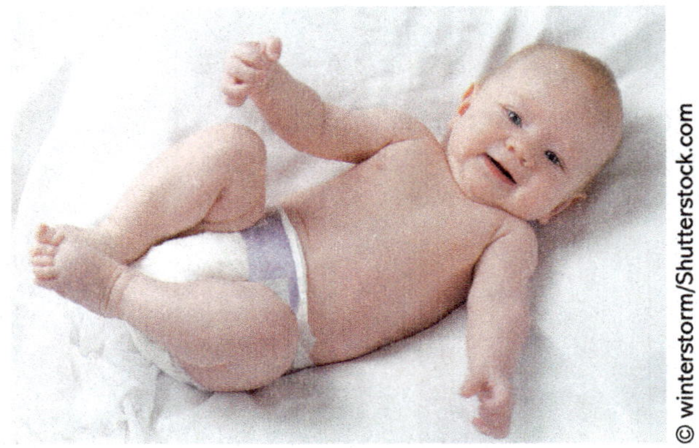


3-month infant loses grasp and holds hands slightly open

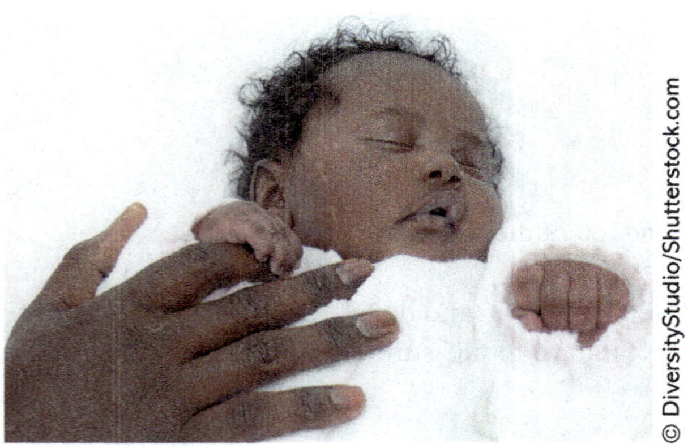


4-month infant grasps

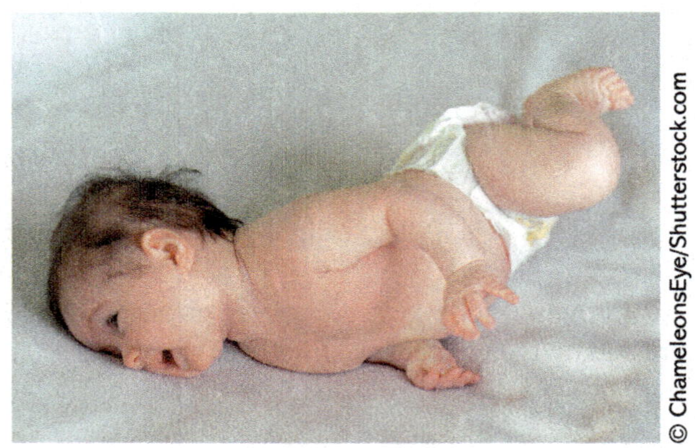


4-month infant rolls back to side

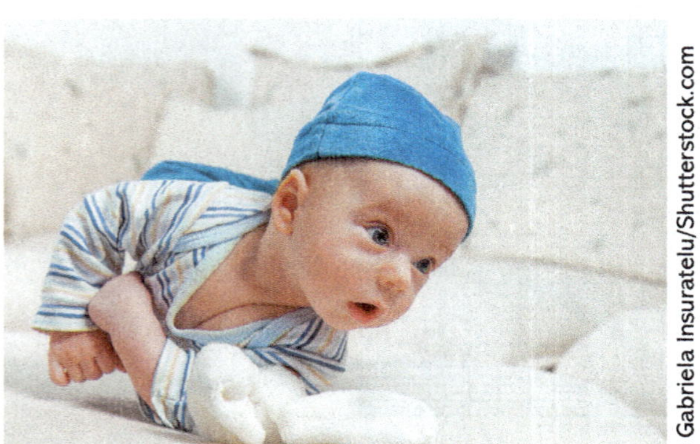


5-month infant rolls front to back

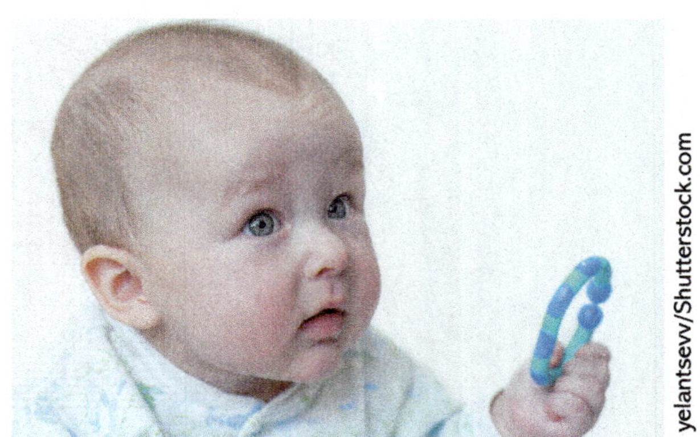


5-month infant dominant palmar grasp

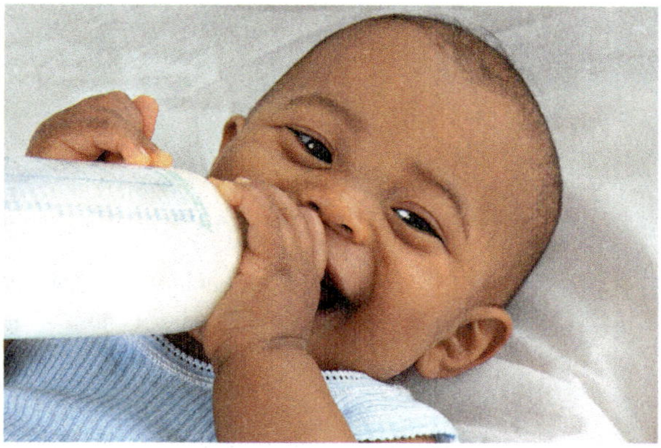


6-month infant holds bottle

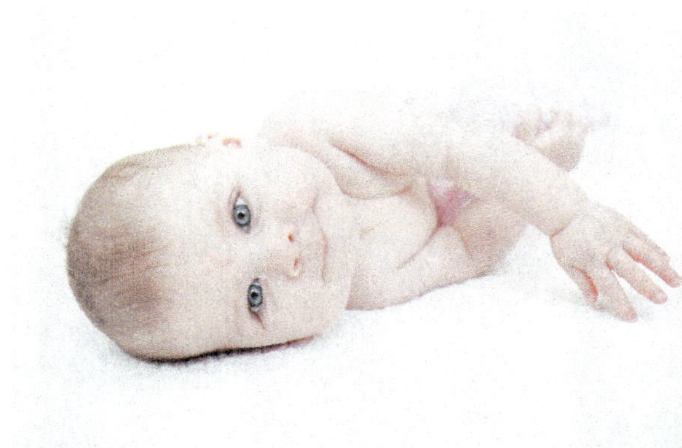


6-month infant rolls back to front

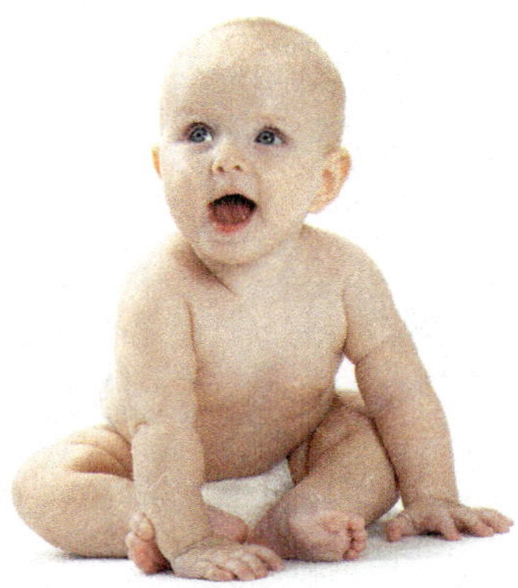


7-month infant sits leaning forward on both hands

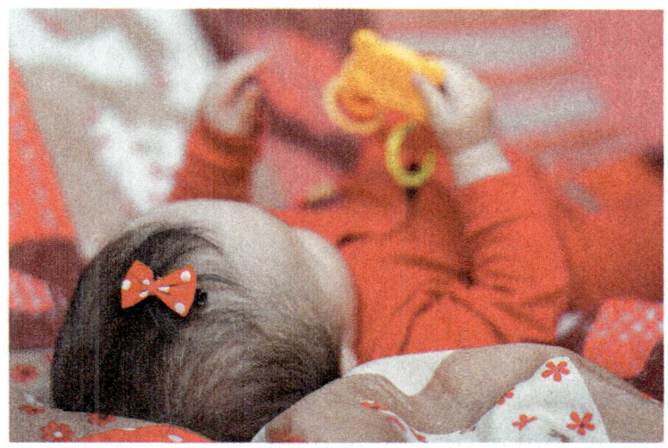


7-month infant moves object from hand to hand

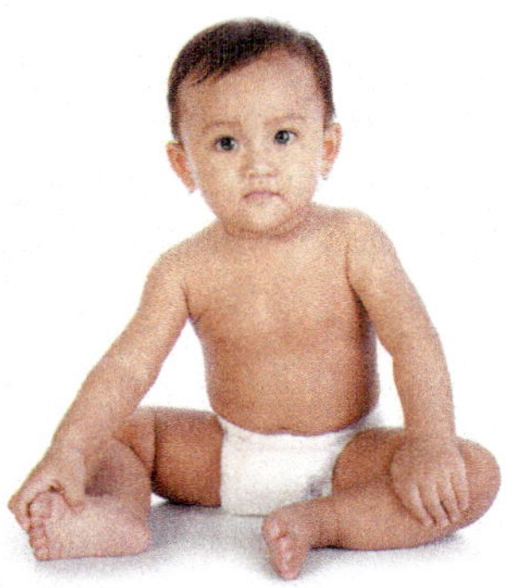


8-month infant sits completely unsupported

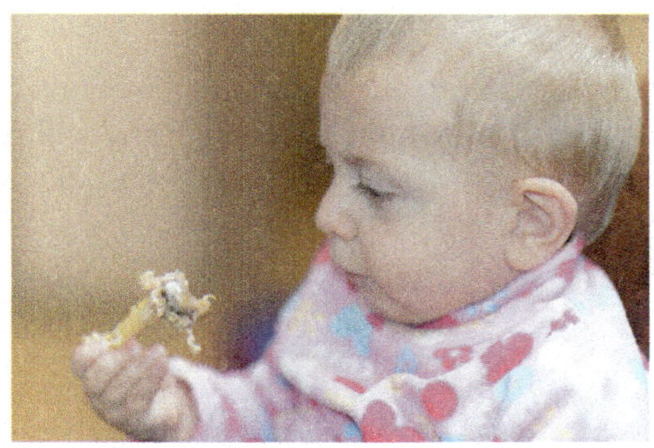


8-month infant pincer grasp

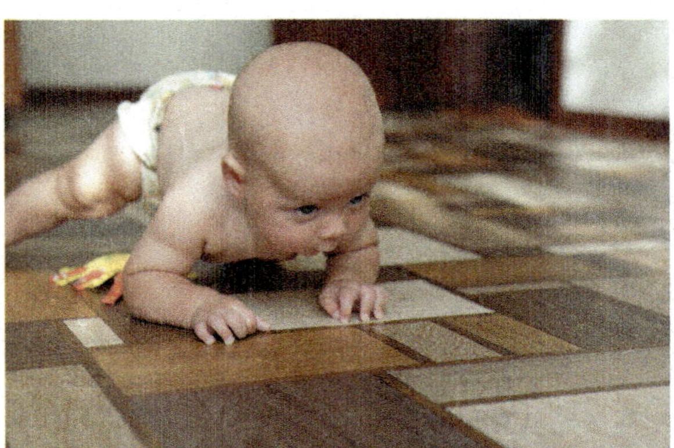


9-month infant creeping

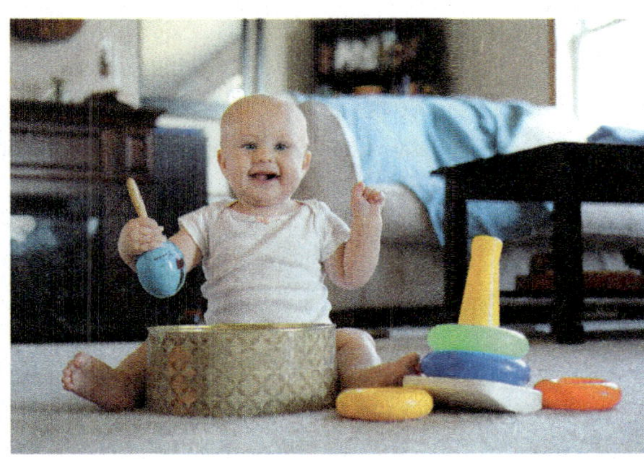


9-month infant shows a hand preference

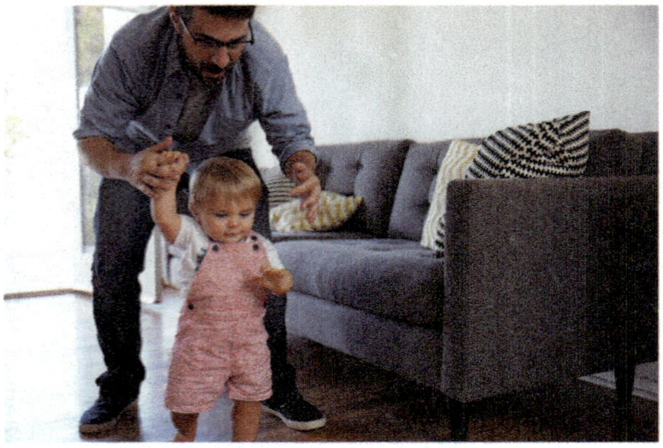



11-month infant cruises or walks with help of one hand

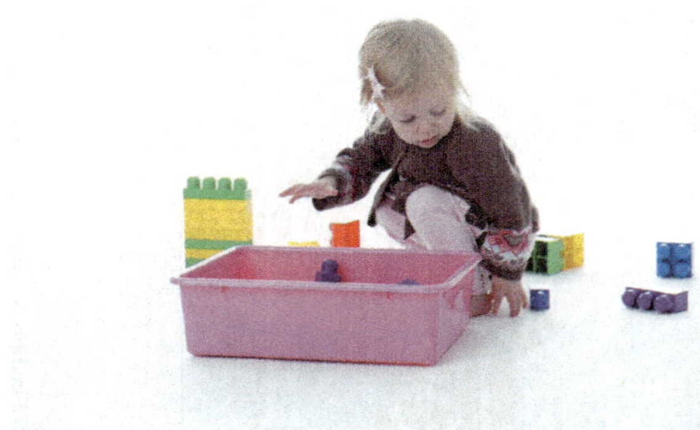



11-month infant places objects in a container

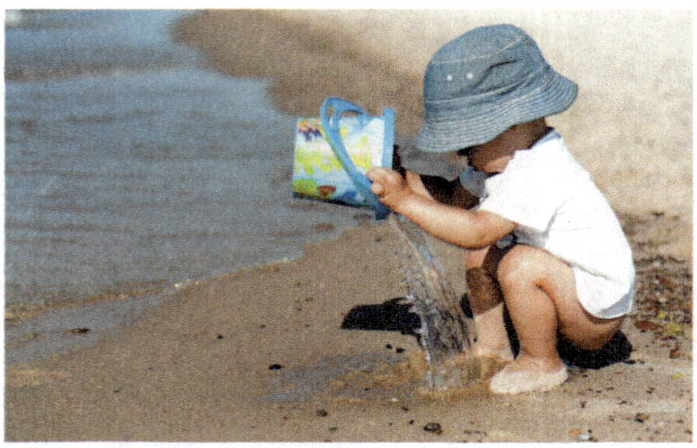



12-month infant standing to sitting

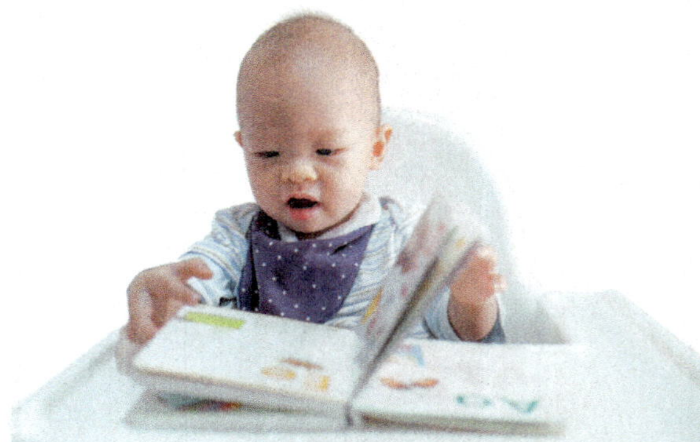



12-month infant turns the pages of a book

## Cognitive Development

Infants must use the one million connections being made in their brains every second. The brain knows which channels were not used enough and will prune them by age three. To survive the pruning process, the use of certain neural pathways for certain skills require practice (Center on the Developing Child at Harvard University 2017).

**Table 2-3** Infant Language Development

| Age | Stage |
|---|---|
| 3 weeks | Crying 1-1 1/2 hours per day |
| 6 weeks | Crying 2-4 hours per day |
| 2 months | Single vowel sounds |
| 3-4 months | Cooing; turns head to sounds and makes consonant sounds |
| 9-10 months | Understands "no"; 2 word to 3 word phrases |
| 1 year | 3-5 words |

Information sourced from ATI Testing. Table courtesy of Sondae Stevens © Kendall Hunt Publishing Company.

## Language Development

Infants learn quickly to process the language around them. This coding of ideas into auditory responses is one of the great wonders of being human. Research suggests that babies hear and to some extent processes language even before they are born. There is behavioral and physiological evidence that infants can hear sounds while in utero by the time they are 8-month-old fetuses (e.g., Birnholz and Benacerraf 1983; Walker, Grimwade, and Wood 1971). Furthermore, newborn infants prefer to hear their mothers' voices over the voice of another woman (DeCasper and Fifer 1980).

This biological framework supports an infant's language acquisition. Newborn cries are not just expressions of discomfort they represent the infants first communication. An infant could be fussy from being hot or cold or might cry like a fire alarm for a diaper change or feeding. They may use a high pitched shriek that could mean pain or irritation, a whiny cry that can mean exhaustion, or a colicky cry which is constant even when the infant is clean, dry, fed, burped, and held. Parents should know typical infants cry for 1 to 1 hour 30 minutes each day up to 3 weeks of age and increases to 2–4 hours by 6 weeks of age (ATI Testing 2016).

Infants will say single vowel sounds by 2 months old and consonants by 3 to 4 months old. Crying decreases typically by 12 weeks of age as vocalizations with cooing noises replace them at 3 to 4 months of age. The infant should also show considerable interest in the environment by 3 months by responding and turning to the sound of a rattle. Laughing and squealing are typically seen by 4 months. An infant's two-word phrases will evolve into three-word phrases. Infants understand the meaning of the word "no" by 9–10 months and obey single word commands that include gestures, such as sign language (ATI Testing 2016).

## Dentition

Teeth develop with the rest of the body in the first trimester. Secondary teeth develop in the second trimester. Therefore, medications ingested during pregnancy, such a tetracycline, can damage infant teeth before they are born (http://www.eapd.eu/804C40C2.en.aspx). Parents can expect six to eight teeth to erupt in the first year of age. The first primary teeth typically erupt between the ages of 6 and 10 months (average age 8 months).

Children may show subtle signs of teething, such as sucking or biting on their fingers or hard objects and drooling. Others show visible signs and are irritable, have trouble sleeping, develop a mild fever, pull on their ears, and have decreased appetite for pureed foods (ATI Testing 2016).

Parents need education about "bottle-rot" or the decay of adult teeth from improper care of the primary teeth (baby teeth). Wiping down teeth with a clean, damp washcloth will dissolve any sugar from breastmilk or formula (ATI Testing 2016).

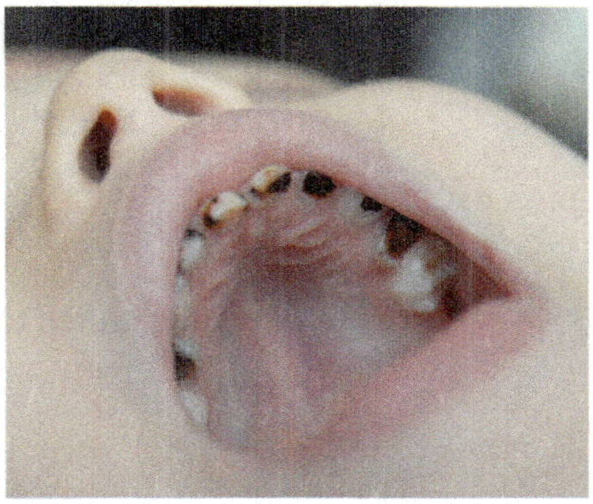



**Fig 2-9** Bottle-rot from not wiping teeth after breast milk or formula

## Psychosocial Development

The infant is in the trust or mistrust stage of Erickson's theory (ATI Testing). As the infant explores the environment, insecurities will begin to manifest as a result of new experiences. For example, touching something hot causes a memory that will cause the infant to hesitate if presented with the same circumstance again. Infants will look to their attachment figure for stability of care. Infants who experience consistent, reliable care develop trust and subsequently hope that experiences may produce a favorable outcome. If care is inconsistent, unreliable or too rigid, the child will develop mistrust. Mistrust can undermine a child's confidence and ability to believe they can affect change in the world. Mistrust disrupts the process of attachment and may have repercussions on a child's potential for healthy relationships in the future (Erickson 2013).

## Social Development

Certainly infant behavior consists of genetically controlled reflexes, action/reaction, and cultural impressions, but infants are beyond physiology. Infants actively participate in social behavior.

Social development occurs during any social behavior the infant experiences. These include attachment, separation, recognition/anxiety, and stranger fear. Social skills develop when the social environment includes healthy parents and children who have positive feeding experiences, and receive adequate rest. By 11–12 months, infants anticipate the mother's imminent departure by watching her behaviors. Stranger fear becomes apparent between 6 and 8 months of age when infants have the ability to discriminate between familiar and unfamiliar people. Reactive attachment disorder originates from maladaptive or absent attachment between the infant and primary caregiver and can last through childhood and adulthood (ATI Testing 2016).

## Age Appropriate Toys

Infants should be given age appropriate toys to encourage brain development and language acquisition. However, appropriate toys must be safe for a particular age group. Infants discover the world through their hands and their mouths. This mechanism leaves infants particularly susceptible to aspiration, bodily harm, burns, drowning, falls, poisoning, falls, and suffocation. A parent must choose designated toys, or children will create them from objects around them. Parents learn to choose toys based on growth and development stages is and requires exploration explore during wellness visits with the nurse (ATI Testing, 2016).

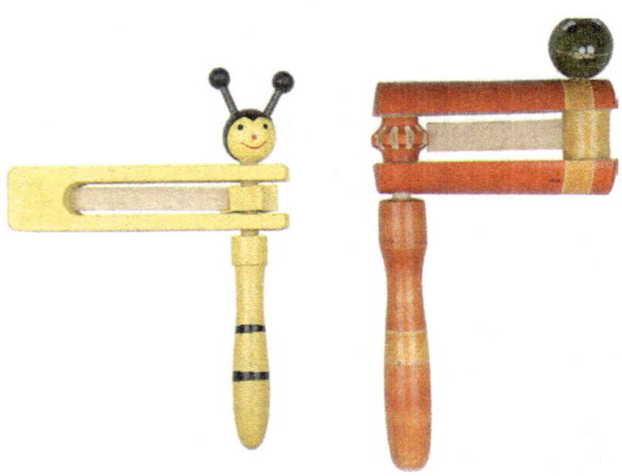



- Rattles

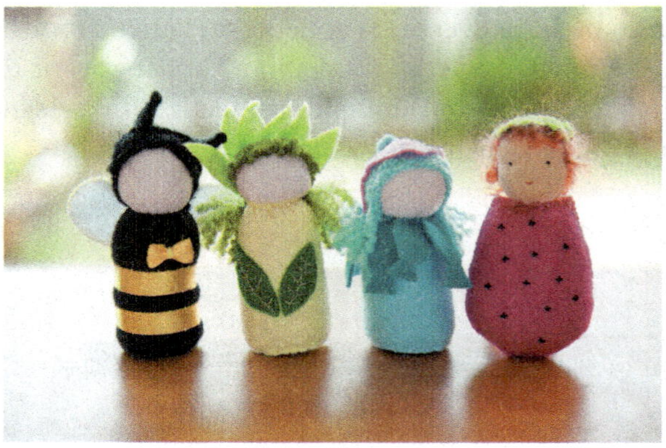



- Soft stuffed toys

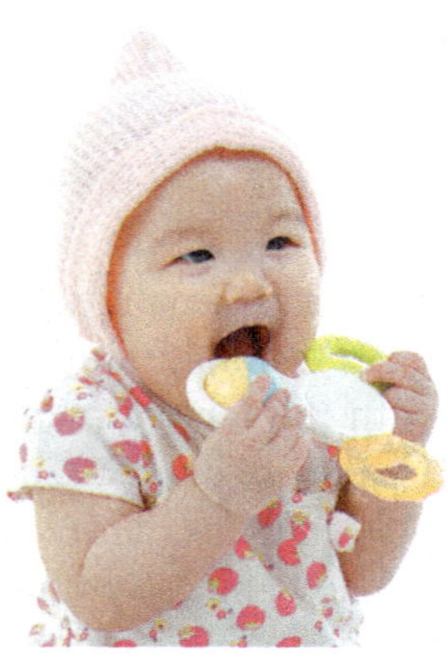



- Teething toys

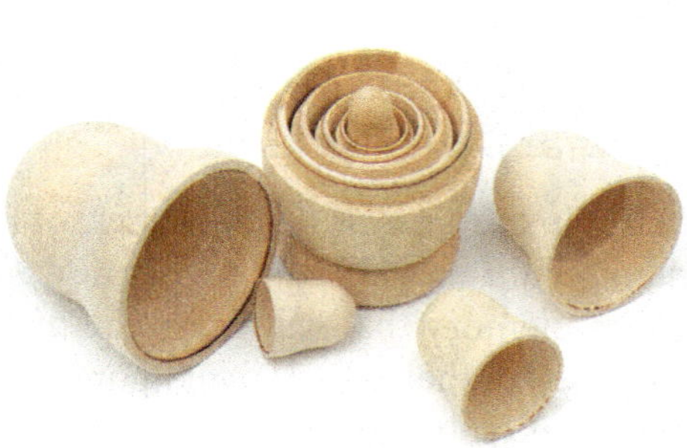



- Nesting toys

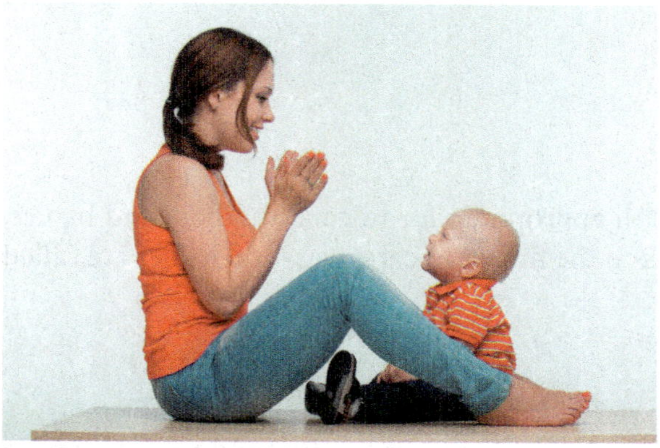



- Playing pat-a-cake

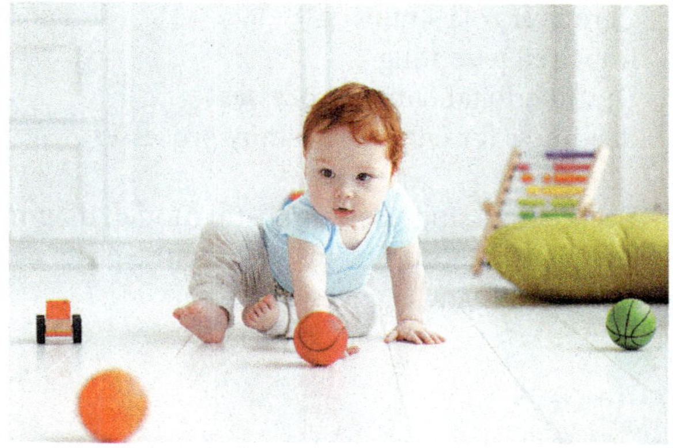



- Playing with balls

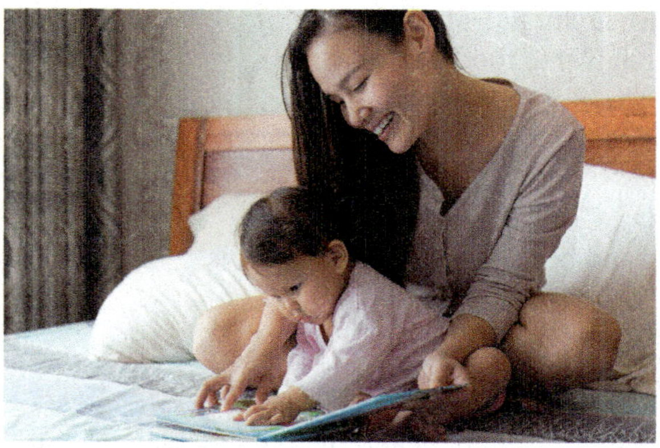



- Reading books

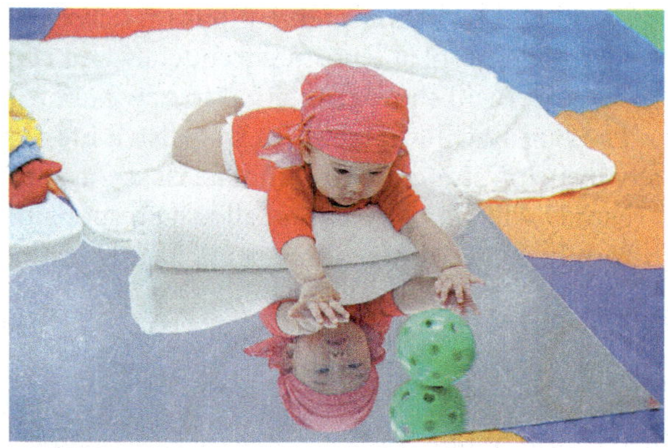



- Mirrors

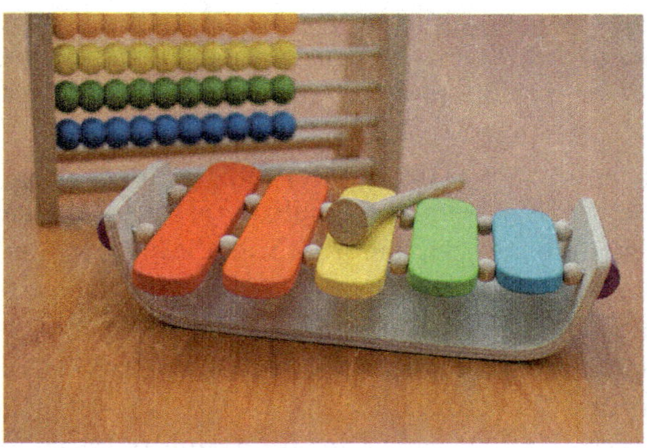



- Brightly colored toys

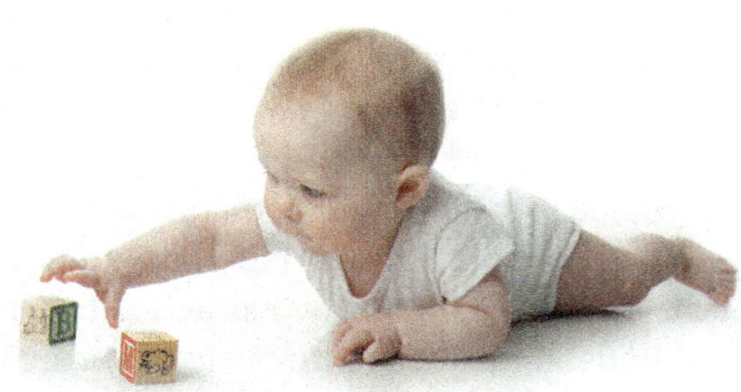



- Playing with blocks

## Nursing Diagnosis

Infants need various nursing diagnoses at different times because they grow in dynamic ways. Some NANDA diagnosis of the typical infant might include:

Interrupted breastfeeding
Impaired Dentition
Sleep deprivation
Constipation

Caregiver role strain
Impaired parenting
Dysfunctional family processes
Readiness for enhanced family processes

Because nursing uses a holistic model, diagnoses are still appropriate for normal mothers and babies, without physiologic problems. During the postpartum time and the first year, caregivers and babies are called upon to make many changes.

## Outcomes

Client will demonstrate behavior that promotes breastfeeding and the use of a breast pump to maintain lactation.

Caregiver will verbalize interventions to deter tooth decay.

Client will verbalize interventions that promote sleep with an infant; a feeling of being well rested.

Client will stool at a normal frequency and consistency relative to food choice.

Caregiver will show adaptation to new parenting role.

The family will define roles and distribute responsibilities fairly. Parent will demonstrate psychosocial safety by using strategies to eliminate risks for abuse.

Family will define roles and allocate responsibilities fairly.

Family demonstrates adoption of healthy eating patterns and healthy coping mechanisms.

## Interventions and Health Promotion

The creation of nursing outcomes makes concrete goals for parents to understand the nursing plan. Nursing diagnoses can be ruled out, as new ones develop. Infants require constant re-evaluation for health promotion. Infant interventions for growth and development foster health promotion and health maintenance.

Interventions must be customized for each family and will vary based on the intersection of circumstances. Interrupted breastfeeding may result from an illness in mother or child that requires separation. Other reasons may include formula supplementation from perceived insufficient milk supply or knowledge deficits about the process of breastfeeding.

Physiology must be the basis for breastfeeding education and serves as the primary nursing intervention for interrupted breastfeeding. Mothers must understand when there is not enough stimulation at the breast; the breast makes no milk. Mothers must also understand that what milk they can pump out with the breast pump is not the same amount a baby has access to through breastfeeding. Formula and the breast pump decrease breast stimulation and can ultimately undermine the breastfeeding process in the first six weeks. The breast pump is an effective intervention, but mothers must understand the stimulation is not equivalent to a baby's suck. Using this tool correctly is essential to breastfeeding success (Flaherman 2016).

Impaired dentition requires an assessment of dietary practices. If infants only drink breast milk or formula, caregivers can wipe their gums with water to remove sugar residues. Breast milk is the optimal nutrition for babies if the mother is eating a balanced diet. A maternal diet high in sugar may leach a significant amount of fructose, a sugar not naturally found in milk, into human milk (Jane 2017). Mothers can approach healthy eating as a process that begins with pregnancy, continues with breastfeeding, and fully develops to incorporate healthy eating for the family.

Sleep and rest for mother and baby can be challenging. Sleep must be thought of as a vitamin to keep mothers and baby's relationship on track. Human milk may contribute to establishing circadian rhythms in the infant, which will help consolidate sleep during night hours (Cohen, Hadash, Shehadah and Pillar 2012; Cubero, Valero, Sanchez, Rivero, Parvez, Rodriguez, and Barriga 2005; Sanchez, Cubero, Sanchez, Chanclon, Rivero, Rodriguez, and Barriga 2009).

Nocturnal sleep patterns typically develop by 3 to 4 months of age. Infants sleep up to 15 hours daily around the age of 4 months. Infants sleep through the night and take 1–2 naps during the day by the age of 12 months. Close contact with the mother and exposure to light/dark cues accelerates the development of baby's circadian rhythms (McGuire 2013).

Normal growth and development benefits from proper nutrition. An elimination assessment can inform future diet choices. If stools are normal per feeding regime, then the diet allows for nutrient absorption. If constipation occurs, then food should be reevaluated. Formula fed babies often experience constipation related to formula consumption. Exclusively breastfed babies rarely exhibit constipation (Quinlan, Lockton, Irwin, and Lucas 1995). Formula fed babies may need a laxative prescribed by a doctor until they can start eating foods that can help with the consistency of the stool. Foods such as pureed solids and fortified-iron baby cereal may also cause constipation.

Caregiver role strain, impaired parenting, dysfunctional family processes, and readiness for enhanced family processes all require a multidisciplinary approach that will include nursing, social services, and behavioral therapy. The nurse's primary responsibility is to connect the child and family to the available resources that will vary depending on the community (ATI Testing 2016).

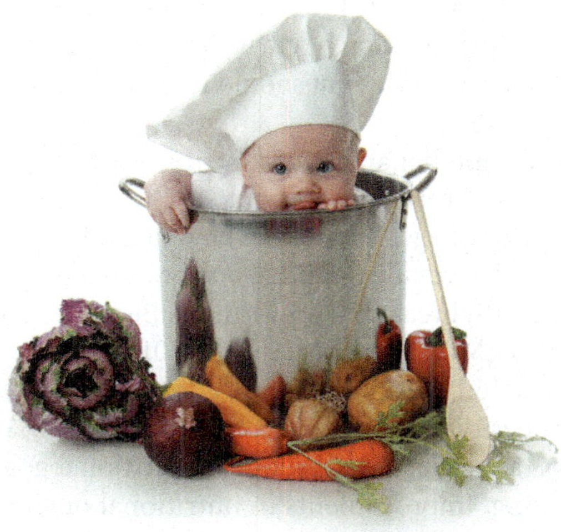



**Fig 2-10** Having a baby is a great time to get healthy

## Nutrition

Breastfeeding provides a complete diet and ideal bonding experience for infants. An iron-fortified formula substitutes for breast milk in certain situations, but it will never be an equivalent replacement. If women choose formula, they will need education on burping, feeding with a slow nipple and how to manage constipation and spitting up. Nurses should encourage a formula feeding mother to provide the colostrum, if possible, for the first few days after birth. Breastfeeding mothers need education about high-quality diets. Women must understand the baby will receive the ingested nutrients before the mother does, which can leave mothers deficient in vitamins and minerals (ATI Testing 2016).

Breastfeeding is contraindicated in certain patient populations. These include infants with galactosemia, those positive for human T-cell lymphotrophic virus type I or II (adult t-cell leukemia/lymphoma), and HIV. It also includes infants whose mothers received antimetabolites or chemotherapy treatments, certain cytotoxic or psychotropic drugs, have active herpes on the breast, hepatitis A or B, cytomegalovirus (CMV), Lyme disease, or active tuberculosis (ATI Testing 2016).

Infant physiology includes a high composition of extracellular water, which leaves them susceptible to fluid shifts moving in and out of the vascular compartment. Alternative sources of fluids, such as juice or water, are not needed during the first 4 months of life. Too much water intake could result in hyponatremia and water intoxication. After the age of 6 months, 100% fruit juice should be offered optionally to families. If so, limit juices to 4–6 oz. per day. The choice to start solid foods should wait for 4–6 months dependent on the indicators for readiness: interest in solid foods, voluntary control of the head and trunk, and disappearance of the extrusion reflex (ATI Testing 2016).

However, research indicates solid food should start at 6 months when infant's produce adequate amylase enzyme, which digests carbohydrates. Recommendations of iron-fortified cereal as a first food due to its high iron content come from pediatricians. However, iron-fortified cereal may not have a positive effect on bone health (Michaëlsson, Wolk, Langenskiöld, Basu, Lemming, Melhus and Byberg, 2014; Feskanich, Bischoff-Ferrari, Frazier and Willett, 2014). White rice cereal may induce obesity as the processed rice cereal has a high-glycemic index that is associated with diabetes (Fabricatore, A. N., Ebbeling, C. B., Wadden, T. A., and Ludwig, D. S. 2011).

New foods should be introduced individually, over a 5- to 7-day period, to observe for signs of allergy or intolerance, such as fussiness, rash, vomiting, diarrhea, and constipation (ATI Testing 2016). Vegetables, fruits, and whole grains are started first between 6 and 8 months of age. Solid foods should not be started before 6 months as infants do not produce salivary amylase, an enzyme that digests starches until this time (Sevenhuysen, Holodinsky and Dawes 1984). After the introduction of fruits vegetables and whole grains, the introduction of meats may follow. The introduction of citrus fruits begins after 6 months of age. Breast milk/formula decreases as intake of solid foods increases but should remain the primary source of nutrition through the first year (Mccarthy & McCarthy 2014).

Appropriate finger foods include ripe bananas, toast strips, graham crackers, cheese cubes, noodles, firmly-cooked vegetables, and raw pieces of fruit (except grapes). Table foods that are well-cooked, chopped, and unseasoned are appropriate by 1 year of age. Infants can be weaned from a bottle when they show signs of readiness and can drink from a cup. Care-providers replace one breastfeeding session or one bottle of formula with an infant cup with handles filled with breastmilk or formula. Bedtime feedings remain as the last feeding until bedtime feedings are unnecessary (Mccarthy & McCarthy 2014).

According to Healthy People 2020, 16.1% of children and adolescents were obese between 2005 and 2008. Healthy People 2020 aims to reduce obesity in children and adolescents by 10% (US Department of Health and Human Services, 2014). Some important strategies to support nutritional goals in children include: a school curriculum that includes healthy eating, improvements in nutritional quality of the food supply in schools, cultural practices that support children eating healthier foods and being active throughout each day, and support for teachers and other staff to implement health promotion strategies and activities, physical activity, increased sessions for physical activity and the development of fundamental movement skills throughout the school week, and body image. At home, parent support home activities that encourage children to be active, eat nutritious foods and minimize screen-based activities to develop healthy eating patterns in children (Waters, de Silva-Sanigorski, Burford, Brown, Campbell, Gao, Armstrong, Prosser, and Summerbell 2011). Children and adults should begin nutrition modification in pregnancy and continue making lifestyle changes as the child develops.

## Vegetarian Diets

All children begin life eating a vegetarian diet based on breast milk or formula. According to the American Dietetic Association, there isn't any reason to change this (Sabat, J. and Wien, M. 2010). Vegetarians maintain a lower BMI and are at less risk for obesity. However, the diet must come from whole foods. The nurse encourages a diverse diet rich in unprocessed foods, and allows parents to choose what diet they wish to follow whether it is meat based, vegetarian or something in between. Children need a healthy adult model to guide them to appropriate vegetarian choices. There is a vegetarian food pyramid nurses can recommend to their families from the Department of Nutrition, School of Public Health, Loma Linda University (Vegetarian Food Pyramid VegSource. n.d.)

## Nutritional Barriers

Parents report many barriers to healthy eating including lack of time, lack of cooking skills, and limited financial resources. Parents report children had limited food preferences and got bored with their diet choices. In addition, parents report a decrease in social programs, like after-school programs, to reinforce and demonstrate healthy food choices. Parents expressed the difficulty of working against the media images that their children saw during screen time (Ling, J., Robbins, L., and Hines-Martin, V. 2016).

To create effective interventions, nurses must use anticipatory guidance to prepare parents to create a healthy lifestyle. Research points to the quality of the mother's health as the determinant of the family's health (Gundersen, C., and Ziliak, J. P. 2014).

The success of the interventions often depends on creating healthy daily habits that begin during pregnancy and continue through the lifespan. With one in five children living with hunger, nurses need practical applications of nutrition that are culturally sensitive. Parents must efficiently work around time constraints through weekly meal planning and budgeting. Supporting typical families to avoid processed foods in favor of whole foods changes the paradigm of American eating to high-quality, nutrient-rich foods instead of low-quality, nutrient-poor diets most Americans eat. When finances are limited a simple diet of legumes, rice or whole grains, vegetables, and water-based drinks such as unsweetened, herbal, fruit-flavored iced teas will contain costs. As finances increase small amounts of meat, fish, dairy and 100% fruit juice is acceptable. Parents who lack cooking skills need education about ingredients and healthy cooking methods. The internet offers many sources for recipes and brings a learning environment to healthy eating. In addition, online groups may provide support and further resources that keep food social and fun. Parents can win the battle on food choice by controlling the foods children eat from the beginning. Children who eat vegetables in infancy will eat vegetables throughout their lives. Children like variety if they always have variety. Variety makes any diet more interesting, which will keep children engaged in the healthy eating process. Finally, eliminating or reducing screen time will reduce the numbers of times parents will have to counter the information and images children see on television. Parents should also be encouraged to create their own groups of their peers in their communities to support their families who want to make lifestyle changes. All of these behaviors work together to create healthy eating habits children can have for a lifetime.

## Preventative Screenings and Interventions

Infant screenings are frequent and parents must understand the importance of wellness visits to enable the timeliness infant screening. These include height and weight, head circumference, vision, hearing, developmental screening, psychosocial and behavioral screenings, immunizations, hemoglobin and hematocrit, TB test, and oral health. Parents should understand screenings are not diagnostic tools, but tools used to find children at risk (Committee on Practice and Ambulatory Medicine and Workgroup, B. F. 2017).

The Denver Developmental screening test identifies children at risk for being behind the growth and development curve. The test measures gross motor, fine motor, language development and social skills. It informs nurses to identify families and children who may need diagnosis and treatment (Frankenburg, W. K., Dodds, J., Archer, P., Shapiro, H., and Bresnick, B. 1992).

## Injury Prevention

Infants experience unintentional injury as the leading cause of death. The implementation of prevention strategies must happen indoors and outdoors. Indoor injury prevention includes: aspiration, bodily harm, burns, drowning, bodily harm, falls, and poisoning.

Infants are prone to aspiration of foreign objects due to a smaller windpipe and the impetus to explore the world through their mouths. To prevent aspiration, hold the infant for feedings, never prop a bottle. In addition, small objects such as grapes, coins, loose buttons, and candy may occlude the throat and are not safe (ATI Testing 2016).

### Bodily Harm

Sharp objects should be stored out of reach of infants. Safety hardware to anchor heavy equipment such as television sets keeps infants from overturning heavy equipment. Infants and animals require constant monitoring (ATI Testing 2016).

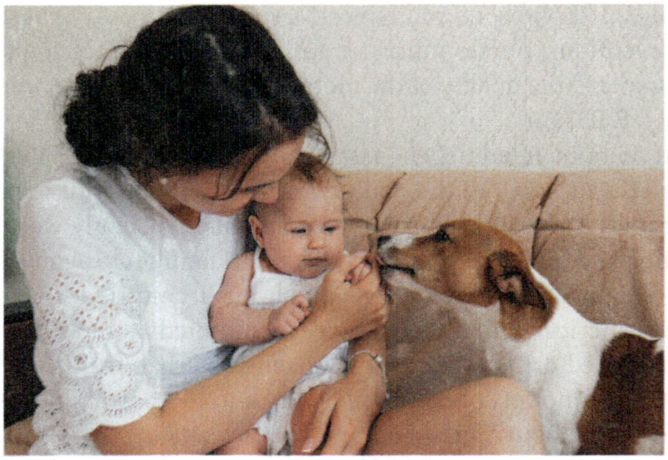

© Romanova Anna/Shutterstock.com

### Burns

Do not use a microwave to heat formula because hot spots can occur, which can burn the infant. The temperature of the formula needs double checking before feeding. The temperature of the bath requires warm and not hot water. Hot water thermostats are set at or below 49° C (120° F) to prevent burns in the shower. The handles of pots and pans should be kept out of reach and turned towards the back of the stove. (ATI Testing 2016).

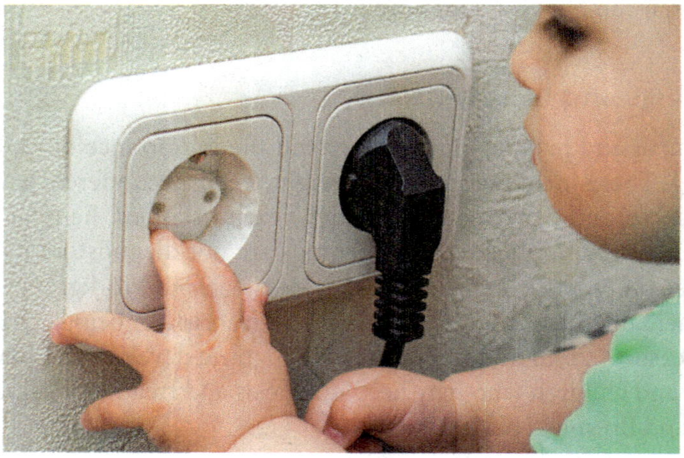

© Krystyna Taran/Shutterstock.com

Working smoke detectors are kept in the home and checked every year for batteries. Electrical outlets need plastic plugs to protect the child from inserting a metal object into the wall (ATI Testing 2016).

### Falls

A tour of the living space down on hands and knees may highlight things easy to miss at adult eye level. Fall prevention includes safety gates placed at the top and bottom of stairs. Cribs are appropriately sized crib mattresses in the lowest position possible with the rails all the way up. In addition, crib slats are no farther apart than 6 cm (2.375 in). Crib mobiles and/or crib gyms are removed by 4–5 months of age in anticipation of the infant sitting up (ATI Testing 2016).

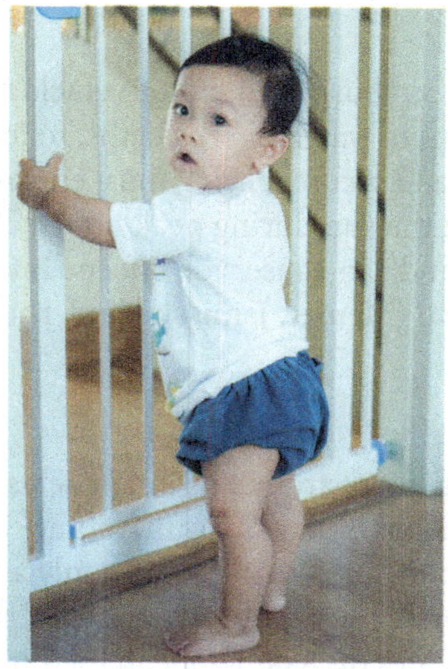

© Photo by MHIN/Shutterstock.com

Fall prevention includes safety gates placed at the top and bottom of stairs. Cribs must have appropriately sized crib mattresses in the lowest position possible with the rails all the way up. In addition, crib slats should be no farther apart than 6 cm (2.375 in). Crib mobiles and/or crib gyms should be removed by 4–5 months of age in anticipation of the infant sitting up (ATI Testing 2016).

Parents can prevent Sudden Infant Death Syndrome (SIDS), by removing pillows and stuffed animals from the crib. Parents place infants on their backs for sleep. Toys with small parts, especially from older siblings, are kept out of reach. Parents must remove drawstrings from jackets and other clothing if children are unsupervised or sleeping (ATI Testing 2016).

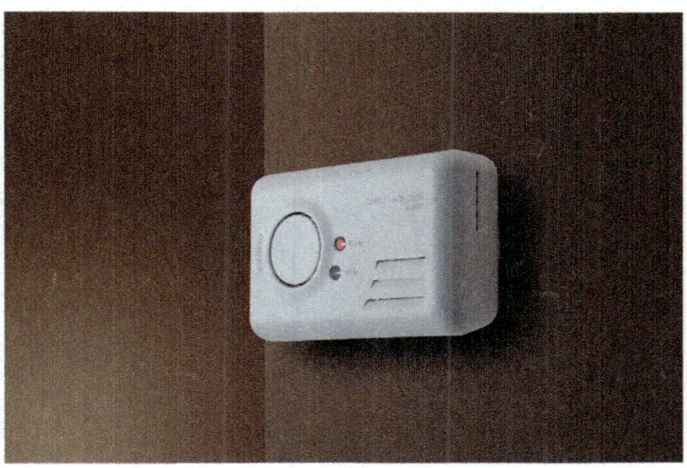

© abimages/Shutterstock.com

### *Poison*

Poisoning prevention includes removing lead paint and making sure paint has not flaked off. Toxins and plants are kept out of reach because they are easily digestible. Cleaners and household chemicals are secured in cabinets with safety locks. Parents should post the phone number for a poison control center near the phone. Medications belong in a childproof container, out of reach of infants. A working carbon monoxide detector identifies toxic emissions. Suffocation prevention includes the removal of plastic bags or balloons around infants (ATI Testing 2016).

### Sun Protection

Outdoor injuries may include drowning, sunburn, and motor vehicle injuries. Drowning prevention includes supervision of infants around any amount of water such as baths, toilets, cleaning buckets, or drainage areas. Caregivers keep bathroom doors closed, and secure fencing must enclose swimming areas. Babies should wear hats, or be placed in the shade and avoid the sun during peak hours. The chemicals in sunscreen at this time are highly absorbable through the skin and can cause side effects. Infants should wear sunscreen when they are 6 months old when exposed to the sun (Meurer, Jamieson and Thurman 2006).

### Car Seat Safety

Car seat accident prevention includes using restraints in infant seats. If infants use car seats indoors, seats must rest on the floor, and direct supervision is necessary. Infants are not safe unattended or on elevated surfaces. Motor-vehicle accident prevention includes using infant-only and convertible infant-toddler car seats. Infants and toddlers ride in a rear-facing car seat until two years of age or the height recommended by the manufacturer. The backseat of the car creates the safest zone in the car for infants. Never place rear-facing car seats in the front seat of vehicles with passenger airbags. Parents cannot leave an infant in a parked car (ATI Testing 2016).

Historically, the first 40 days of infancy are a time for mother and baby to build a solid foundation for a lifetime relationship. The modern woman faces challenges from every angle to make this transition seamless. Nursing can best support woman and babies by recognizing the diversity of women and their experiences and giving them support and respect as they take on the hardest job in the world. Nursing can continue to support mother and child as they expand into familial roles through wellness attainment and maintenance. If the measure of the health of a nation is the health of its women and children, then the United States needs a renewed commitment to the health of women and children. Pediatric nurses can support families build their health literacy and in turn their family's health on a daily basis. (Ou, Heng 2016).

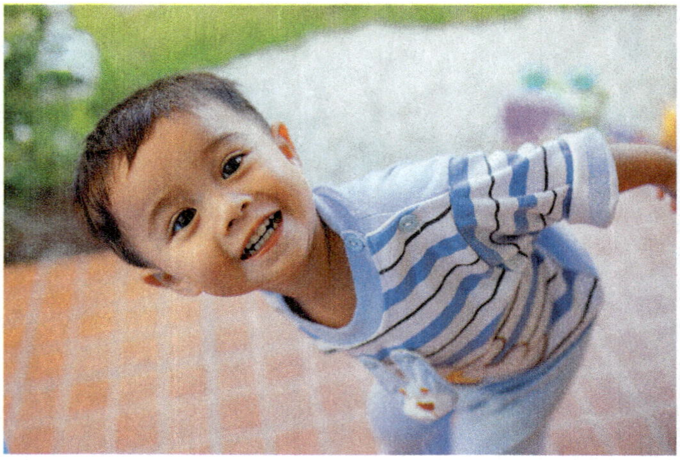



## TODDLERS

### Assessment

This growth period compared with an infant moves slower as the toddler learns to move their body through space. The typical toddler weights four times their birth weight by the time they are 30 months old. Toddlers height will increase about 7.5 cm (3 in) per year. A toddler's head circumference and chest circumference are usually equal, by 1 to 2 years of age (ATI Testing 2016).

## Communication with Toddlers

There is a surge of language skills in the toddler. However, toddlers still use nonverbal language to communicate. Nurses should get down to the toddler's eye level and speak directly to them, like any adult patient. Nurses should aim for a positive but realistic tone. Sing-song tones can quickly become patronizing. The nurse engages the toddler in the assessment, asks them to hold something or help in some way, and makes sure to spend time listening as the child's story and nonverbal communication are important assessments in themselves (Chambers 2013).

Nurses should speak in short, clear sentences, and set healthy boundaries. One way to accomplish this is through choices. Choices foster autonomy in the toddler. Toddlers need time to process and to respond to information. Nurses can explain everything they do as the assessment unfolds. Toddlers may cry during the assessment, if they do, acknowledge their feelings and validate them as real. Validation works equally well with parents who are frightened by the sudden loss of control (Westwood, C 2007).

Toddlers can respond to blood draws and immunizations with anxiety and fear. Effective communication from the nurse minimizes trauma to the toddler. Nurses can use simple words and explanations such as "we need to give you some medicine, so you're not sick." Nurses should refrain from using yes or no questions as toddlers love to say "no."

Toddlers commonly use negativism, or negative responses, to express themselves. Toddlers hear the word "no" and express the word "no," countless times per day. Parents and toddlers can best keep communication open in a therapeutic learning environment (ATI Testing 2016).

Nurses have the opportunity to build the relationship between child and health-care providers by being honest, knowing what to expect, and reassuring children especially during painful or bloody procedures. Toddlers can have an adverse reaction to seeing blood, so using a band-aid after an intervention may soothe them. Toddlers may respond to a reward such as a sticker and praise them for their cooperation.

## Cognitive Development

The preoperational stage arrives at 19 to 24 months, and the concept of object permanence develops to maturity. Toddlers recall memories of events they experience. Pretend play or domestic mimicry (playing house) predominates play activities. Children can be encouraged to learn simple cleaning tasks or cooking jobs. Children in the preoperational exhibit egocentrism and the understanding and use of symbols to imitate activities in their environment. Toddlers can make a wooden block into a car or quickly engage in role play as parents or older siblings. The interest in the world is robust and makes this time especially important in the child's development (ATI Testing 2016).

## Language Development

Toddlers at 1 year of age use one-word sentences, or **holophrases** such as "up" for "lift me up," or "cup" for "bring me my cup." The child's vocabulary increases to 300 words by 2 years of age. At 2 years of age, toddlers also use multi-word sentences by combining two to three words. Toddlers will say "go up" and "my cup." By three years old, they can combine several words to create simple sentences using grammatical rules (ATI Testing 2016).

Toddlers might say "the cat, and the doggie went to school." Toddlers will explore language through their imaginations in this way; free play supports language development.

## Psychosocial Development

Toddlers are in the Erikson stage of **autonomy** versus shame and doubt (ATI Testing. 2016). They need an environment that fosters independence while also being safe. Toddlers can be a challenging age for parents because a safe toddler environment can feel limiting to the toddler.

Toddlers enjoy kid-friendly environments where an adult will have to use the word "no," very sparingly. Small knick-knacks and other adult objects toddlers will inevitably want will most likely will break and cause hurt feelings. Creating an environment meant for exploration with the senses promotes psychosocial development and makes parenting more enjoyable.

Toddler daily activities naturally fall into a rhythm when sleeping, eating and playtimes occur at fixed times in the daily schedule. Toddlers respond to a predictable day, so they know what is coming and when.

Toddlers use **negativism**, or negative responses, to express their independence. Toddlers hear the word "no" and express the word "no" countless times per day. "No" may simply mean, "I'll figure it out by myself". Parents and toddlers can best keep communication open in a therapeutic learning environment (ATI Testing 2016).

Toddlers begin to learn **ritualism** or a rhythm to the day (ATI Testing 2016). Mothers or caregivers establish a rhythm that is congruent with the family lifestyle. Once an established rhythm materializes, moments of transition unfold uneventfully. Toddler daily activities naturally fall into a rhythm when sleeping, eating, and playtimes occur at fixed times in the daily schedule. Toddlers respond to a predictable day, so they know what is coming and when.

A typical toddler's behavior tends toward the egocentric, which makes them unable to see things from another point of view. Punishment and orientation to rules begin with a sense that good behavior reaps rewards and bad behavior reaps consequences. Learning about actions and reactions helps toddlers to sequentially develop a self-concept separate from their parents and eventually feel autonomous (ATI Testing 2016).

Toddlers have a curiosity about the environment and their body parts. They benefit from learning anatomical names so they can communicate clearly to adults in case they experience abuse. This is a safety technique to protect the child from potential sexual abuse.

Typical toddlers develop gender identity by 3 years of age. If parents report a **transgendered** child, then referrals to family counseling for the child and family occur. Currently, in the medical community, the diagnosis of Gender Dysmorphia applies to transgendered people in the Diagnostic and Statistical Manual of Mental Disorders (DSM-5). Transgendered feelings may be a biological or a psychological phenomenon. Regardless, nursing must create a therapeutic environment to deepen the relationship between the family and the medical community. Transgendered people are at risk for risky behaviors related to the stress of living an openly transgendered life (Gibson, B., and Catlin, A. J. 2010). Many families experience a turmoil phase that leaves a void for support and encouragement. There is an opportunity to provide the family holistic health care and a healthy relationship with the health-care team (Gregor, C., Davidson, S., and Hingley-Jones, H. 2016). A healthy relationship facilitates access to resources and referrals. Effective initial care can make the difference between a family having access to resources and not (ATI Testing 2016).

## Age Appropriate Activities

The solitary play of infants evolves into parallel play in toddlers. Toddlers observe other children and then might engage in a similar, yet separate activities nearby. (One chart with Age appropriate Activities and one chart with milestones)

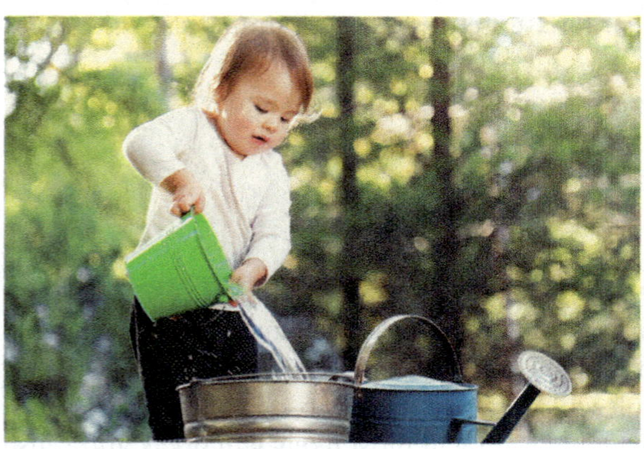



Filling and emptying containers

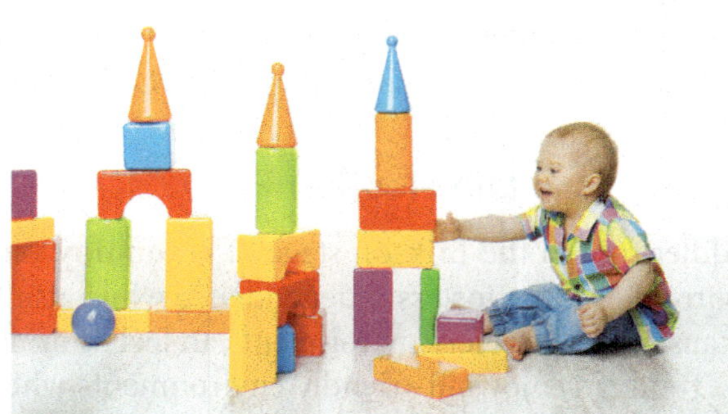



Playing with blocks

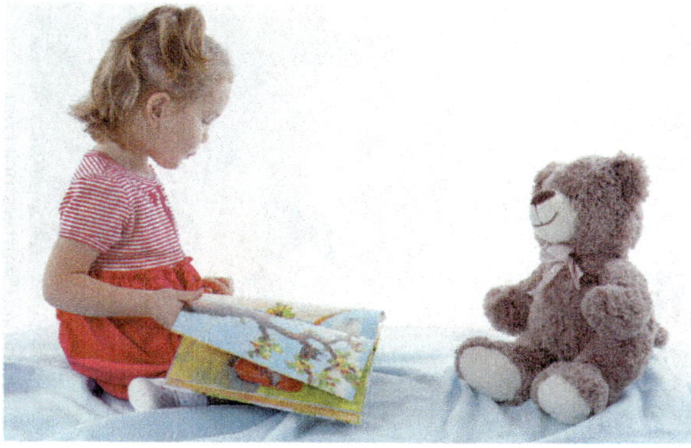


Looking at books

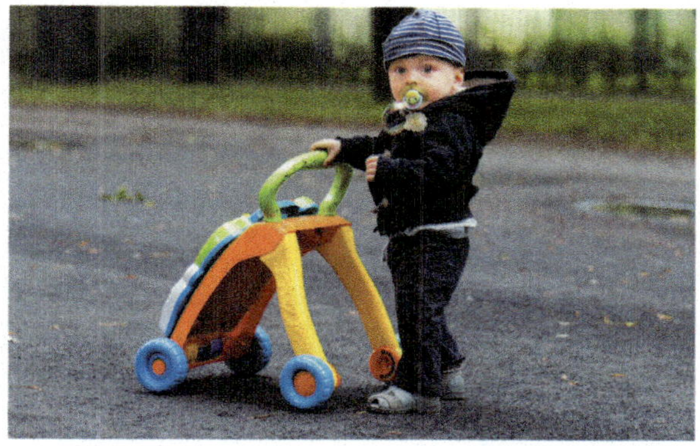


Push-pull toys

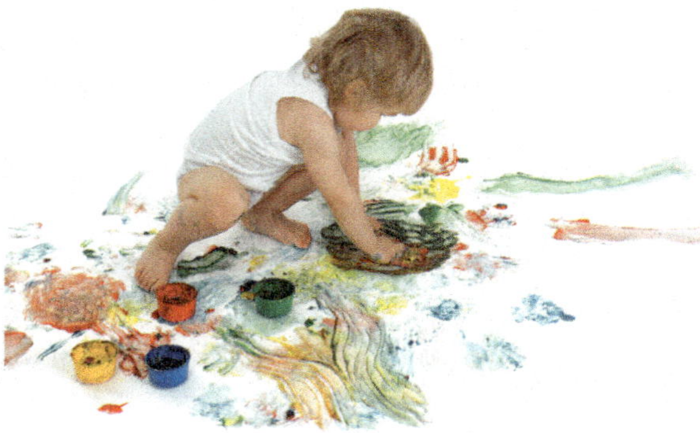


Fingerpainting

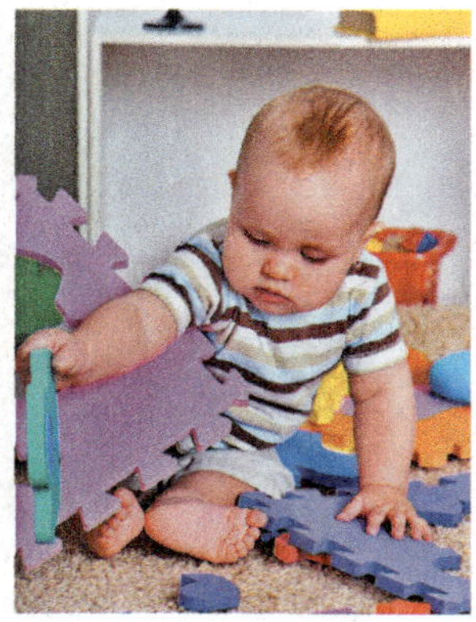


Large-piece puzzles

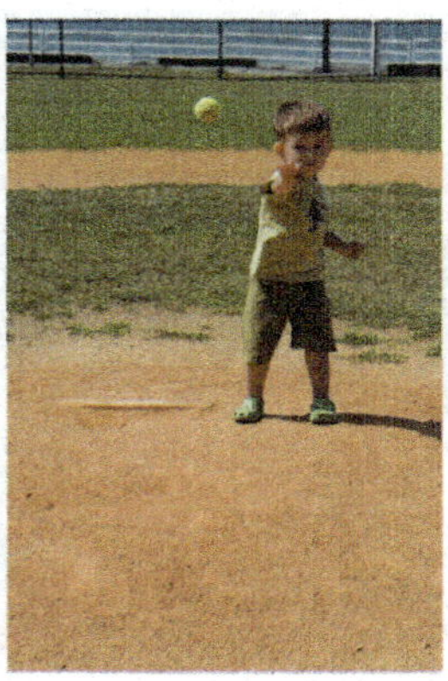


Throwing a Ball

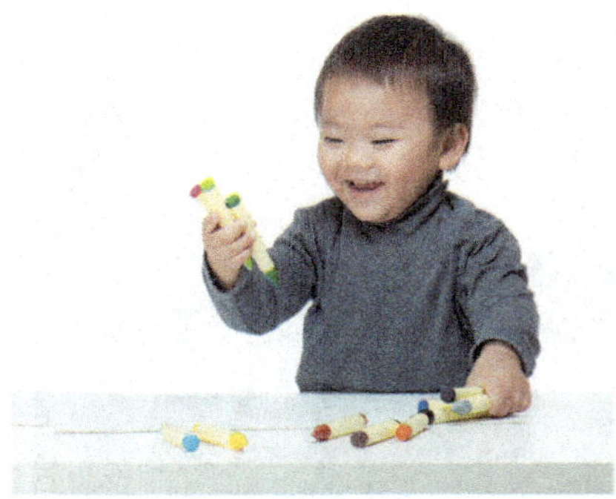


Thick crayons

## Toddler Milestones

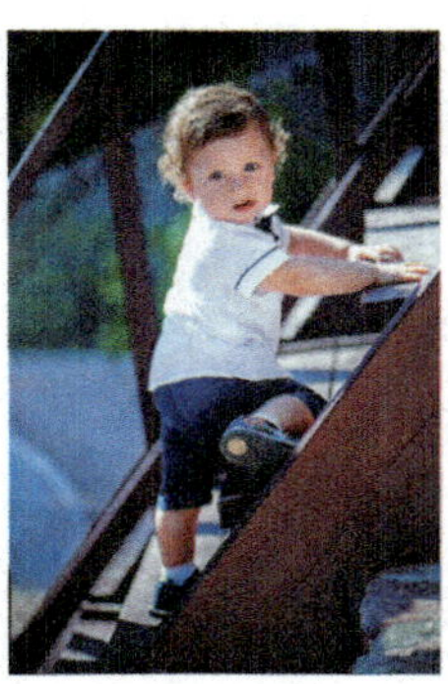


15-month infant walk up stairs unassisted

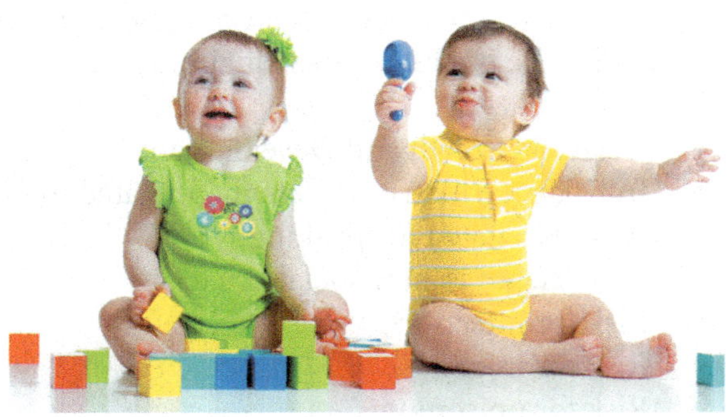

15-month infant builds a two block tower

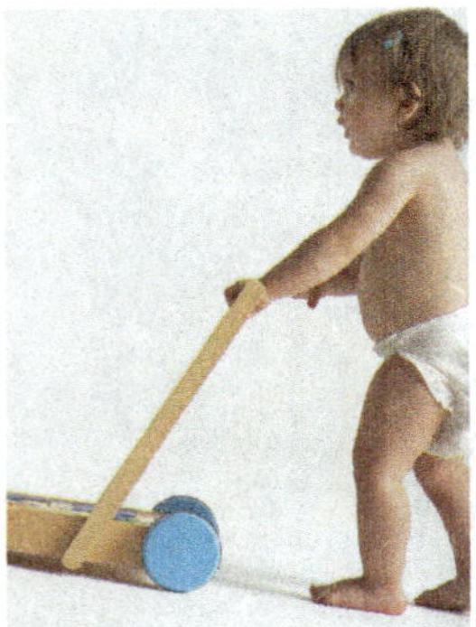

18-month infant pull-push toys

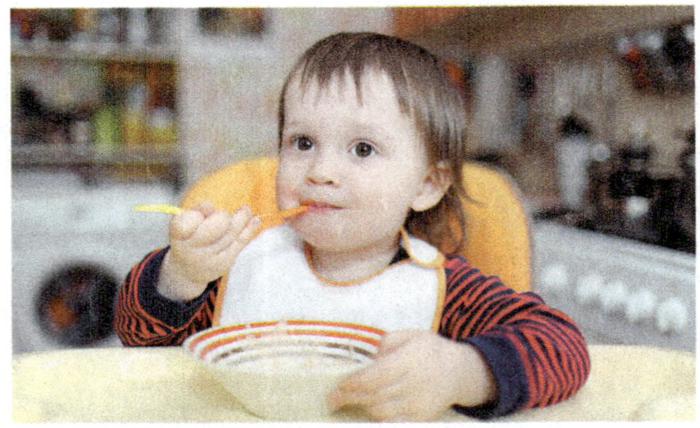

18-month infant manages a spoon

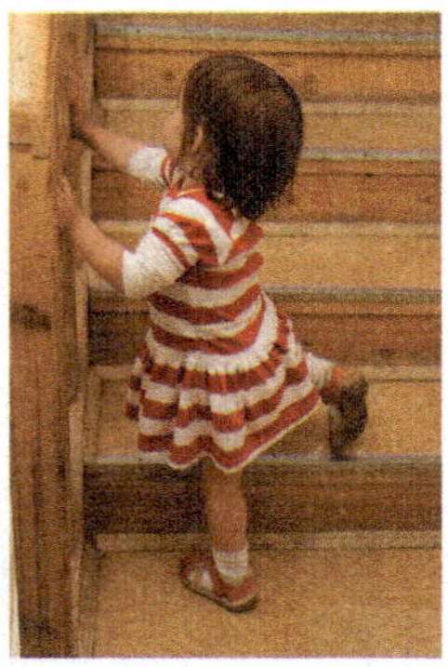

A 2-year-old goes up stairs with both feet on each step

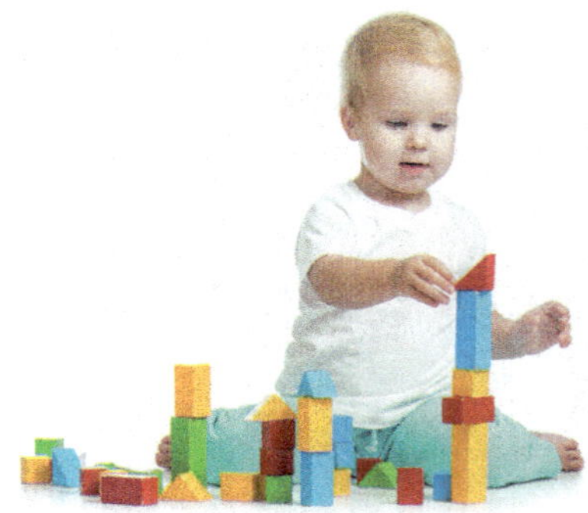

A 2-year-old builds 6–7 block tower

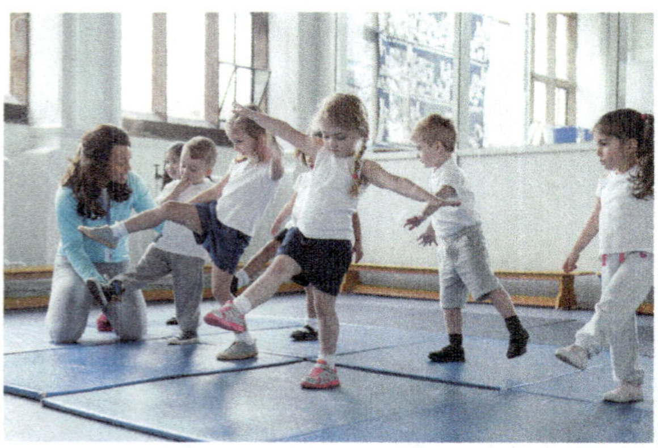

A 2-and-half-year-old stands on one foot momentarily

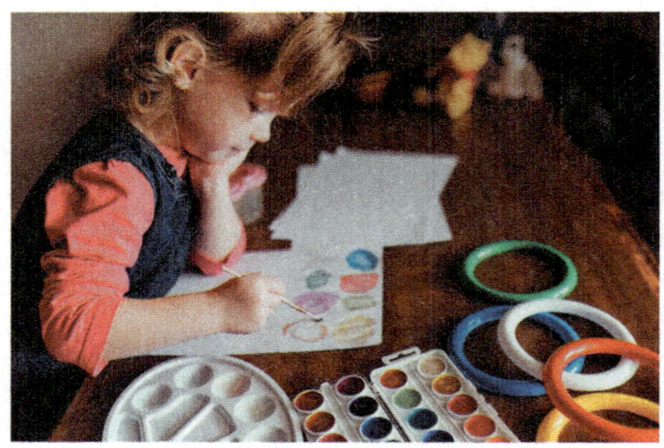

A 2-and-a-half year old draws circles

## Nursing Diagnosis

Healthy toddlers have many applicable nursing diagnoses including those that affect infants. Some NANDA diagnosis for the typical toddler might include:

- Delayed Growth and Development
- Imbalanced Nutrition, less than related to picky eating and poor dietary variety
- Anxiety related to speaking
- Fear related to new social situations
- Risk for infection
- Risk for injury
- Risk for poisoning

### *Outcomes*

The child will demonstrate increased age-appropriate behaviors in the following measures:

- Cognitive skills
- Balanced nutrition
- Knowledge deficit related to dental care and flouride as evidence by parents verbalizing concern about flouride in the water supply and in toothpastes
- Language
- Socialization
- Child is up-to-date on vaccinations
- Motor skill development and limit setting
- Child will remain poison free

## Interventions and Health Promotion

Delayed growth and development requires early intervention. The quick identification of children can facilitate outside therapies such as speech, physical therapy, and occupational therapy. If the child is inpatient, continuity of care is stressed. The nurse can help the child work at their highest potential, which may include enlisting Child Life for support based on patient acuity.

## Nutrition

Children that continue with a healthy diet have an opportunity to establish lifetime healthy eating habits during early childhood. Toddlers begin developing taste preferences based on the foods mothers ate in utero and gave as infants as their first foods (Clark-Gambelunghe and Clark 2015). Toddlers repeatedly request their favorite foods, known as a food jag, and is quite common.

Growth rates slow in the toddler and their appetite will decline and exhibit **physiologic anorexia**. Therefore, toddlers do not require the constant nutrition parents become accustomed to in infancy. Toddlers appear as fussy eaters, but it's probably more to do with adult expectations than contrariness (ATI Testing 2016).

Toddlers can now consume cow milk, but it is an unnecessary food item (Lanou, A. J., Berkow, S. E., and Barnard, N. D. 2005). If chosen as a food source, toddlers should consume no more than 24–28 oz of milk per day to prevent iron deficiency and loss of appetite for food. Toddlers may switch from drinking whole milk to drinking low-fat milk after 2 years of age. Cow's milk is not recommended at this time and is optional at other times. There are concerns about elevated estradiol and progesterone levels from drinking cow milk in causing early sexual maturation (Maruyama, Oshima and Ohyama 2010). As well as concerns about estrogen-sensitive cancers such as breast and ovarian cancers (Ganmaa, D., and Sato, A. n.d.; Brinkman, Baglietto, Krishnan, English, Severi, Morris, Hopper and Giles 2010; Genkinger, J. M., Hunter, D. J., Spiegelman, D., Anderson, K. E., Arslan, A., Beeson, W. L., Smith-Warner, S. A. 2006; Chan, J. M., and Giovannucci, E. L. n.d.; Giovannucci, E.1998; Chan, J. M., Stampfer, M. J., Ma, J., Gann, P. H., Gaziano, J. M., and Giovannucci, E. L. 2001; Qin, L. Q., Xu, J. Y., Wang, P. Y., Tong, J., and Hoshi, K. n.d.; Qin, L. Q., Xu, J. Y., Wang, P. Y., Kaneko, T., Hoshi, K., and Sato, A., n.d; Tate, P. L., Bibb, R., and Larcom, L. L. 2011; Ganmaa, D., Li, X. M., Wang, J., Qin, L. Q., Wang, P. Y., and Sato, A. 2002). Estrogens in milk can decrease testosterone in men, and soy may not have a feminizing effect on men as previously thought (Maruyama, K., Oshima, T., and Ohyama, K. 2010).

New evidence on cow milk's impact on bone health shows more detrimental effects than once thought. Milk also exposes drinkers to antibiotic and pesticide residues. In addition, new research indicates overestimations of daily calcium in the past; the current recommendation is 500–750 mg/day instead of the 1,200 mg previously recommended (Hunt and Johnson 2007).

Vitamin D supplements should begin within the first few days of life to prevent rickets and vitamin D deficiency in mothers who are deficient. Research indicates high dose vitamin D of 6400IU/day raises the vitamin D levels of mothers, not the recommended 400IU/day (Wagner, C.L., Hulsey, T.C., Fanning, D., Ebeling, M, and Hollis, B. 2006).

Iron supplements are recommended for exclusively breastfed infants after the age of 4 months, especially in cases of food insecurity. However, mothers with a robust hemoglobin value give birth to babies with a robust hemoglobin, so maternal diet cannot be emphasized enough in the health of the child (Marques, R. V., Taddei, J. C., Konstantyner, T., Marques, A. V., and Braga, J. P. 2016).

Toddlers do not require juice in their diets. If parents choose to give juice, they must limit it to 4–6 oz per day. Toddlers should drink only 100% fruit juice, not fruit juice drinks, beverages or cocktails (ATI Testing 2016).

The family should avoid trans fatty acids and minimize saturated fats. Common childhood foods such as cookies, pizza rolls, and fruit rolls contain trans fat. Read the labels for hydrogenated or partially hydrogenated oils. The entire family should minimize fast foods, and snacks or desserts that are high in sugar, fat, or sodium (ATI Testing 2016).

Serving sizes are small compared to adult standards. One tbsp for each year of age, or 1/4–1/3 of an adult portion. A healthy diet should include 1 cup of various fruits daily for nutrition and development of taste buds. Toddlers prefer finger foods because they like to eat on the go. Regular meal times and nutritious snacks best meet nutrient needs and develop a routine for well-being (ATI Testing 2016).

Foods are choking hazards to toddlers. Avoid nuts, whole grapes, hot dogs, peanut butter, raw carrots, tough meats, and popcorn at this stage. Toddlers need adult supervision during snack and meal times to minimize choking risks. Cutting foods into small, bite-size pieces to makes them easier to swallow. Toddlers should not drink or eat during play activities or while lying down, to minimize choking and ear infections from liquid leaking into the ears (ATI Testing 2016).

Familiarize parents with the US Department of Agriculture's guidelines for nutrition (US Department of Agriculture 2017). However, educate parents that a better model comes from Harvard's Healthy Eating Plate. This plate provides complete nutrition recommendations. It emphasizes lean protein, and eschews processed foods especially meats. Harvard Healthy Eating Plate specifies good fats to meet the fat requirement. Olive, coconut, avocado, walnut and flaxseed oils should take the place of all trans fats and a low-fat high-carbohydrate diet that promotes weight gain. This plate limits dairy, unlike MyPlate that encourages it with every meal. Fruit juice counts as a fruit on the MyPlate menu, on the Harvard Plate water is a suggested beverage. Juice is very similar in sugar content to soda and should be limited to a small glass a day or eliminated. Finally, the Harvard plate proposes exercise as one of its elements, MyPlate does not mention exercise (Tagtow, A., Haven, J., Maniscalco, S., Johnson-Bailey, D. Bard, S. 2015)

## Clinical Pearl

If a toddler learns to eat healthy foods, they will eat healthy foods over a lifetime. Although tasting of different foods beings in utero, toddlers have an opportunity to develop their culinary palettes at this stage. Adults must model healthy eating and ensure healthy foods are available, while children must decide which healthy foods they will consume and how much (Brawley, L., and Henk, J., 2014). Parents should think of this as a process that builds toward the ultimate goal of a healthy family.

Toddlers should establish the habit of seeing a dentist by the age of 1 year. Brushing and flossing are maintained by the adult caregiver to remove plaque. Brushing after meals and at bedtime is optimal. At bedtime, food and drink cease except for water to prevent bottle rot. Early childhood caries, or bottle-rot, refers to decaying teeth from going to bed with a bottle of juice or milk. Consumption of cariogenic foods (such as candy) should not start, and extra care of the teeth initiated if children are eating these foods (ATI Testing 2016).

Doctors may prescribe fluoride supplementation for children living in areas without adequate levels in drinking water. Parents may raise the issue of fluoride toxicity from the fluoridation of public water. Fluoride is proven to reduce caries (Schaffer and Adair 2000).

Concerned parents should supervise brushing and refrain from fluoride rinses and gels to assuage their fears as they balance the pros and cons of this supplement.

## Language

Learning language is a continuous process and continues in the toddler. Oral language must be heard and repeated to be learned, talking, reading, singing, and making up stories are all beneficial activities. Oral communication builds language skills used in later years to create literacy in children. (Chambers 2013)

Children need language nutrition, a term coined by Head-Zauche et al. 2017, to describe a process where children are immersed in language experiences that are full of stimulation and happen in the context of social situations. Language nutrition is strongly associated with future literacy, academic achievement, and health (Head Zauche, Lauren; Darcy Mahoney, Ashley E.; Thul, Taylor A.; Zauche, Michael S.; Weldon, Arianne B.; Stapel-Wax, Jennifer L. 2017).

Toddlers need socialization, experiences to support integration into the family, community and eventually school environments. Social skills are learned through play and conflict, as these two things inevitably intersect. Sharing is not age-appropriate at this time and adults should not overregulate the child's play experience (ATI Testing 2016).

Parents must let children experience consequences to figure out who they are. If a child takes a toy from another child, a parent might take it back and return to the original child. Adult intervention decreases the child's experience to know if they would accept losing the toy, decide to take the toy back, maybe the child would not mind and return to the toy later, or some children may cry. These responses are the socialization that should occur to let the child know where they belong in the world.

## Immunizations

"The Centers for Disease Control and Prevention immunization recommendations for healthy toddlers 12 months to 3 years of age include: 12–15 months: inactivated poliovirus (third dose between 6 and 18 months); Haemophilus influenzae type B; pneumococcal conjugate vaccine; measles, mumps, and rubella; and varicella. From 12 to 23 months: hepatitis A (Hep A), given in two doses at least 6 months apart" (Immunization Schedules 2017). From 15 to 18 months: diphtheria, tetanus, and acellular pertussis. Toddlers, 12 to 36 months receive yearly seasonal trivalent inactivated influenza vaccine. After 2 years of age, toddlers may receive the live, attenuated influenza vaccine by nasal spray (Immunization Schedules 2017; ATI Testing 2016).

## Toddler Screenings

Toddlers begin screenings for BMI and dyslipidemia by 2 years of age. They are also given an autism screening at 18 months of age. Lead screenings begin between 1 and 2 years of age (Committee on Practice and Ambulatory Medicine, and Workgroup, B. F. 2017).

## Aspiration

Toddlers commonly aspirate foreign objects. Toddlers frequently aspirate batteries, grapes, coins, candy, and clothing buttons. Older children's toys with small parts are hazards. Parents should use only age-appropriate toys to increase safety and development. Toddlers need supervision around balloons to avoid aspiration. Parents should know emergency procedures for choking and Cardiopulmonary Resuscitation (ATI Testing 2016).

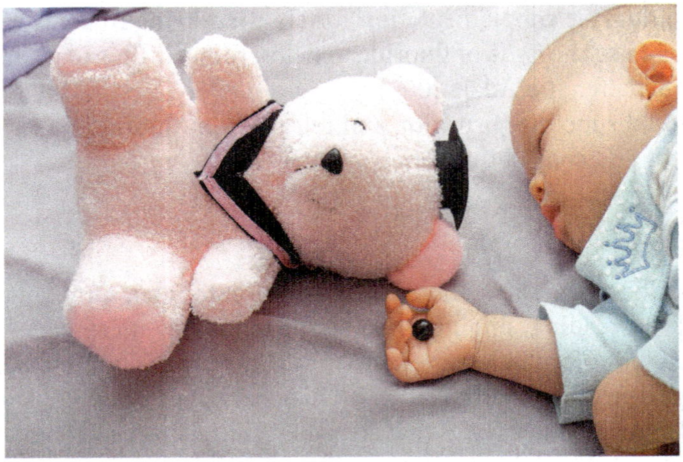

© Yaoinlove/Shutterstock.com

# Injury Prevention

## Bodily Harm

Parents should secure toddler areas by keeping sharp objects locked away. Parents must also place firearms in a locked box or cabinet. Toddlers need supervision with any animal to prevent injuries. Toddlers should learn stranger safety as well as communication skills to indicate any danger they feel at any time (ATI Testing 2016).
Burns

The caregiver must check the temperature of bath water should before exposing the child. The thermostat is set to less than 49° C (120° F) to prevent burns. A working smoke detector, tested yearly, should be kept in the home. Pot handles are not left turned toward the front of the stove; they are set toward the back to prevent an accidental spill on to the toddler. Adults must cover electrical outlet to avoid an electric shock to the toddler with specially fitted plugs. Toddlers also wear sunscreen when outside, reapplied as needed (ATI Testing 2017).

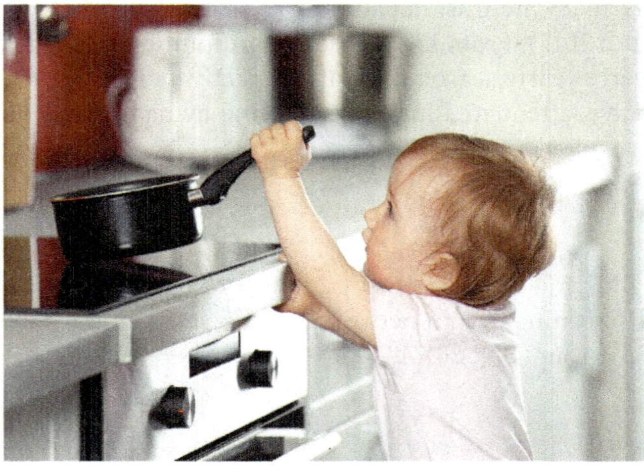

© Africa Studio/Shutterstock.com

## Drowning

Toddlers are never left unattended in bathtubs. Toilet lids should be kept closed, and toddlers are closely supervised when near pools or any other body of water. Toddlers can begin swimming lessons if they have not already (ATI Testing 2016).

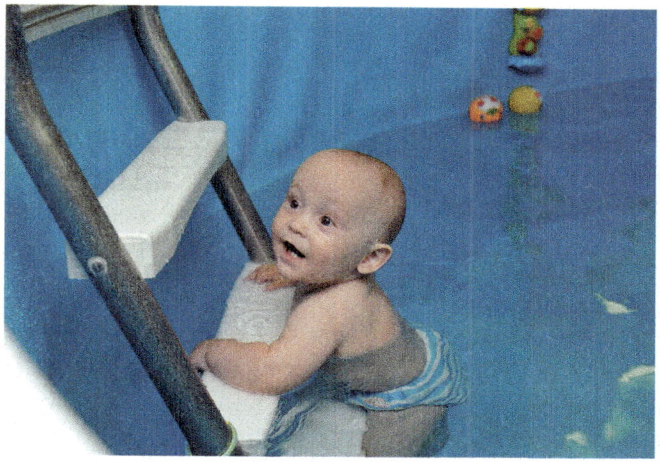

© Alex Bard/Shutterstock.com

## Falls

Doors and windows are kept locked. Crib mattresses are placed in the lowest position with the rails all the way up. Safety gates at the top and bottom of stairs prevent falls (ATI Testing 2016).

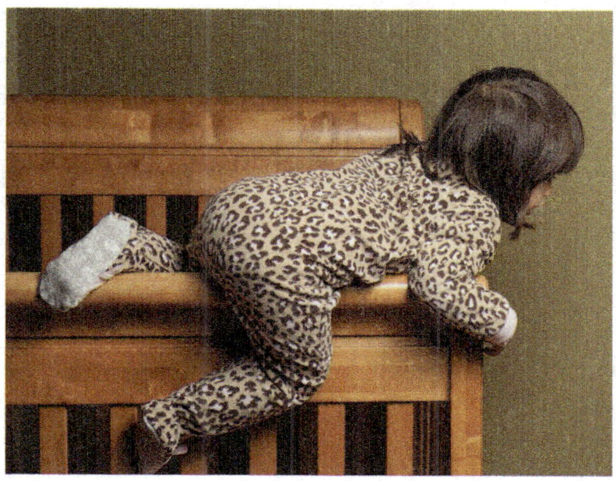

© Michael Pettigrew/Shutterstock.com

## Motor-Vehicle Injuries

Parent place infants and toddlers in a rear-facing car seat until 2 years of age or the height recommended by the manufacturer, as this is the safest area. Once the toddler is over 2 years of age, or meets the height recommendations for a rear-facing seat, parents can move them to a forward-facing car seat. A child should never sit in a rear-facing car seat in the passenger seat of vehicles with deployable passenger airbags (ATI Testing 2016).

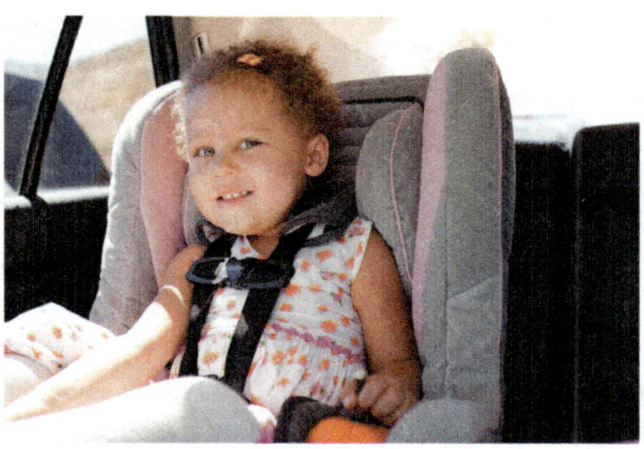

© pixelheadphoto digitalskillet/Shutterstock.com

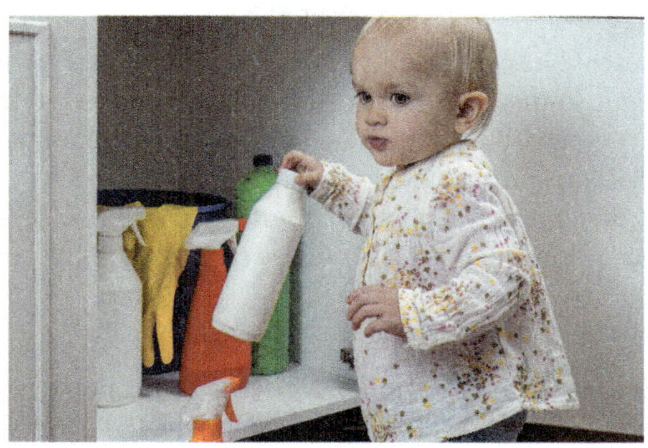

© Red pepper/Shutterstock.com

### Poisoning

Exposure to lead paints negatively impacts the brain of the developing toddler, as the element lead is a neurotoxin. Parent must place safety locks on cabinets that contain cleaners and other household chemicals. Parents should post the phone number for a poison control center somewhere easily accessible, and keep medications in childproof containers, out of the reach of toddlers. A working carbon monoxide detector can indicate toxic emissions (ATI Testing 2016).

### Suffocation

Plastic bags are eliminated from the toddler's environment and kept out of reach in the rest of the house. Crib mattresses should fit tightly to prevent the toddler's head from getting caught underneath the mattress. Crib slats are no farther apart than 6 cm (2.375 in), and parents should remove pillows from cribs. Parents should remove drawstrings from jackets and other clothing (ATI Testing 2016).

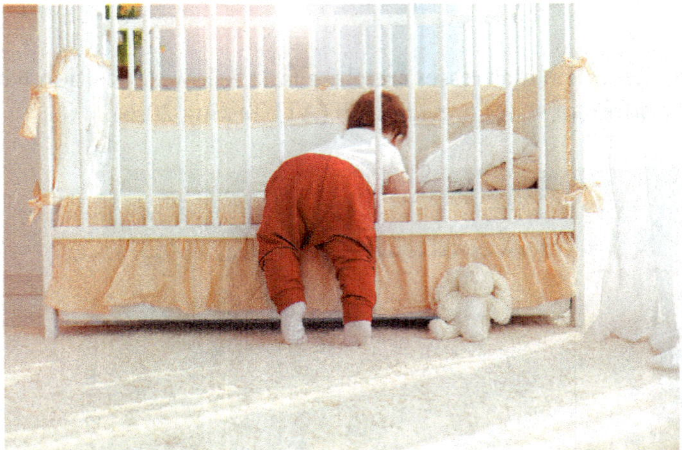

© Olesia Bilkei/Shutterstock.com

Toddlers desire the opportunity to use their senses during play. Their engagement in free play helps develop language and social skills. Toddlers require direction but do not need to be kept busy. Toddlers are busy all by themselves. Creating a therapeutic environment will support the toddler's development, and help parents "be the good guy" in the toddler's eyes, and not just glorified disciplinarians. This will help children and parents enjoy this exciting time. Never again will a child have the curiosity and wonder that a toddler brings. Pediatric nurses can remind parents of wellness appointments to be mindful of this stage. Inpatient pediatric nurses can rejoice with the family when the toddler is well enough to engage in typical toddler behaviors.

## PRESCHOOL

### Assessment Preschoolers

Preschoolers are 3–to 6 years of age. This growth period continues to slow compared with toddlers. Preschoolers begin to display their personality in new and dynamic ways. Children learn new rules, and may vacillate between willful independence and demands for attention. The typical preschooler gains about 2 to 3 kg (4.5 to 6.5 lb) every year, and grows approximately 6.5 to 9 cm (2.5 to 3.5 in) every year. Preschoolers must learn how to manipulate their bodies around their environment and other children, developing gross and fine motor skills that follow a set of sequences as each skill builds on the last skill (ATI Testing 2016).

### Communication with Preschoolers

Preschoolers have similar concerns about invasive procedures. However, they can express themselves better and are very literal. Allow time for the child to understand directions and explanations. Make sure to use anatomical names for body parts and incorporate a doll or toy to explain care. Children may create drawings to show how they feel. Allow reasonable choices, and encourage preschoolers to make them (ATI Testing 2016).

## Cognitive Development

According to Piaget, preschoolers continue in the preoperational period. Now, the preconceptual thought of toddlers, transitions into intuitive ideas at approximately 4 years old. Intuitive thought lasts from 4 to 7 years old. The preschooler thoughts shift from egocentric thoughts to a social awareness that enables them to consider the viewpoints of other people. Preschoolers intuitively make judgments based on visual appearances. Preoperational thinking includes phenomenon such as magical thinking, animism, centration, and understanding the sequence of time. Magical thinking causes preschoolers to experience thoughts as all-powerful forces that cause events to happen. Preschoolers use animism to give lifelike qualities to inanimate objects such as teddy bears and dolls. **Centration** leads preschoolers to focus on one aspect of an object instead of considering possible alternatives. Preschoolers do not yet understand time, but they understand a sequence of events. Parents who have ritualized, or use a rhythm, to their days facilitates learning that preschoolers now understand. Using time in relation to an event, best promotes preschooler understanding. By 5 years of age, children should know their full name, address, and phone number. By 6 years of age, children understand time-oriented words such as their birthday or Christmas (ATI Testing 2016).

## Language Development

Language development explodes in the preschool years. Preschoolers can sing songs and say nursery rhymes. Listening to oral language readies the preschool mind for reading. When children listen to oral stories, they create pictures of the events in their minds. These images mark the decoding of language, where words now equal pictures. Pictures give way to ideas and literacy as children grow into students. Parents will notice that delaying or omitting screen time creates space for natural, analog experiences. The integration of oral storytelling throughout the day builds literate children (Isbell, R., Sobol, J., Lindauer, L., and Lowrance, A. n.d.). Preschooler vocabularies increase to more than 2,100 words by 6 years old. They speak in three to four-word sentences by the age of 3 to 4 years of age, and four to five words between 4 to 5 years of age. Preschoolers mark the primary use of language as communication (ATI Testing 2016).

## Psychosocial Development

Preschoolers are in the third Erikson stage of initiative vs. guilt. Preschoolers need to exert themselves in the world to find where they fit. That may take the form of numerous questions about every subject imaginable. Preschoolers become vivacious learners, despite not having all of the motor skills or social skills necessary to complete the phase. If the preschooler feels stifled, they feel guilt for being in the way. Guilt can also occur when preschoolers believe they have misbehaved or when they are not successful at a task. Preschoolers need guidance to attempt activities within their capabilities, without dampening their will to learn (ATI Testing 2016).

## Moral Development

Early preschoolers continue in the reward or punishment model from toddlerhood. Older preschoolers seek to satisfy personal needs but understand the concepts of justice and fairness. Preschoolers develop a self-concept and feel good about themselves when mastering skills that allow independence like dressing and feeding. If stress occurs in the family or hospitalization, insecurity, or illness, preschoolers can regress to previous immature behaviors or develop immature habits such as nose picking, bed-wetting, and thumb sucking (ATI Testing 2016).

## Body-Image Changes

Preschoolers identify differences in appearances and identify socially acceptable and unacceptable norms. Preschoolers begin comparing themselves with peers by age five. Parents that project a positive body image help children reconcile this in the adolescent period. Preschoolers have a poor understanding of anatomy that makes invasive experiences, such as injections or cuts, frightening to preschoolers. If they bleed, they may think all of their blood will come out. Pediatric nurses understand the importance of using bandages after an injury or vaccination (ATI Testing 2016).

## Social Development

Preschoolers generally leave behind stranger and separation anxiety in the toddler years. Changes in daily routine are tolerated, but imaginary fears may develop. Preschoolers still benefit from routine. Prolonged separation from the family, such as during hospitalization, can produce anxiety. Favorite toys and appropriate play can assuage preschoolers' fears. **Pretend play** helps preschoolers determine the difference between reality and fantasy that continues into the school-aged years. Pretend play promotes self-regulation, problem-solving, and empathy (Kaufman 2013).

## Age Appropriate Activities

**Parallel play** in toddler-hood shifts to **associative play** during the preschool years. Playtime is not highly organized, but cooperation does exist between children. The following age appropriate activities promote development in preschoolers.

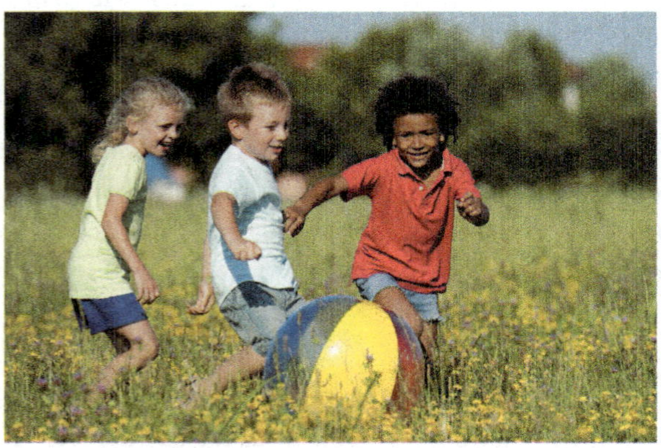


- Playing ball

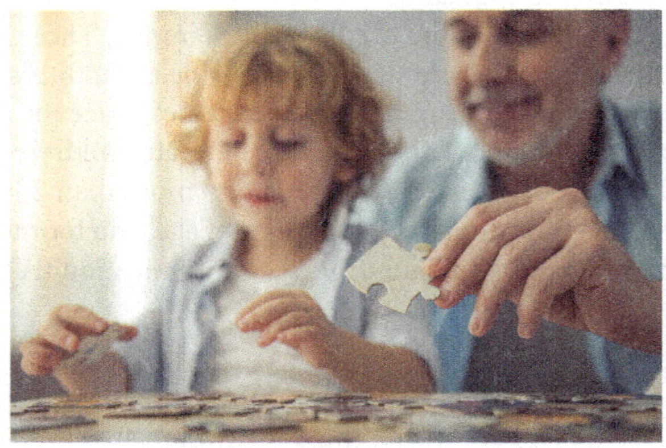


- Putting puzzles together

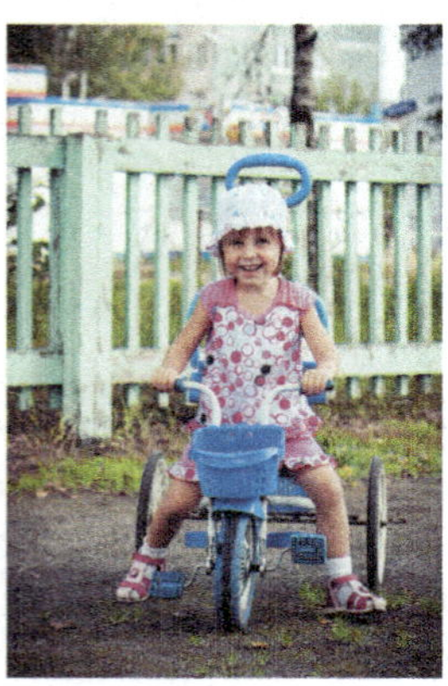


- Riding tricycles

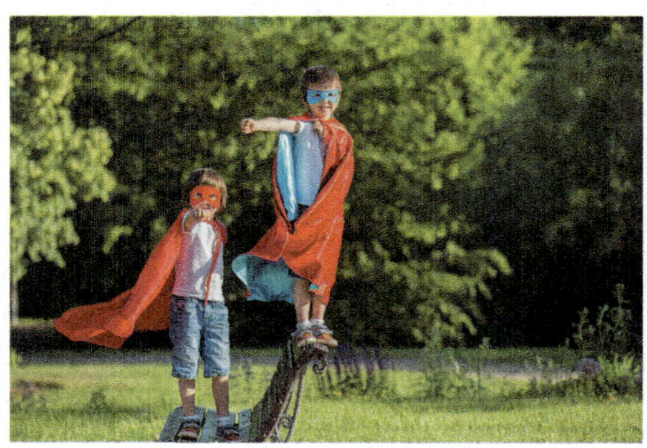


- Playing pretend and dress-up activities

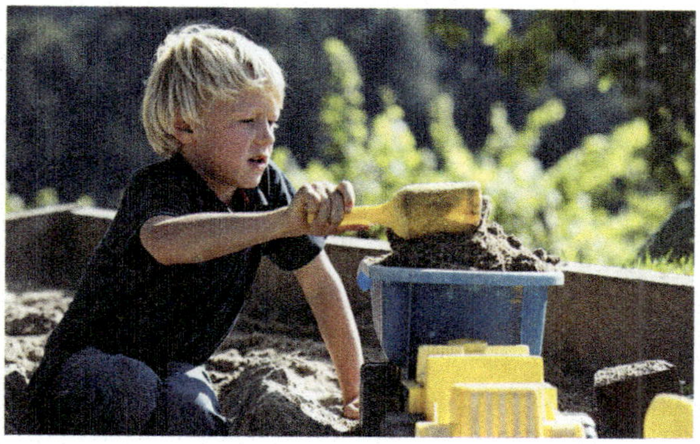
© OtmarW/Shutterstock.com

- Sand play

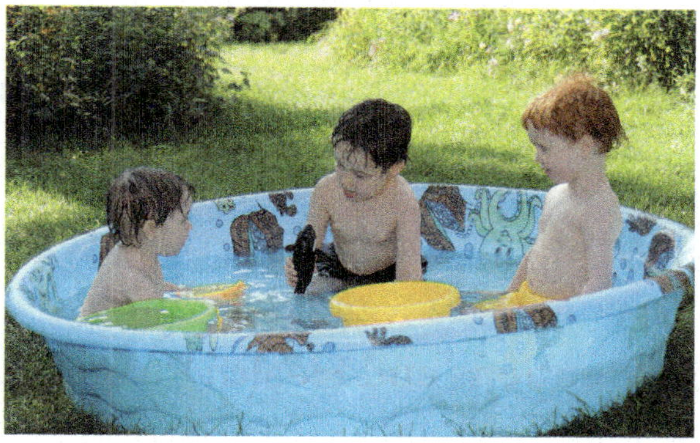
© Rossario/Shutterstock.com

- Wading pools

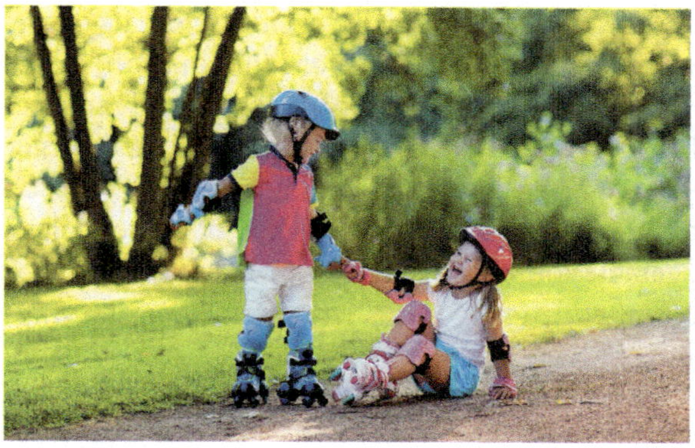
© FamVeld/Shutterstock.com

- Skating

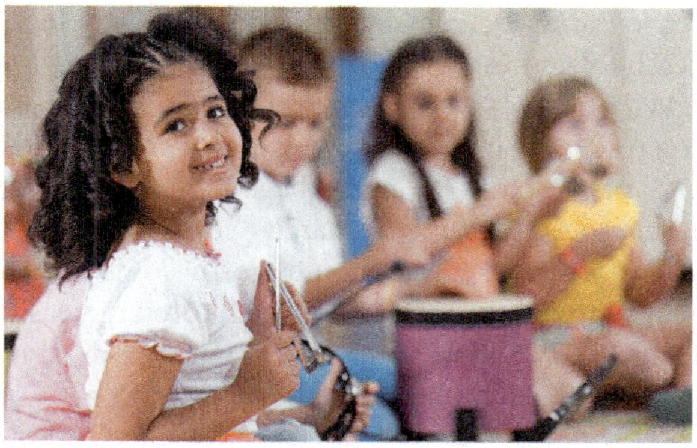
© Fh Photo/Shutterstock.com

- Musical toys

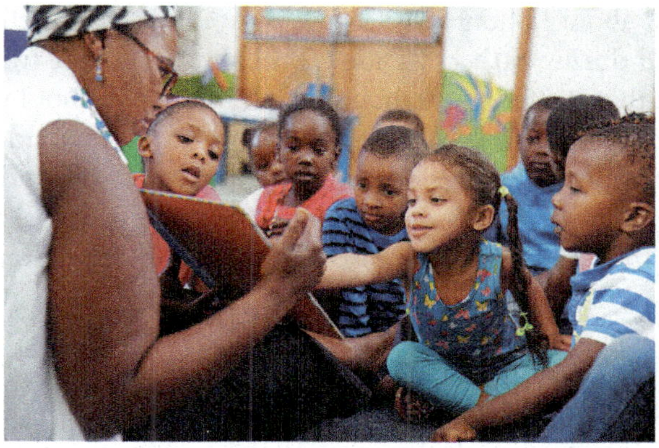
© Monkey Business Images/Shutterstock.com

- Reading books

## Nursing Diagnosis

Healthy preschoolers have many applicable nursing diagnoses because they grow in dynamic ways. Some NANDA diagnosis for the typical preschooler might include:

Imbalanced nutrition, more than body requirements
Disturbed sleep patterns
Risk for dental trauma
Risk for infection
Risk for injury

### Outcomes

Caregiver will verbalize understanding of giving nutritious food to prevent further weight gain
Client will wake up refreshed
Caregiver will verbalize steps to follow if tooth is injured
Client will be up-to-date on vaccinations
Motor skill development and limit setting

## Interventions and Health Promotion

### Nutrition

Preschoolers continue with taste exploration with an emphasis on whole foods in different colors (Ramsay, S. A., Shriver, L. H., and Taylor, C. A. 2017). Preschoolers can consume up to 1,800 kcal if they are very active. Finicky eating can remain a behavior in preschoolers, but given a diversity of foods will subside by 5 years of age. Preschoolers need 13 to 19 g/day (0.45 to 0.67 oz/day) of protein and adequate intake of calcium, iron, folate, and vitamins A and C. Meat protein should not comprise all of the protein requirement, and vegetable sources are a viable option for protein. Healthy proteins from vegetable sources include lentils (18g/cup), veggie burger (13g/1 patty), bagel (10 grams/bagel), Pinto beans (15g/cup), spaghetti (8g/cup), spinach (5g/cup), and broccoli (4g/cup) (Agricultural Research Service n.d.). Saturated fats should comprise less than 10% of preschoolers' total caloric intake. Fats should mostly come from healthy vegetable sources such as olive, sunflower, and avocado. With obesity rates in young children increasing, the recommendations for prevention include: 5 servings of fruits and vegetables per day for vitamins and protein, 2 hours or less of screen time for psychosocial health, 0 servings of sugar-sweetened beverages to minimize sugar intake, and 1 hour of physical activity per day to promote health and wellness (ATI Testing 2016).

### Sleep and Rest

Preschoolers typically need about 12 hours of sleep per day and infrequently take daytime naps. Sleep disturbances can frequently occur during early childhood. Problems can range from difficulty going to bed to night terrors. A bedtime routine that started in infancy pays off in the preschool years as it will minimize struggles over bedtime. Night terrors may begin earlier in childhood. Parents should not wake the child, and the child may not remember the experience. Parents should report night terrors and other sleeping difficulties to the health-care provider. Parents can promote sleep hygiene if they keep a consistent bedtime routine, use a night-light in the room, provide the child with a comforting toy, and leave a covered container of water by the bed (ATI Testing 2016).

### Dental Health

The eruption of deciduous (primary) teeth finalizes by the beginning of the preschool years. Parents need to assist and supervise brushing and flossing to ensure it is performed correctly to prevent dental caries and excess fluoride consumption. Children are accident prone in the preschool years, if they experience trauma to their gums or teeth, parents should take the child to see a dentist as soon as possible (ATI Testing 2016).

### Immunizations

The Centers for Disease Control and Prevention (CDC) immunization recommendations for healthy preschoolers 3–6 years of age (Immunization Schedules, 2017) include:

From 4 to 6 years of age: Diphtheria and tetanus toxoids and pertussis (DTaP); measles, mumps, and rubella (MMR); varicella; and inactivated poliovirus (IPV).

From 3 to 6 years of age: Yearly seasonal influenza vaccine; trivalent inactivated influenza vaccine; or live, attenuated influenza vaccine by nasal spray (ATI Testing 2016).

## Injury Prevention

### Bodily Harm

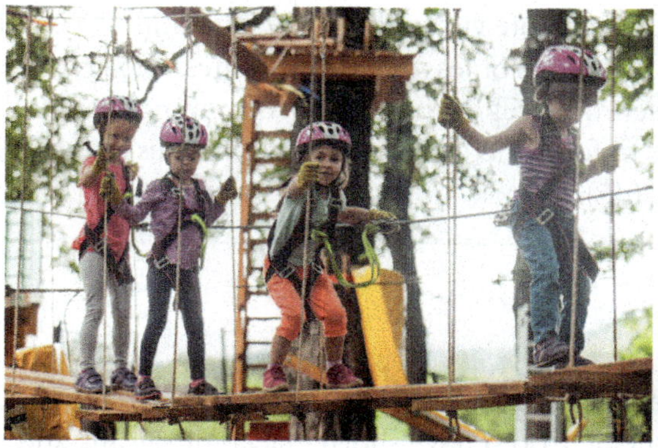

© Oksana Shufrych/Shutterstock.com

Preschoolers use intuitive reasoning not logical thinking and need injury prevention strategies in their homes. Items such as firearms, stranger safety, and sports safety require logical thinking. Therefore, adult supervision is necessary. Firearms are locked in cabinets or containers. Preschoolers learn about stranger safety and know to report adults who ask them to keep secrets or make them feel uncomfortable. Preschoolers are also taught to wear protective equipment such as helmets and protective pads to protect their bodies during playtime (ATI Testing 2016).

### Burns

Parents keep hot water thermostats set at or below 49°C (120°F) and continue to check water temperature before allowing the preschooler to enter. Parents should test smoke detectors each year for new batteries. Preschoolers should have sunscreen applied when outside (ATI Testing 2016).

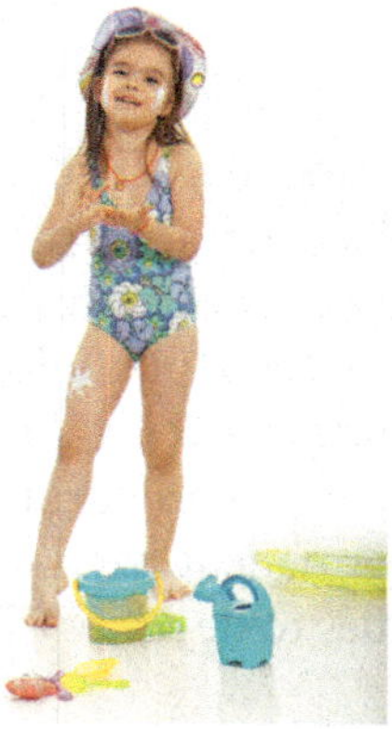

Blaj Gabriel/Shutterstock.com

### Drowning

Parents must supervise preschoolers in bathtubs, and do not allow them to play near a pool or any other body of water. Preschoolers should be taught to swim (ATI Testing 2016).

### Motor-Vehicle Injuries

Parents are required to use a federally approved car seat with preschoolers who ride in a car. Once the forward-facing car seat is too small, the preschooler needs a booster seat. The recommendation is to use an approved car restraint system until the child's height is 145 cm (4 feet, 9 in). The safest area for children remains in the backseat of the car (ATI Testing 2016).

## Clinical Pearl

Preschool children are vulnerable to the negative effects of media exposure. Excessive screen time can impair language development, precipitate violent behavior, and inhibit a child's self-concept. Preschoolers screen time should be limited to 2 hours or less per day. Families who receive support during health maintenance visits to decrease screen time report increased communication and decreased violent behavior. Nurses can encourage families to form media rules for their houses and peer groups (Yilmaz, G., Demirli Caylan, N., & Karacan, C. D. 2015).

### Screen Time

Preschoolers who have an increased BMI are likely to be overweight adults. Children exposed to increased screen time and a television in the bedroom have shorter sleep durations and promote overweight preschool children (Sijtsma, A., Koller, M., Sauer, P., and Corpeleijn, E. 2015).

Parents should refrain from any screen time for children under 2 years of age. If parents do not create a strategy to meet this goal, then success is unlikely. To achieve this recommendation a cultural change is necessary for most Americans. Parents should strive to create a developmentally appropriate environment for their preschooler, and form groups for support in the community.

Preschoolers experience executive brain function development at 4 years of age. Executive brain function can predict early school success. Executive brain functions may include task persistence, impulse control, emotion regulation, and creative, flexible thinking (Radesky, J. S., and Christakis, D. A. 2016).

Preschool-age children need supervision. Supervise children when playing and do not allow them to play near a curb or parked cars. Parents should teach pedestrian safety rules to preschooler children including standing back from the curb while waiting to cross the street, and before crossing the street, look left, then right, then left again. At night, children should wear light-colored clothing with fluorescent materials to promote safety.

## SCHOOL AGE

The school-age period spans from 6 to 12 years of age. School-age children experience growth spurts in this growth period by 10 or 11 years old. Typical school-age children gain about 2 to 3 kg (4.4 to 6.6 lb) per year and about 5 cm (2 inches) per year. Prepubescence activates in preadolescence, around 9 years of age for girls and later for boys. Prepubescence marks the onset of physiologic changes that will result in adulthood. During growth spurts, rapid weight and height changes occur. The sexual differentiation between boys and girls emerges. Visible sexual maturation is minimal in boys during preadolescence (ATI Testing 2016).

School-age children start to get their permanent teeth. Bladder capacity matures but remains greater in girls than boys. The immune system continues to develop. Children's bones continue to ossify.

### Communication with School-Age Children

School-age children like concrete examples of diagrams and pictures to explain their care to them. Nurses should assess the child to determine what knowledge they have and build upon that. Children should understand procedures before they occur. Nurses can use counting or sing a song to manage uncomfortable interventions. Honestly discuss the plan of care with the child and family present (ATI Testing 2016).

### Cognitive Development

School-age children are in the third stage of Piaget's concrete operational stage. Thinking transitions from perceptual thinking to conceptual thinking. Perceptual thinking means an understanding of the environment that comes through the senses. School-age children move from using perceptual thinking to more abstract, conceptual thinking. School-age children understand the concept of conservation. Conservation of mass makes sense first, followed by conservation of weight, and then conservation of volume. Children learn to tell time on their own. They can also integrate a lot of complex information and can see problems from another point of view. School-age children can solve mathematical problems and other concrete operations (ATI Testing 2016).

## Psychosocial Development

School-age children are in the fourth Erikson stage of industry vs. Inferiority. School-age children achieve a sense of industry is obtained through the development of skills and knowledge. Children gain a sense of accomplishment through cooperating and competing with others. Children should be challenged with practical tasks and allowed to work through individual differences to complete the tasks. Children respond to systems that reward successful mastery of skills and tasks, however not completing the task can create a sense of inferiority. Children learn they will not master every skill and develop an appreciation for a balance of individual strengths and weaknesses (ATI Testing 2016).

## Moral Development

Early school-age children do not know the reasoning behind rules and expectations for behavior. They make judgments from previous experience about rewards and punishment. They can occasionally interpret accidents as punishment for past behaviors. By the end of the school-age years, children can judge the intentions of an act rather than just its consequences. They move beyond the dichotomy of right and wrong and understand different points of view. School-age children cultivate the ability to treat other people with respect (ATI Testing 2016).

## Self-Concept Development

In addition to moral development, school-age children develop personal values, abilities, and physical characteristics. The self-concept has many aspects and may include confidence, self-ideals, and relationship to peers. Confidence originates from a positive self-concept, which leads children to provide significant contributions to their lives. Parents continue to influence the early school-age child's self-ideals, but by late school age, the opinions of peers and teachers become more valuable (ATI Testing 2016).

## Body-Image Changes

School-age children gain an awareness of their body image. Parents provide a positive framework to see the body as a well-oiled machine that needs maintenance for life. Children take more responsibility for the care of the body. Parents should praise intrinsic qualities in children to promote self-worth. Parents must transform negative self-talk into a positive affirmation while eliminating negative influences such as overexposure to the media. Curiosity naturally develops about sexuality, and scientific education regarding sexual development and the reproductive process begins. School-age children change quickly showing more modesty than preschoolers. Adolescents place an emphasis on privacy issues (ATI Testing 2016).

## Social Development

Peer groups emerge as the next step in social development, and peer pressure begins. Children take an interest in different clubs and form new relationships. School-age children may even designate a best friend. School-age children experience bullying actions and must learn to ask for help when necessary. Teach children to support the child subject to bullying and to also ask an adult for help. Early school-age children prefer the company of same-gender companions, but a developing an interest in the opposite sex typically occurs toward the end of the school-age years (ATI Testing 2016).

Children find comfort in conformity. Most relationships come from school associations, so a good fit between child and school eases this stage of development.

## Age Appropriate Activities

**Competitive play** and **cooperative play** is predominant in school-age children.

Young school-age children from 6 to 9 years of age engage in the following age appropriate activities to promote development.

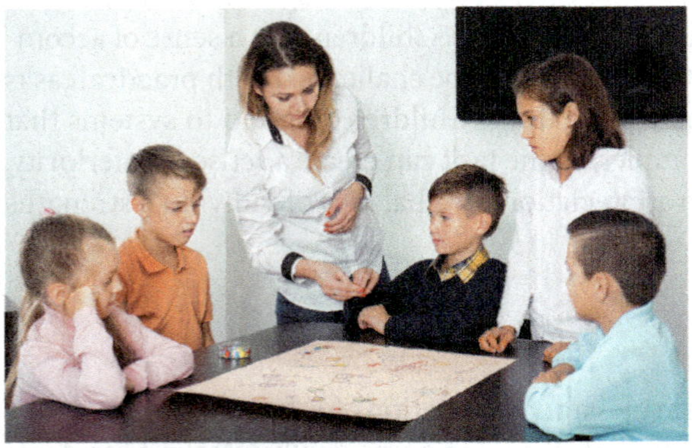
© Iakov Filimonov/Shutterstock.com

- Play simple board and number games

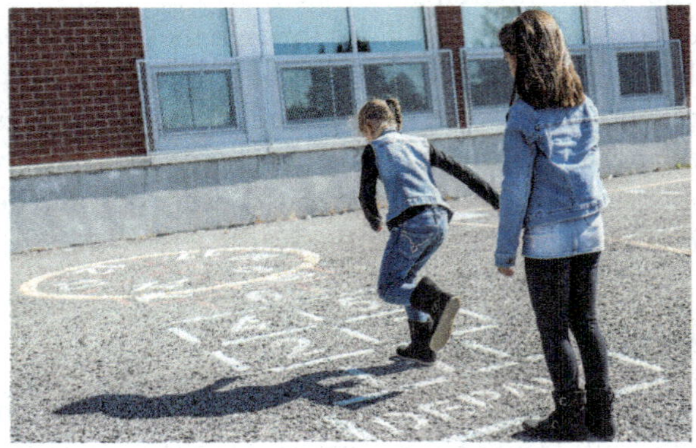
© Lopolo/Shutterstock.com

- Play hopscotch

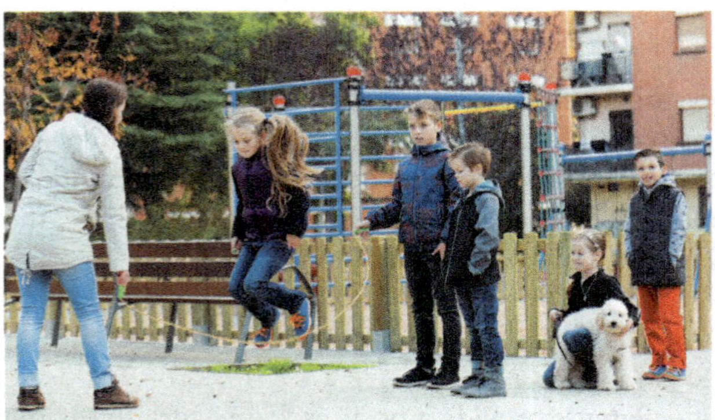
© Iakov Filimonov/Shutterstock.com

- Jump rope

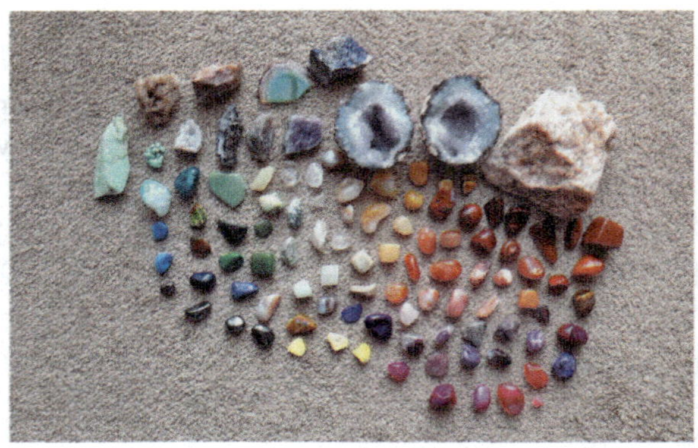
© Holly Christopher 17/Shutterstock.com

- Collect rocks, stamps, cards, coins, or stuffed animals.

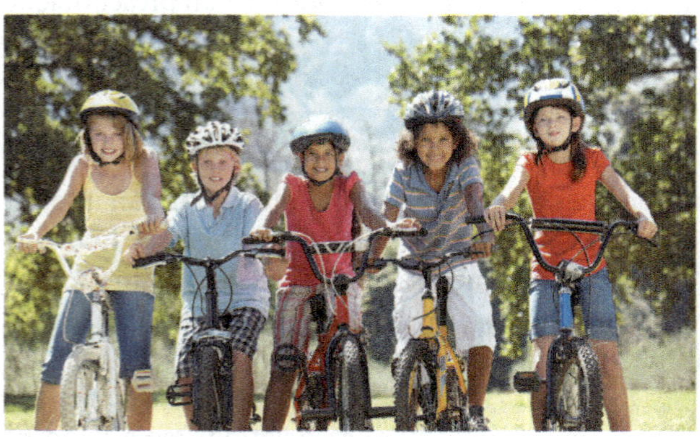
© Monkey Business Images/Shutterstock.com

- Ride bicycles

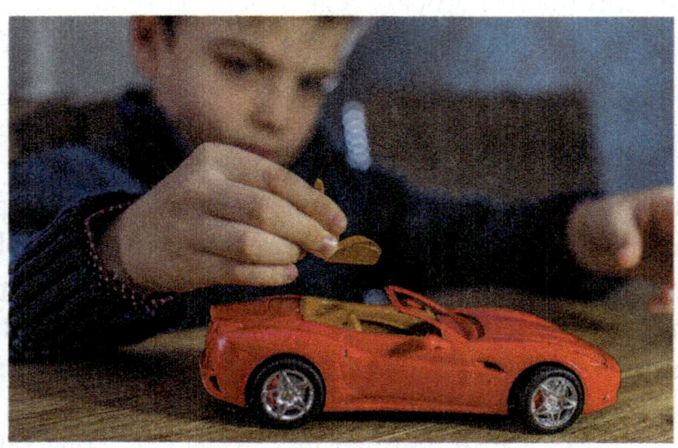
© mike mols/Shutterstock.com

- Build simple models

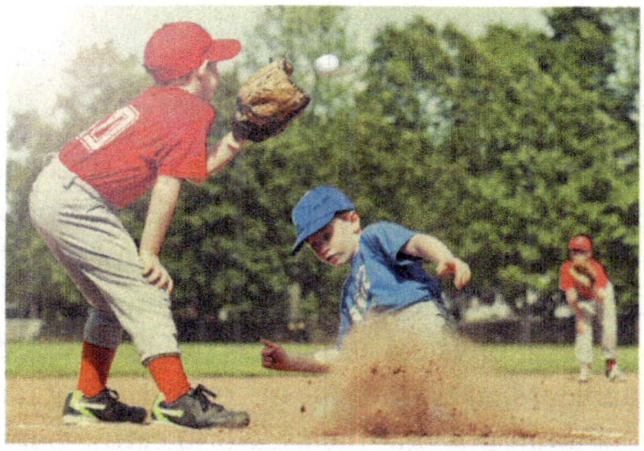
Stuart Monk/Shutterstock.com

- Join organized sports (for skill building)

Older School-Age children from 9 to 12 years old engage in age appropriate activities to promote development

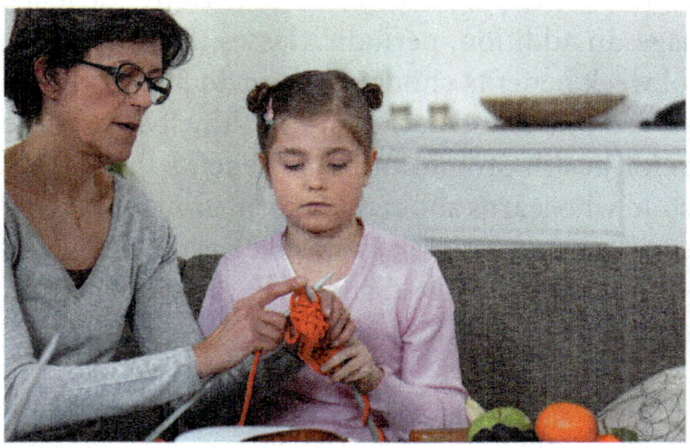
© Phovoir/Shutterstock.com

- Make crafts

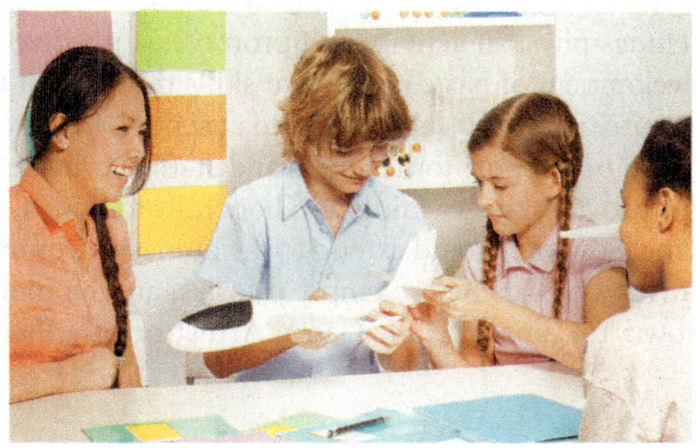
© Sergey Novikov/Shutterstock.com

- Build models

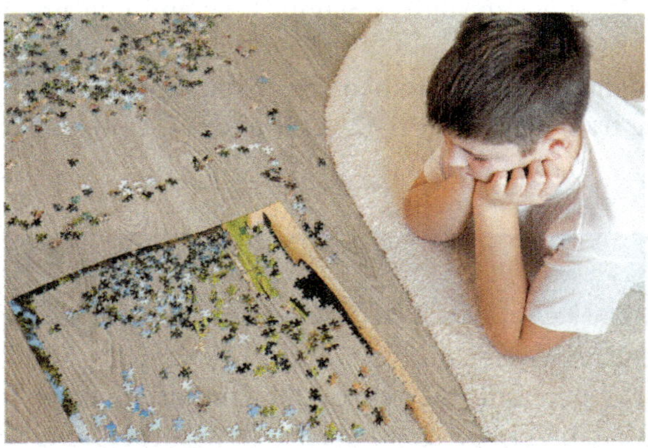
© BestPhotoPlus/Shutterstock.com

- Solve jigsaw puzzles

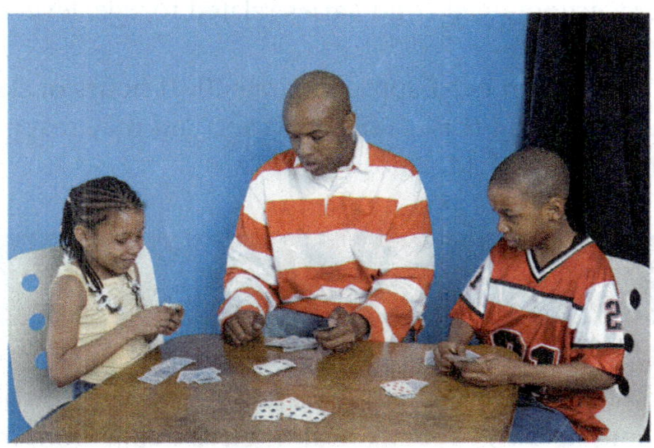
© Karen Struthers/Shutterstock.com

- Play board and card games

## School-Age Screenings

School-age children receive screenings for scoliosis. An examination of the spine before and during growth spurts that reveals a lateral curvature of the spine may be scoliosis. Screenings can take place at schools or health-care facilities. Screenings will identify children who may have scoliosis. Children who do not pass the screening need a referral to a pediatrician for diagnostic testing (Greydanus 2008).

Children receive screenings for drugs and alcohol that includes teaching about the research of addiction. Screenings for Sexually Transmitted Infections and additional screenings Girls receive screening for cervical dysplasia through a pap-smear test, and boys receive screening for testicular cancer (ATI Testing 2016).

## Interventions and Health Promotion

### Nutrition

By the late school-age years, children should eat three meals and a snack of mainly whole foods. Children should learn to only eat they are hungry and learn to listen to this cue. School-age children should help make meals in the kitchen and nutritious snacks for after school periods. School-age children can battle obesity. This predisposes children to low self-esteem, diabetes, heart disease, and high blood pressure. Parent must refrain from using food as a reward, and emphasize physical activity. School-age children should avoid fast food or make healthier options if it is unavoidable. Meal planning can combat using fast food as a default option due to poor planning. School-age children should not skip meals. Good eating habits come from the modeling of good eating habits from parents. Good eating habits established in the toddler and preschool years continue into the school-age years and adulthood (ATI Testing 2016).

There is strong evidence to support certain interventions to prevent obesity in children 6–12 years of age. This evidence is international evidence that means these findings can have applications in many geographical locations. The evidence is clear that a school curriculum that teaches children to eat foods high in nutrients, includes physical activity and promotes a positive body image. In addition, periodic classes that allows the development of basic movement skills throughout the school week benefits children. The evidence also calls for nutritious foods being offered at school, improving the environment and culture for healthy living. There should be support for teachers and staff to provide activities for health promotion. This benefits the teacher who provides the teaching, and hopefully follows it, and the child who learns about the information for healthy living. Support should extend to the home environment to decrease screen time (if applicable), eat high-quality nutritious foods before empty calories, and be more active (Waters E., de Silva-Sanigorski A., Burford B. J., Brown T, Campbell K. J., Gao Y, Armstrong R., Prosser L., and Summerbell C. D. 2011).

### Sleep and Rest

Children frequently do not get enough sleep in this age group. The tendency to over-schedule, coupled with large amounts of homework balanced with family life can tire a school-age child. The amount of sleep necessary for a school-aged child varies related to, age, level of activity, and health status ((Schub, T. B., and Pilgrim, J. M. 2016).

Children need approximately 10–11 hours of sleep per night. Resistance to bedtime is sometimes experienced around the age of 8–9 years, and may reappear at the transition from 11-12 years of age (Schub, T. B., and Pilgrim, J. M. 2016).

#### Clinical Pearl

School-age children who have a short sleep duration or behavioral sleep problems impair executive brain function and result in academic under-performance as well as increasing the risk for unintentional injuries and obesity. Creating healthy sleep habits from infancy help children get good quality sleep through the later stages of childhood. Children who establish healthy sleep routines that include consistent bedtimes and wake times, cool, dark and quiet sleeping environments without television sets, and that participate in daily exercise establish a routine carries into later childhood and adolescence. Maintenance of a sleep routine helps children deal with periods of instability and stress, making sleep more important in times of family crisis (Koulouglioti, C., Cole, R., Moskow, M., Mcquillan, B., Carno, M., and Grape, A. 2014).

### Dental Health

The first permanent, adult teeth erupt around 6 years of age. Children should brush after meals and snacks, and at bedtime, and floss daily. Children should have checkups every 6 months.

If determined necessary, children should have regular fluoride treatments. If a child experiences trauma to one or more teeth contact a dentist immediately (ATI Testing 2016).

### Immunizations

The Centers for Disease Control and Prevention (CDC) immunization recommendations for healthy school-age children 6 to 12 years of age (Immunization Schedules 2017) include:

A catch-up schedule for the following vaccinations by 6 years of age: diphtheria and tetanus toxoids and pertussis (DTaP); inactivated poliovirus; measles, mumps, and rubella (MMR); and varicella. In addition, a yearly seasonal influenza vaccine either the trivalent inactivated influenza vaccine (TIV) or live, attenuated influenza vaccine (LAIV) by nasal spray are administered.

For 11–12 year olds: tetanus and diphtheria toxoids and pertussis vaccine (Tdap); human papillomavirus vaccine: HPV2 or HPV4 in three doses for females, HPV4 for males; and meningococcal (MCV4).

School-age children become more self-directed and peer-focused. They experience meaningful friendships while still enjoying time with their families. School-age children feel peer pressure and benefit from open communication with parents to manage the new pressures. Therefore, open parental communication developed in the toddler and preschool years becomes a foundation for communication in the school-age years. School-age children try many different things to find their purpose in life.

## Injury Prevention

### Bodily Harm

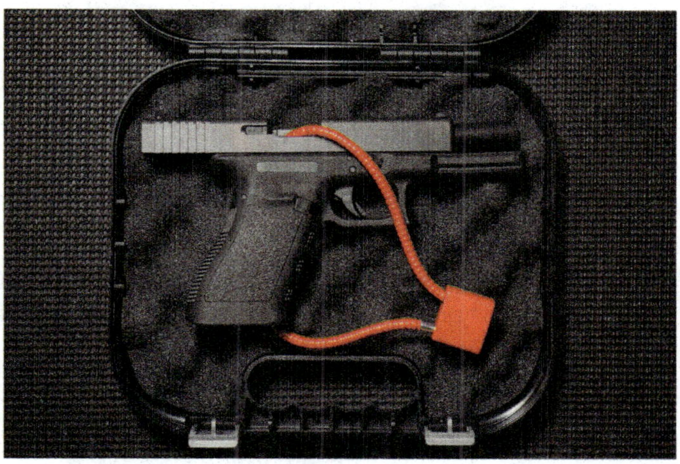

© Nic Neufeld/Shutterstock.com

Firearms are kept out of reach of children, have a trigger lock and placed in locked cabinets or boxes. If guns are kept in the home, then children need education about gun safety. Parents must identify developmentally appropriate safe play areas for school-age children.

Parent must teach stranger safety to children, in addition to good communication about adults who ask them to keep secrets or make them feel uncomfortable (ATI Testing 2016).

Parents must teach and reinforce the use of safety equipment when climbing, roller skating, skateboarding, bicycling, riding scooters, skiing, or snowboarding (ATI Testing 2016).

### Burns

Parents will teach fire safety and potential burn hazards in the home. Parents need an escape route to run mock fire drills. Parents must place working smoke detectors in the home. Children should use sunscreen when outside and reapply every few hours. Children should learn safety precautions while cooking, especially around younger siblings (ATI Testing 2016).

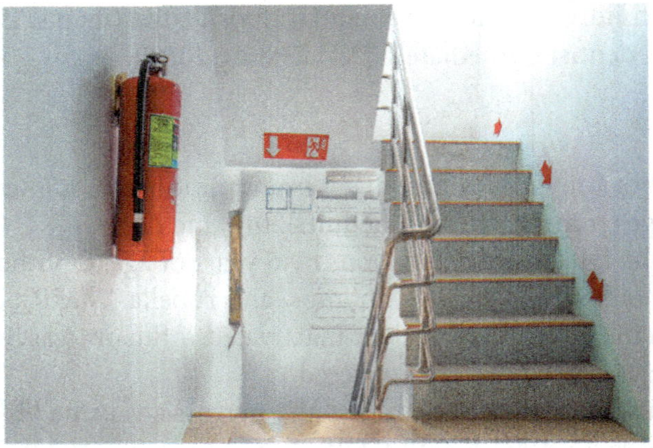

© Mr.Yotsaran/Shutterstock.com

## Drowning

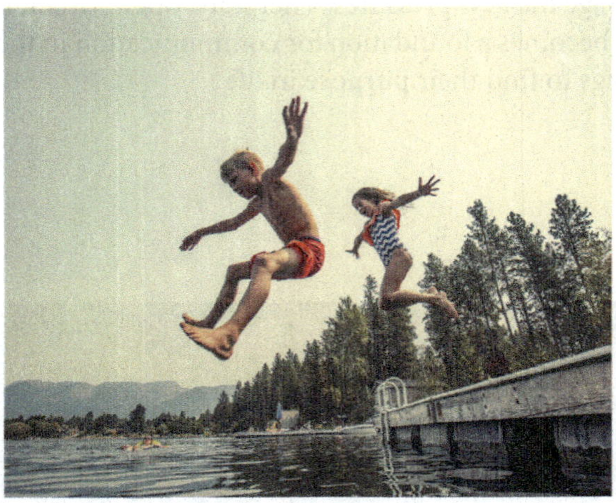

© Brocreative/Shutterstock.com

Children need supervision when swimming or when near a body of water. Children should learn to swim or increase their swimming skills. Always check the depth any water before allowing children to dive. Parents should encourage breaks from swimming to prevent children from becoming over-tired (ATI Testing 2016).

## Motor-Vehicle Injuries

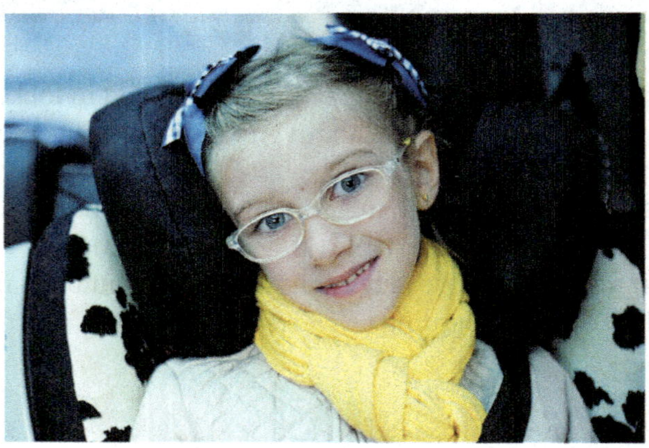

© Alinute Silzeviciute/Shutterstock.com

Children should use an approved car seat until they reach a height of 145 cm (4 feet, 9 inches). Children must use a seat belt use when a car restraint system or booster seat becomes unnecessary. Children ride most safely in backseat of the car. Parents can never let children ride in the bed of a pickup truck or in the front seat before they are tall enough. Parents should also reinforce safe pedestrian behaviors when walking with the child across streets (ATI Testing 2016).

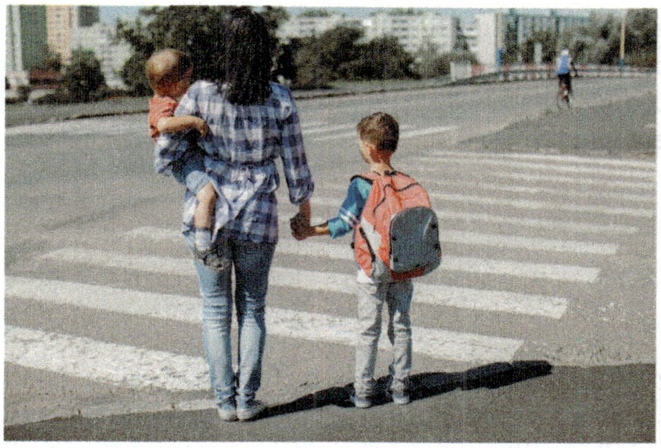


## Poisoning/Substance Abuse

Household cleaners and chemicals stay in locked cabinets and out of reach of younger children. Children who mow lawns or do yard work may experience inhale pesticides or toxins from the plants and soil. Any rashes or respiratory signs are reported to a health-care provider (ATI Testing 2016).

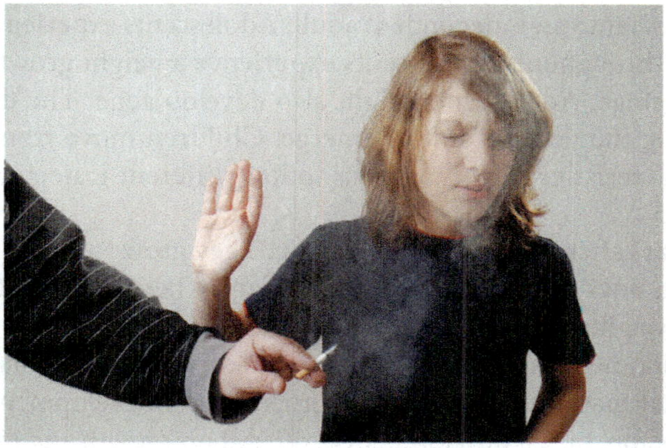


Parents should teach children to say "no" to all substances, but also teach children the dangers of substance abuse especially in a developing body. The best education comes from modeling behavior of the adults the child sees every day (ATI Testing 2016). Parents who smoke should do so away from children (DeSafey 2012).

## Nursing Diagnosis

Healthy school-age children have many applicable nursing diagnosis because they grow in dynamic ways. Some NANDA diagnosis for the typical school-age child might include:

- Imbalanced nutrition, more than body requirements
- Disturbed sleep patterns
- Risk for dental trauma
- Risk for infection
- Risk for scoliosis
- Risk for injury

### Outcomes

- Caregiver will verbalize understanding of giving nutritious food to prevent further weight gain
- Client will wake up refreshed
- Caregiver will verbalize steps to follow if tooth is injured
- Client will be up-to-date on vaccinations
- Client will receive screening for scoliosis
- Motor skill development and limit setting

# ADOLESCENT

## Adolescent Assessment

The pace of adolescence growth ranks second only to the increase in infancy. Brain growth includes the myelination of neurons that increases the speed of neural impulses and can accommodate abstract thinking. Adolescents mature physically and sexually, take on adult roles, and diversify their peer groups to include the opposite sex. Social skills that support more mature relationships develop. Adolescence can stereotypically indicate a pathological state to some adults. However, the adolescent period does not necessarily consist of a series of trouble-making events. Issues during this period should not be considered "normal" and dismissed. Research suggests a holistic model of prevention and health maintenance that includes social institutions, health-care providers and their communities (Institute of Medicine and National Research Council 1999).

Adolescence spans from 12 to 18 years of age. Adolescents experience the final stage of childhood where the once dependent child grows into an independent adult. Adolescents experience many changes physically, cognitively and emotionally throughout. Adolescents experience a height growth spurt as 20%–25% of the final height happens in this stage. Adolescents might also develop acne. The dynamic process of puberty unfolds individually, allowing the young adult to emerge. Children move from sexual immaturity to the development of sexual characteristics. Boys and girls follow different trajectories of development in this stage (ATI Testing 2016).

Girls grow until 2–2.5 years after the onset of menarche. They grow 5–20 cm (2–8 in) in weight and gain 7–25 kg (15.5–55 lb) in weight. Boys grow until 18–20 years of age. They grow 10–30 cm (4–12 in) in height and gain 7–30 kg (15.5–66 lb) in weight (ATI Testing 2016).

The stage of sexual development informs the stage of adolescence more reliably than chronological age. The assessment of girls' sexual maturation follows the order: breast development, pubic hair growth (some girls experience hair growth before breast development) axillary hair growth and menstruation. In boys, sexual maturation occurs in the following order: testicular enlargement, pubic hair growth, penile enlargement, the growth of axillary hair, facial hair growth, and vocal changes (ATI Testing 2016).

## Communication with Adolescents

Communication with adolescents must originate from a place of privacy. An environment of privacy fosters trust and builds rapport. Direct questions to the teenager and then, the parent. Provide written materials as well as talking through topics. Arrange support from other teens in situations of noncompliance. Sensitive information such as STD testing and birth control options do not need parental approval (ATI Testing 2016).

## Cognitive Development

Adolescents are in the fourth Piaget stage of the formal operational stage. Adolescents move from manipulating objects in concrete operations to manipulating ideas in formal operations. Thinking transitions from concrete thinking to abstract thinking. Adolescents think abstractly. They can plan for the future and extrapolate outcomes to various decisions. Formal operations enable adolescents to manipulate more than two categories of variables at the same time. Adolescents can also maintain focus for longer periods of time. Adolescents can now understand how the actions of an individual can influence others.

## Psychosocial Development

Adolescents are in the fifth Erikson stage of identity vs. role confusion. Adolescents seek a sense of self through the integration of experimentation with personas that form an integrated personality. Adolescents develop a sense of personal identity, as they become unique individuals. Adolescents also seek to form a group identity with their peers.

Early adolescence, can involve sexual experimentation driven by curiosity. Friendships transition from friendships to intimate relationships. In late adolescence, the integration of sexual experiences, feelings, and knowledge develops into a sexual identity.

Adolescents typically view themselves as invincible to adverse outcomes of risky behaviors. Adolescents solve moral dilemmas based on earlier experiences in childhood, but also challenge the relevance of existing moral values to society and individuals. Adolescents take pride in the unique characteristics they develop as the adolescent years progress. However, they vacillate in comparing themselves to their peers (ATI Testing 2016).

## Social Development

Peer relationships develop, and act as a support system for adolescents. Friendships increase in number, and a "best friend" may emerge. Parent–child relationships change to allow a greater sense of independence (ATI Testing 2016).

## Age Appropriate Activities

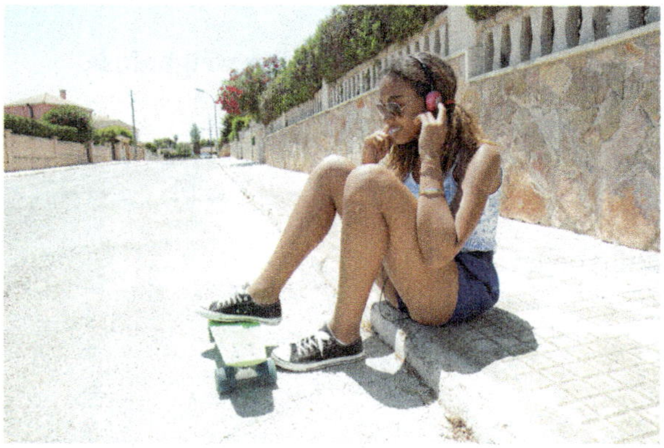

© MJTH/Shutterstock.com

Nonviolent music

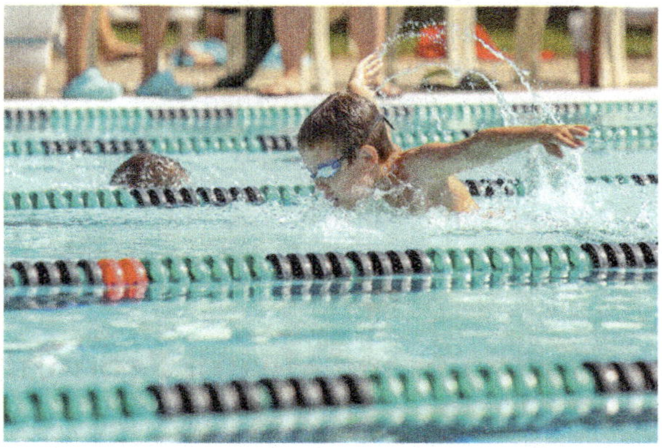

© Suzanne Tucker/Shutterstock.com

Sports

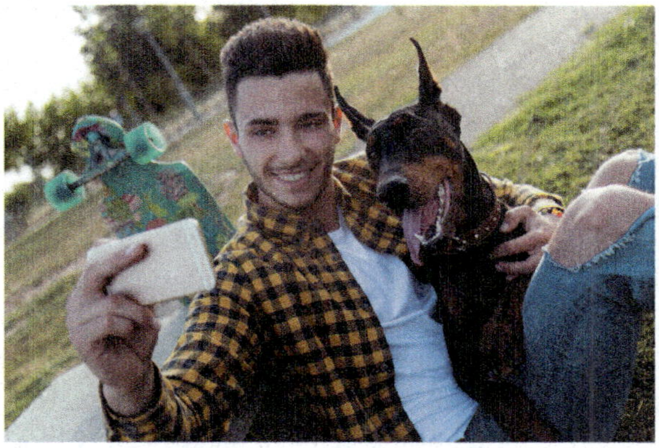

© nenetus/Shutterstock.com

Caring for a pet

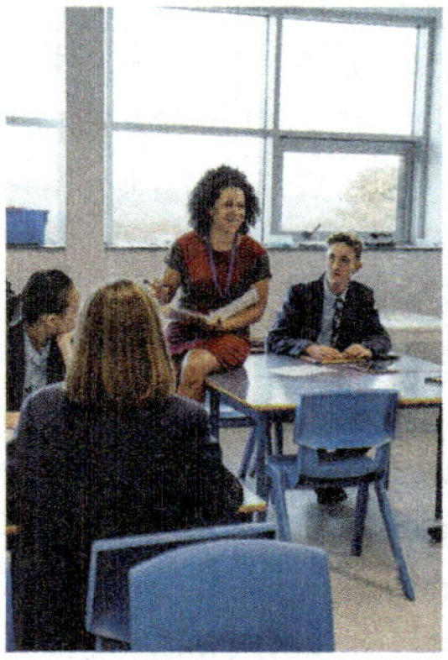

© DGLimages/Shutterstock.com

Career-training programs

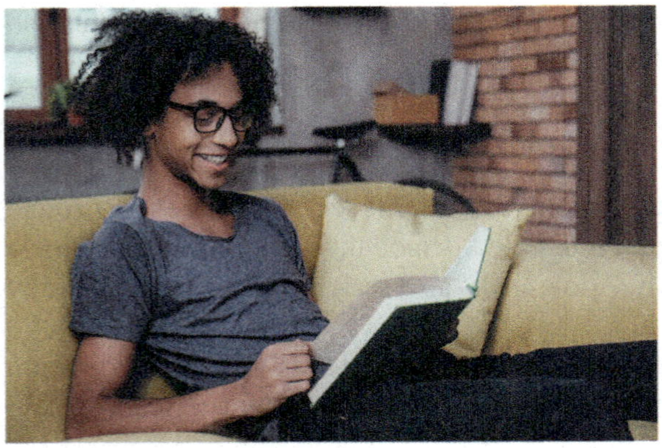

© g-stockstudio/Shutterstock.com

Reading

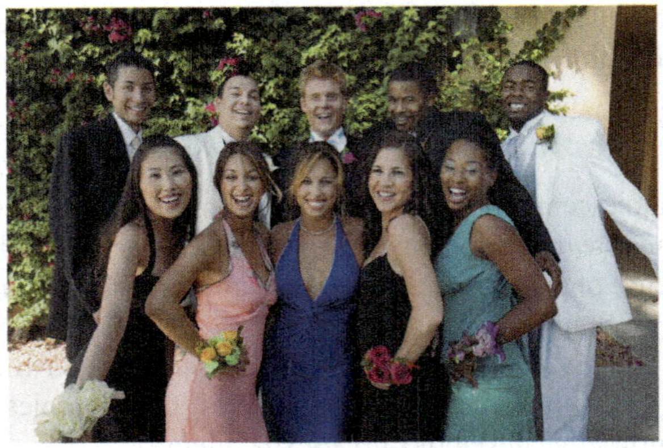

© sirtravelalot/Shutterstock.com

Social events (going to movies, school dances)

## Nursing Diagnoses

Healthy preschoolers have many applicable nursing diagnoses because they grow in dynamic ways. Some NANDA diagnosis for the typical school-age child might include:

- Imbalanced nutrition, less than body requirements
- Disturbed sleep patterns related to increased need for sleep
- Disturbed body image related to corrective dental devices
- Risk for infection
- Readiness for health seeking behavior
- Risk for injury

### *Outcomes*

- Adolescent will verbalize understanding of eating nutritious food to prevent further weight loss.
- Client will wake up refreshed.
- Adolescent will integrate temporary change of self-concept and increase self-esteem.
- Client will be up-to-date on vaccinations.
- Client will verbalize safe sex practices.
- Develops realistic goals and plans to minimize risk taking behavior.

# Interventions and Health Promotion

## Nutrition

Adolescents struggle with both perceived weight issues and actual weight problems. The prevention of these issues begins with instilling healthy eating patterns in early childhood, preferably from infancy. Teen nutrition education should emphasize the importance of getting enough vitamin C, calcium, magnesium, and iron. Carbonated soda has high levels of phosphorus that displaces magnesium and can cause depletion. In addition, children who consume sugar-sweetened carbonated beverages at age 5 decrease the nutrient concentration of protein, calcium, phosphorus, magnesium, potassium, fiber, and Vitamin D in their bodies through adolescence (Ballew, C., Kuester, S., Gillespie, C. 2000). The teenage years are particularly stressful, and adolescents need stress management strategies that do not include stress eating. Regardless of their perception, adolescents struggle with not consuming enough fruits, vegetables and whole grains, and consuming excessive sugar-sweetened drinks and fast foods (Adolescent Nutrition 2009). Their rapid growth and high metabolism require increases in quality nutrients. During growth spurts, additional protein, calcium, iron, and zinc are required. Adolescents are typically deficient in folic acid, vitamin B6, vitamin A, iron, calcium, and zinc. Overeating and under-eating present challenges during the adolescent years. Encourage adolescents to make healthy food choices on a daily basis, and allow for sweets and sodas for celebrations or special occasions. The provider evaluates children for weight, height, and BMI annually for the risk for obesity.

## Sleep and Rest

Sleep gives the brain time to restore the body, the brain will demand sleep even when the adolescent does not. Sleep times shift toward later times during puberty due to the natural delay of the circadian rhythm. Adolescents may also need more sleep during growth spurts. Teenagers sleep more than in the school-aged years. They sleep until later in the morning and go to bed later in the evenings. During periods of active growth, the need for sleep increases (Hagenauer, Perryman, Lee, and Carskadon 2009).

## Dental Health

Adolescents experience dental caries more than any other childhood group. This may be related to new sites for caries to form, low prioritization of dental health, and racial disparities in access to dental care, and issues with access. Positive self-concept and self-esteem support compliance of a regular oral hygiene regimen. Dental therapists deliver dental care in public schools in many places such as New Zealand, Australia, and Canada. The United States is slow to adopt this idea but dental therapists are in Alaska and Minnesota. The likelihood of increasing the utilization of oral health care will not happen without a policy change to make dental care accessible to all Americans (Friedman, J. W., and Mathu-Muju, K. R. 2014).

Positive self-concept and self-esteem support compliance with a regular oral hygiene regimen. Adolescents may need corrective appliances that affect self-concept and self-esteem. Teenagers should brush like an adult, in the morning, after meals, and before bedtime. Adolescents may still benefit from fluoride treatments (Macgregor, I. D. M., Regis, D. and Balding, J. 1997).

## Sexuality

Adolescent sexuality changed in the past 50 years where adolescents reach puberty at an earlier age and marry later in life. Adolescents need education about sexually transmitted diseases, unplanned pregnancy, and emotional ramifications aspects of the sexual act. Provide adolescents with accurate information, and discuss information shared among peers (Sexuality, Contraception, and the Media 2001).

### Clinical Pearl

Adolescents emulate images they see all around them. Media images are particularly powerful to the adolescent mind. An adolescent needs time to create their own self-concept and self-image. Teens have access to sexually explicit content on the internet. The media has become the leading sex educator of children and teenagers. Adolescents need support to find themselves, minimizing media exposure supports this process by increasing self-esteem and developing a healthy self-concept. These concepts support healthy intimate relationships (Sexuality, Contraception, and the Media 2001).

Pediatric nurses emphasize using safe sex practices and manage peer pressure. The nurse communicates this through the utilization of a private space where both parties can safely ask questions. Adolescents need support to problem-solve creatively and make complex decisions. Sex education and parental-child discussion may delay sexual activity and promotes consistent contraception control if the teen regularly engages in sex. Parents must also include sex-positive topics such as love, pleasure, and healthy relationships to improve understanding of the complexity of relationships. Adolescents feel invincible, yet vulnerable. Adolescents need a delicate balance of support and distance during the teen years. Therapeutic, supportive environments, instead of punishment, appear most developmentally appropriate (Ashcraft, A. M., and Murray, P. J. 2017).

## Immunization

The Center for Disease Control and Prevention (CDC) recommends healthy adolescents 13–18 years old catch-up on any doses of missed immunizations not received at 11–12 years of age. In addition, adolescents receive the Trivalent inactivated influenza vaccine or live, attenuated influenza vaccine by nasal spray each year. If adolescents received the Meningococcal (MCV4) vaccination between 13 and 15 years of age, then adolescents receive a Meningococcal (MCV4) booster shot between the ages of 16 and 18 years. Adolescents do not need a booster dose of the vaccination when given after 16 years of age (ATI Testing 2016).

## Health Screenings

Screenings for scoliosis continue during the adolescent years. These screenings include an examination for a lateral curvature of the spine before and during growth spurts. Screenings can take place at school or a health-care facility and identifies adolescents who need a referral to a health-care provider for confirmation of the diagnosis. Drug and alcohol screenings and STI screenings continue into adulthood (ATI Testing 2016).

## Injury Prevention

Adolescents benefit from a community of parents, peers, policy-makers, clinicians, and teachers who work together to reinforce safe lifestyles for adolescents (ATI Testing 2016).

## Bodily Harm

Parents must understand the importance of keeping firearms unloaded and in a locked cabinet or box (ATI Testing 2016).

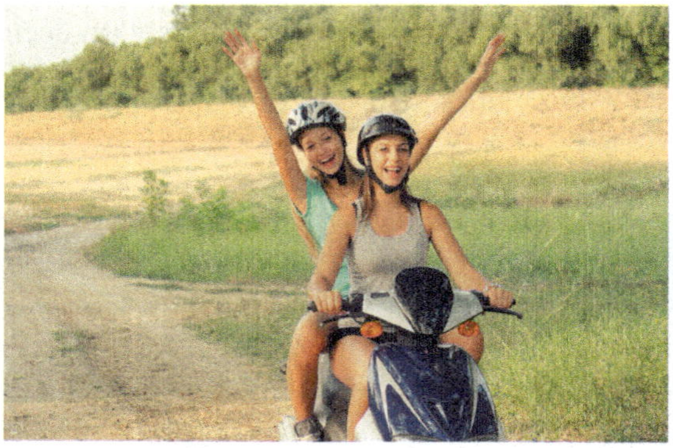



Helmet use and/or pads when roller skating, skateboarding, bicycling, riding scooters, skiing, and snowboarding (ATI Testing 2016).

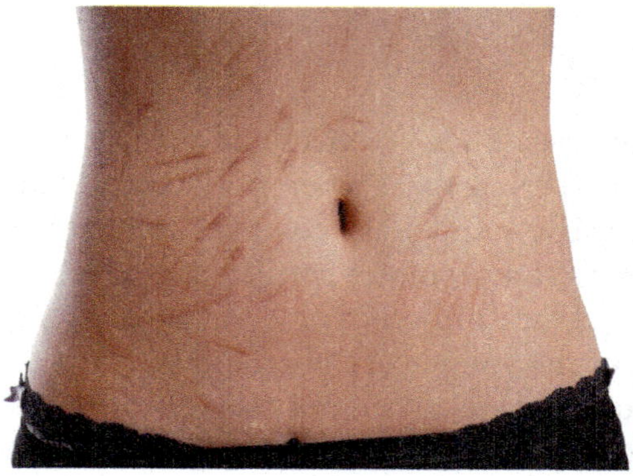

Parents must stay aware of changes in mood or behavior and monitor for self-harm in adolescents who are at risk. Risk factors include poor school performance, lack of interest in things that were of interest to the adolescent in the past. Parents can look for signs of social isolation and disturbances in sleep or appetite. If an adolescent expresses of suicidal thoughts, they need an evaluation by a doctor immediately (ATI Testing 2016).

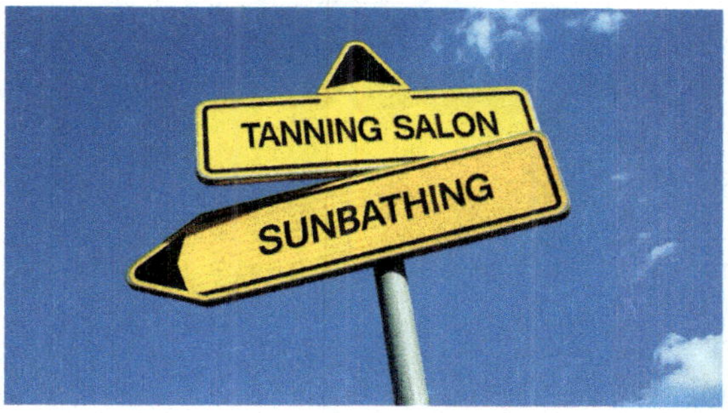

© M-SUR/Shutterstock.com

## Burns

Adolescents may need training to avoid burns in the workplace. Many entry-level jobs come with hazards unfamiliar to adolescents (Schub, T. B., and Pilgrim, J. M. 2016). Parents should reinforce fire safety and escape routes in the home.

Adolescents should apply sunscreen when outside and avoid tanning beds. The World Health Organization classified tanning beds as high-level carcinogens in 2009 (Ban the Tan 2015).

## Drowning

Adolescents can abuse substances, and that may precipitate adolescent near-drownings. Teach adolescents to swim, but also teach safety precautions to minimize risk and supervise swimming when possible (ATI Testing 2016).

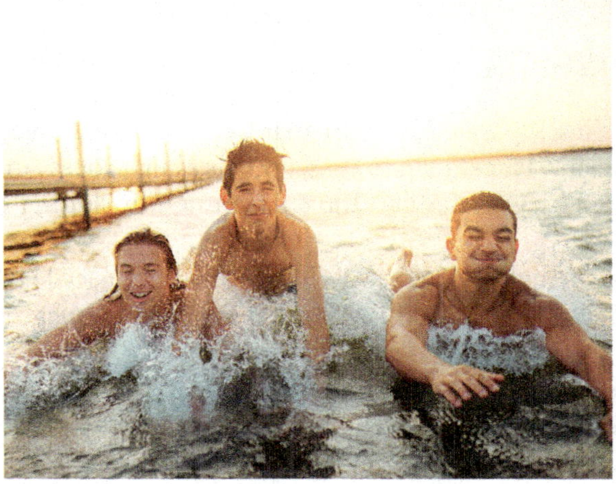
© Uber Images/Shutterstock.com

Teach adolescents not to swim alone.

## Motor-Vehicle Injuries

Adolescents benefit from drivers' education courses that emphasize good safety practices such as wearing seat belts and minimizing distractions in the car (ATI Testing 2016).

Parents must provide helmets for use with bicycles, motorcycles, skateboards, roller skates, and snowboards (ATI Testing 2016).

Parents must emphasize the importance of not using cell phones while driving and enforce the laws regarding their use. Adolescents must understand the dangers of combining substance abuse with driving. Adolescents benefit from positive role models in their parents (ATI Testing 2016).

© ml/Shutterstock.com

## Substance Abuse

The best model to combat substance abuse in teenagers is the promotion of resilience (LaRusso, M., Romer, D., and Selman, R. 2007). Adolescents must learn to persist in their endeavors especially when they experience inevitable failures. A holistic model to enrich the school climate reduces risks for teenagers (Jaynes, S. 2014).

Adolescents should receive education about tobacco use and referrals for smoking cessation if necessary. The evidence shows family intervention in addition to school-based education prevents children and adolescents from becoming smokers. Such interventions include counseling and telephone support for mothers, and school education programs including videos and books (Thomas R. E., Baker P. R. A., Thomas B. C., and Lorenzetti D. L. 2015).

Adolescents experience many changes in a short period. Privacy and trust provide a basis for a productive professional relationship with adolescents. Adolescents develop abstract thought but do not yet have good judgment. Temptations are plentiful, and personal image plays a large part of social interactions. The adolescent must sort out many contradictions in the world as they realize the complications of the world. Parents must balance limit setting and support of their adolescent. The practice of this dynamic prepares the adolescent to move into adulthood.

# CHAPTER HIGHLIGHTS

- Growth and development are separate processes that follow a predictable pattern toward adulthood.
- Major theories of Erikson and Piaget help to direct the nursing process in pediatric patients.
- Development is influenced by genetics and the environment including culture and is individual for each child and family.
- Infants are impressionable beings between 1 month and 1 year of age. They engage in rapid growth and learn basic gross motor and fine motor skills. They begin to use language and develop higher cognitive functions.
- Toddlers are curious beings between the ages of 1 year and 3 years of age. Toddlers become mobile, learn to talk, and learn to use the bathroom by themselves.
- Preschoolers are creative beings between the ages of 3 years and 6 years of age. Preschoolers master physical coordination and language. Social skills should be stressed and developed with only as much parental interference as necessary.
- School-age children are industrious beings between the ages of 6 years and 12 years of age. The school-age years are marked by puberty where sexual maturation begins to occur.
- Adolescents are individuals finding their place in the world. They range in age between 12 years and 18 years of age. Teens cognitively and socially develop. The peer group holds influence over the adolescent.
- Nurses review growth and development at each stage and provide anticipatory guidance to the child and family.

# REFERENCES


Adolescent Nutrition. 2009. Retrieved May 31, 2017, from http://pedsinreview.aappublications.org/content/30/12/494.

Agricultural Research Service. n.d. Retrieved May 30, 2017, from https://ndb.nal.usda.gov/ndb/search/list?qlookup=broccoli&qt=&manu=&fgcd=&SYNCHRONIZER_URI=%2Fndb%2Fsearch%2Flist&SYNCHRONIZER_TOKEN=7a22f49c-4868-4a49-b8f2-911d6cfb1249&ds=Standard%2BReference.

Ashcraft, A. M., and Murray, P. J. 2017. Talking to Parents about Adolescent Sexuality. *Pediatric Clinics of North America,* 64(2), 305–20. doi: 10.1016/j.pcl.2016.11.002.

Association of Women's Health, Obstetric and Neonatal Nurses (AWHONN) (2015). Breastfeeding Support: Preconception Care Through the First Year : Evidence-Based Clinical Practice Guideline.

ATI Testing. 2016. Nursing Care of Children. Retrieved from http://www.atitesting.com/ati_next_gen/DisplayResources.aspx?Name=rm_rn_ncc_2016_ebook_20170417.pdf.

Ballew, C., Kuester, S., Gillespie, C. 2000. "Beverage choices affect adequacy of children's nutrient intakes." *Arch Pediatr Adolesc Med.*, 154, p. 1148–52

Ban the Tan. 2015. *Scientific American*, 312(4), 10.

Bernstein, H. (2014). Baby bottle tooth decay. In Harvard Health Publications (Ed.), Harvard Medical School commentaries on health. Boston, MA: Harvard Health Publications. Retrieved from https://chamberlainuniversity.idm.oclc.org/login?url=http://search.credoreference.com/content/entry/hhphoh/baby_bottle_tooth_decay/0?institutionId=8802

Bernstein, H. (2014). Take care of your child's oral health. In Harvard Health Publications (Ed.), Harvard Medical School commentaries on health. Boston, MA: Harvard Health Publications. Retrieved from https://chamberlainuniversity.idm.oclc.org/login?url=http://search.credoreference.com/content/entry/hhphoh/take_care_of_your_child_s_oral_health/0?institutionId=8802

Birnholz, J. C. and Benacerraf, B. R. 1983. The development of human fetal hearing. Retrieved July 20, 2017, from https://www.ncbi.nlm.nih.gov/pubmed/6623091.

Brawley, L. and Henk, J. 2014. "Encouraging healthy eating behaviors in toddlers." *Dimensions of Early Childhood*, 42(2), 18–22.

Brinkman, M. T., Baglietto, L., Krishnan, K., English, D. R., Severi, G., Morris, H. A., Giles, G. G. et al. 2010. "Consumption of animal products, their nutrient components and postmenopausal circulating steroid hormone concentrations." Retrieved May 29, 2017, from http://www.ncbi.nlm.nih.gov/pubmed/19904296.

Brooker, R. J., Buss, K. A., Lemery-Chalfant, K., Aksan, N., Davidson, R. J., & Goldsmith, H. H. (2013). The development of stranger fear in infancy and toddlerhood: normative development, individual differences, antecedents, and outcomes. Developmental Science, 16(6), 864-878.

Center on the Developing Child at Harvard University. 2017. "Brain Architecture." Retrieved from http://developingchild.harvard.edu/science/key-concepts/brain-architecture/.

CDC Health Disparities & Inequalities Report (CHDIR). 2015. Retrieved June 08, 2017, from https://www.cdc.gov/minorityhealth/CHDIReport.html.

Chambers. 2013. *Cognitive and Language Development: The Child's Journey*. Dubuque, IA: Kendall Hunt.

Chan, E. S., & Cummings, C. (2013). Dietary exposures and allergy prevention in high-risk infants. Paediatrics & Child Health (1205-7088), 18(10), 545–549.

Chan, J. M., Stampfer, M. J., Ma, J., Gann, P. H., Gaziano, J. M., and Giovannucci, E. L. 2001. "Dairy products, calcium, and prostate cancer risk in the Physicians' Health Study." Retrieved May 29, 2017, from http://www.ncbi.nlm.nih.gov/pubmed/11566656.

Chan, J. M. and Giovannucci, E. L. n.d. Dairy products, calcium, and vitamin D and risk of prostate cancer. Retrieved May 29, 2017, from http://www.ncbi.nlm.nih.gov/pubmed/11588859.

Clark-Gambelunghe, Melinda B.; Clark, David A. In *The Healthy and Sick Newborn, The Pediatric Clinics of North America.* April 2015 62(2), 367–84 Language: English. doi: 10.1016/j.pcl.2014.11.003.

Committee on Practice and Ambulatory Medicine and Workgroup, B. F. 2017. "2017 Recommendations for Preventive Pediatric Health Care." Retrieved June 08, 2017, from http://pediatrics.aappublications.org/content/139/4/e20170254.

Crenshaw, K. 1991. "Mapping the Margins: Intersectionality, Identity Politics, and Violence Against of Women of Color." Retrieved from http://socialdifference.columbia.edu/files/socialdiff/projects/Article__Mapping_the_Margins_by_Kimblere_Crenshaw.pdf.

Crowley S. J., Acebo C., Fallone G., and Carskadon M. A. 2006. "Estimating dim light melatonin onset (DLMO) phase in adolescents using summer or school-year sleep/wake schedules." *Sleep*, 29, 1632–41.

Cohen Engler, A., Hadash, A., Shehadeh, N., and Pillar, G. 2012. "Breastfeeding may improve nocturnal sleep and reduce infantile colic: potential role of breast milk melatonin." *European Journal of Pediatrics*, 171(4), 729–32. doi: 10.1007/s00431-011-1659-3.

Rodriguez A. B. and Barriga C. 2005. "The circadian rhythm of tryptophan in breast milk affects the rhythms of 6-sulfatoxymelatonin and sleep in newborn." *Neuro Endocrinol Lett*, 26(6): 657–61.

Cubero J., Sanchez J., Chanclon B., Rivero M., Rodriguez A. B., and Barriga C. 2009. "The circadian rhythm of tryptophan in breast milk affects the rhythms of 6-sulfatoxymelatonin and sleep in newborn." *Neuro Endocrinol Lett*, 26(6): 657–61.

DeCasper, A. J. and Fifer, W. P. 1980. Of human bonding: newborns prefer their mothers' voices. Retrieved July 20, 2017, from https://www.ncbi.nlm.nih.gov/pubmed/7375928.

DeSafey, L. K. (Ed.). (2012). Injury prevention for children and adolescents : research, practice, and advocacy. Retrieved from https://ebookcentral-proquest-com.chamberlainuniversity.idm.oclc.org

Elfrink, M., Moll, H., Kiefte-de Jong, J., El Marroun, H., Jaddoe, V., Hofman, A., & ... Veerkamp, J. (2013). Is Maternal Use of Medicines during Pregnancy Associated with Deciduous Molar Hypomineralisation in the Offspring? A Prospective, Population-Based Study. Drug Safety, 36(8), 627–633. doi:10.1007/s40264-013-0078-y

Erikson Institute. 2013. Erik H. Erikson. Retrieved from http://www.erikson.edu/about/history/erik-erikson/.

Ferguson, S. L., and Campinha-Bacote, J. 1997. "Cultural competence: A critical factor in child health policy." *Journal of Pediatric Nursing*, 12(4), 260–2. doi: 10.1016/s0882-5963(97)80013-9.

Feskanich, D., Bischoff-Ferrari, H.A., Frazier, L. and Willett, W.C. 2014. "Milk Consumption During Teenage Years and Risk of Hip Fractures in Older Adults." *JAMA Pediatr.*, 168(1): 54–60.

Flaherman, V. J., Hicks, K. G., Huynh, J., Cabana, M. D., and Lee, K. A. 2016. "Positive and negative experiences of breast pumping during the first 6 months." *Maternal & Child Nutrition*, 12(2), 291–8. doi: 10.1111/mcn.12137.

Frankenburg, W. K., Dodds, J., Archer, P., Shapiro, H., and Bresnick, B. 1992. The Denver II: a major revision and restandardization of the Denver Developmental Screening Test. Retrieved July 16, 2017, from **https://www.ncbi.nlm.nih.gov/pubmed/1370185.**

Friedman, J. W. and Mathu-Muju, K. R. 2014. "Dental Therapists: Improving Access to Oral Health Care for Underserved Children." *American Journal of Public Health*, 104(6), 1005–9.

Fowler, P. A. 2016. *Foundations of Nursing Practice: Growth and Development*. Dubuque, IA: Kendall Hunt.

Ganmaa, D., Li, X. M., Wang, J., Qin, L. Q., Wang, P. Y., and Sato, A. 2002. Incidence and mortality of testicular and prostatic cancers in relation to world dietary practices. Retrieved May 29, 2017, from http://www.ncbi.nlm.nih.gov/pubmed/11857417.

Ganmaa, D. and Sato, A. n.d. The possible role of female sex hormones in milk from pregnant cows in the development of breast, ovarian and corpus uteri cancers. Retrieved May 29, 2017, from http://www.ncbi.nlm.nih.gov/pubmed/1612532.

Genkinger, J. M., Hunter, D. J., Spiegelman, D., Anderson, K. E., Arslan, A., Beeson, W. L., Smith-Warner, S. A. et al. 2006. Dairy products and ovarian cancer: a pooled analysis of 12 cohort studies. Retrieved May 29, 2017, from http://www.ncbi.nlm.nih.gov/pubmed/16492930.

Gibson, B. and Catlin, A. J. 2010. "Care of the child with the desire to change gender--Part I." *Pediatric Nursing*, 36(1), 53–9.

Giovannucci, E. 1998. Dietary influences of 1, 25(OH)2 vitamin D in relation to prostate cancer: a hypothesis. Retrieved May 29, 2017, from http://www.ncbi.nlm.nih.gov/pubmed/10189042.

Gray, Peter. 2013. *Free to Learn*. New York, New York: Basic Books.

Gregor, C., Davidson, S., and Hingley-Jones, H. 2016. The experience of gender dysphoria for pre-pubescent children and their families: a review of the literature. *Child & Family Social Work*, 21(3), 339–46. doi: 10.1111/cfs.12150.

Greydanus, Donald E. The Pediatric Diagnostic Examination New York : McGraw-Hill Professional. 2008. eBook., Database: eBook Collection (EBSCOhost)

Gundersen, C. and Ziliak, J. P. 2014. "Childhood Food Insecurity in the U.S.: Trends, Causes, and Policy Options." *Future of Children*, 1–19.

Hagenauer, Perryman, Lee, and Carskadon. 2009. "Adolescent Changes in the Homeostatic and Circadian Regulation of Sleep." *Developmental Neuroscience*, 31(4), 276. doi: 10.1159/000216538.

Harvard Health Publications (Ed.), Prevent accidental poisonings! (2014). Harvard Medical School commentaries on health. Boston, MA: Harvard Health Publications. Retrieved from https://chamberlainuniversity.idm.oclc.org/login?url=http://search.credoreference.com/content/entry/hhphoh/prevent_accidental_poisonings/0?institutionId=8802

Hasinuddin, M.& Fitriah, F. (2017). ANTICIPATORY GUIDANCE MODULE CHANGES THE AUTHORITARITATIVE PARENTING OF PARENTS IN STIMULATING CHILDREN DEVELOPMENT. Jurnal Ners, Vol 6, Iss 1, Pp 50-57 Retrieved November 24, 2017, from https://doaj-org.chamberlainuniversity.idm.oclc.org/article/a19ed0c86b164cb6b37ebacc5e292df7

Head Zauche, Lauren; Darcy Mahoney, Ashley E.; Thul, Taylor A.; Zauche, Michael S.; Weldon, Arianne B.; Stapel-Wax, and Jennifer L. 2017. In *Journal of Pediatric Health Care*, 31(4):493–503.

Hunt, C. D. and Johnson, L. K. 2007. "Calcium requirements: new estimations for men and women by cross-sectional statistical analyses of calcium balance data from metabolic studies [electronic resource]." *American Journal of Clinical Nutrition AJN*, 86(4), 1054–63.

Immunization Schedules. (2017, February 06). Retrieved September 01, 2017, from https://www.cdc.gov/vaccines/schedules/hcp/imz/child-adolescent.html.

Institute of Medicine and National Research Council. 1999. *Adolescent Development and the Biology of Puberty: Summary of a Workshop on New Research*. Washington, DC: The National Academies Press. doi: https://doi.org/10.17226/9634.

Isbell, R., Sobol, J., Lindauer, L., and Lowrance, A. n.d. The Effects of Storytelling and Story Reading on the Oral Language Complexity and Story Comprehension of Young Children. Retrieved May 30, 2017, from https://link.springer.com/article/10.1023%2FB%3AECEJ.0000048967.94189.a3?LI=true.

Jane, H. 2017. Fructose in breast milk 'unhealthy' for babies. *Daily Telegraph, The (Sydney)*. p. 107.

Jovanovic, J. 2011. "Saying Goodbye: An Investigation into Parent-Infant Separation Behaviours on Arrival in Childcare." *Child Care in Practice*, 17(3), 247–69.

Jaynes, S. 2014. "Using Social Disorganization Theory to Guide Substance Abuse Prevention among Adolescents: Implications for Educators." *Journal of at-Risk Issues*, 18(1), 35.

Kassing, D. 2002. "Bottle-feeding as a tool to reinforce breastfeeding." *J Hum Lact*, 18(1), 56–60.

Kaufman, S. B. 2013. The Need for Pretend Play in Child Development. Retrieved May 30, 2017, from https://blogs.scientificamerican.com/beautiful-minds/the-need-for-pretend-play-in-child-development/.

Koren, M.R. (2016). Health Promotion for Children and Adolescents. Springer Science+Business media: New York, New York

Koulougliotti, C., Cole, R., Moskow, M., Mcquillan, B., Carno, M., and Grape, A. 2014. "The Longitudinal Association of Young Childrens Everyday Routines to Sleep Duration." *Journal of Pediatric Health Care*, 28(1), 80–7. doi:10.1016/j.pedhc.2012.12.006.

Lanou, A. J., Berkow, S. E., and Barnard, N. D. 2005. Calcium, dairy products, and bone health in children and young adults: a reevaluation of the evidence. Retrieved August 30, 2017, from https://www.ncbi.nlm.nih.gov/pubmed/15741380/.

LaRusso, M., Romer, D., and Selman, R. 2007. "Teachers as builders of respectful school climates: Implications for adolescent drug use norms and depressive symptoms in high school." *Journal of Youth and Adolescence*, 37(4), 386–98.

Ling, J., Robbins, L., & Hines-Martin, V. 2016. "Perceived Parental Barriers to and Strategies for Supporting Physical Activity and Healthy Eating among Head Start Children." *Journal of Community Health*, 41(3), 593–602. doi: 10.1007/s10900-015-0134-x.

Loftin, R. W., Habli, M., Snyder, C. C., Cormier, C. M., Lewis, D. F., & DeFranco, E. A. (2010). Late Preterm Birth. Reviews in Obstetrics and Gynecology, 3(1), 10–19.

Marcel, C. B. (2016). Nutrition in Healthy Toddlers. CINAHL Nursing Guide,

Marques, R. V., Taddei, J. C., Konstantyner, T., Marques, A. V., and Braga, J. P. 2016. "Correlation between hemoglobin levels of mothers and children on exclusive breastfeeding in the first six months of life." *Jornal De Pediatria, 92,* 479–85. doi: 10.1016/j.jped.2015.11.006.

Maruyama, K., Oshima, T., and Ohyama, K. 2010. "Exposure to Exogenous Estrogen through Intake of Commercial Milk Produced from Pregnant Cows." *Pediatr Int*; 2010 Feb; 52(1):33–8. Available here: http://www.ncbi.nlm.nih.gov/pubmed/19496976.

Macgregor, I. D. M., Regis, D. and Balding, J. 1997. "Self-concept and dental health behaviours in adolescents." *Journal of Clinical Periodontology*, 24: 335–9. doi: 10.1111/j.1600-051X.1997.tb00766.x.

Mccarthy, C., & McCarthy, C. (2014). Introducing solid foods: Eight keys to success. In Harvard Health Publications (Ed.), Harvard Medical School commentaries on health. Boston, MA: Harvard Health Publications. Retrieved from https://chamberlainuniversity.idm.oclc.org/login?url=http://search.credoreference.com/content/entry/hhphoh/introducing_solid_foods_eight_keys_to_success/0?institutionId=8802

McCarthy, C. (2014). Prevent drowning - Four keys to protect your child. In Harvard Health Publications (Ed.), Harvard Medical School commentaries on health. Boston, MA: Harvard Health Publications. Retrieved from https://chamberlainuniversity.idm.oclc.org/login?url=http://search.credoreference.com/content/entry/hhphoh/prevent_drowning_four_keys_to_protect_your_child/0?institutionId=8802

McGuire, E. 2013. "Maternal and infant sleep postpartum." *Breastfeeding Review*, 21(2), 38–41.

Meurer, L. N., Jamieson, B., and Thurman, C. 2006. "Clinical inquiries. What is the appropriate use of sunscreen for infants and children?" *The Journal of Family Practice*, 55(5), 437.

Michaëlsson, A. Wolk, S. Langenskiöld, S. Basu, E. W. Lemming, H. Melhus and L. Byberg. 2014. "Milk Intake and Risk of Mortality and Fractures in Women and Men: Cohort Studies." *BMJ*. 349:g6015.

National Research Council (US); Institute of Medicine (US). Children's Health, The Nation's Wealth: Assessing and Improving Child Health. Washington (DC): National Academies Press (US); 2004. 3, Influences on Children's Health. Available from: https://www.ncbi.nlm.nih.gov/books/NBK92200/.

Noel-Weiss, J., Woodend, A. K., Peterson, W. E., Gibb, W., and Groll, D. L. 2011. "An observational study of associations among maternal fluids during parturition, neonatal output, and breastfed newborn weight loss." *International Breastfeeding Journal*, 6, 9. http://doi.org/10.1186/1746-4358-6-9.

Ou, Heng (2016). The First Forty Days: The Essential Art of Nourishing the New Mother. Steart, Tabouri & Chang: New York, New York

Qin, L. Q., Xu, J. Y., Wang, P. Y., Kaneko, T., Hoshi, K., and Sato, A. n.d. Milk consumption is a risk factor for prostate cancer: meta-analysis of case-control studies. Retrieved May 29, 2017, from http://www.ncbi.nlm.nih.gov/pubmed/15203374.

Qin, L. Q., Xu, J. Y., Wang, P. Y., Tong, J., and Hoshi, K. n.d. Milk consumption is a risk factor for prostate cancer in Western countries: evidence from cohort studies. Retrieved May 29, 2017, from http://www.ncbi.nlm.nih.gov/pubmed/17704029.

Quinlan P. T., Lockton S., Irwin J., and Lucas A. L. 1995. "The relationship between stool hardness and stool composition in breast- and formula-fed infants." *J Pediatr Gastroenterol Nutr*. 20: 81–90.

Radesky, J. S. and Christakis, D. A. 2016. "Increased Screen Time." *Pediatric Clinics of North America,* 63(5), 827–39. doi: 10.1016/j.pcl.2016.06.006.

Ramsay, S. A., Shriver, L. H., and Taylor, C. A. 2017. "Variety of fruit and vegetables is related to preschoolers' overall diet quality." *Preventive Medicine Reports, 5,* 112–7. doi: 10.1016/j.pmedr.2016.12.003.

Sabat, J. and Wien, M. 2010. "Vegetarian diets and childhood obesity prevention." *American Journal Of Clinical Nutrition*, 91(5), 1525s–1529s.

Sanchez, Cubero, Sanchez, Chanclon, Rivero, Rodriguez, and Barriga. 2009. "The possible role of human milk nucleotides as sleep inducers." *Nutr Neurosci*, 12(1): 2–8

Schafer, T. E. and Adair, S. M. 2000. Prevention of dental disease. The role of the pediatrician. Retrieved July 26, 2017, from https://www.ncbi.nlm.nih.gov/pubmed/11059348.

Schafer, T.E. and Adair, S.M., 2006. Prevention of Dental Disease: The Role of the Pediatrician. Retrieved from https://doi-org.proxy.chamberlain.edu:8443/10.1016/S0031-3955(05)70256-X.

Schub, T. B. and Pilgrim, J. M. 2016. Burns: Prevention—an Overview. *CINAHL Nursing Guide.*
Schub, T. B. and Pilgrim, J. M. 2016. "Parent Teaching: Teaching Parents about Sleep in Infants and Children." *CINAHL Nursing Guide.*

Shields L, Zhou H, Pratt J, Taylor M, Hunter J, and Pascoe E. 2012. "Family-centred care for hospitalised children aged 0–12 years." *Cochrane Database of Systematic Reviews* 2012, Issue 10. Art. No.: CD004811. doi: 10.1002/14651858.CD004811.pub3.

Sevenhuysen, G. P., Holodinsky, C., and Dawes, C. 1984. "Development of salivary alpha-amylase in infants from birth to 5 months." *The American Journal of Clinical Nutrition*, 39(4), 584–8.

Sexuality, Contraception, and the Media. 2001. *Pediatrics*, 107(1), 191.

Siantz, M. L. 2008. Leading Change in Diversity and Cultural Competence. *Journal of Professional Nursing*, 24(3), 167–71. doi: 10.1016/j.profnurs.2008.01.005.

Sijtsma, A., Koller, M., Sauer, P., and Corpeleijn, E. 2015. "Television, sleep, outdoor play and BMI in young children: the GECKO Drenthe cohort." *European Journal of Pediatrics*, 174(5), 631–639. doi: 10.1007/s00431-014-2443-y.

Smith, L. n.d. Jean Piaget Society. Retrieved October 16, 2017, from http://www.piaget.org/aboutPiaget.html.

Smith, N. C., & Mennella, H. A. (2017). Parent-Newborn Bonding: Evaluating and Encouraging. CINAHL Nursing Guide.

Tagtow, Angela; Haven, Jackie; Maniscalco, Shelley; Johnson-Bailey, Donna; Bard, and Sasha. 2015. *Journal of the Academy of Nutrition & Dietetics*, 115(7): 1039–40. 2p.

Tate, P. L., Bibb, R., and Larcom, L. L. 2011. Milk stimulates growth of prostate cancer cells in culture. Retrieved May 29, 2017, from http://www.ncbi.nlm.nih.gov/pubmed/22043817.

Thomas R. E., Baker P. R. A., Thomas BC, Lorenzetti D. L. 2015. "Family-based programmes for preventing smoking by children and adolescents." *Cochrane Database of Systematic Reviews 2015*, Issue 2. Art. No.: CD004493. doi: 10.1002/14651858.CD004493.pub3.

US Department of Agriculture. 2017. 10 Tips: Build a Healthy Meal. Retrieved July 27 2017, from https://www.choosemyplate.gov/ten-tips-build-healthy-meal.

Vegetarian Food PyramidVegSource. n.d. Retrieved from http://www.vegsource.com/nutrition/pyramid.htm.

Wagner, C. L., Hulsey, T. C., Fanning, D., Ebeling, M., and Hollis, B., 2006. Breastfeeding Medicine. July 2006, 1(2): 59–70. doi: 10.1089/bfm.2006.1.59.

Walker, D., Grimwade, J., and Wood, C. 1971. Intrauterine noise: a component of the fetal environment. Retrieved July 20, 2017, from https://www.ncbi.nlm.nih.gov/pubmed/5538977.

Waters E., de Silva-Sanigorski A., Burford BJ, Brown T, Campbell KJ, Gao Y, Armstrong R, Prosser L, and Summerbell C. D. 2011. Interventions for preventing obesity in children. *Cochrane Database of Systematic Reviews*, 12. CD001871. doi: 10.1002/14651858.CD001871.pub3.

Westwood, C. 2007. "Connecting with children." *Nursing Standard*, 21(31), 62–3.

World Health Organization. 2014). Ten facts on breastfeeding. Retrieved from http:// www.who.int/features/factfiles/breastfeeding/en/

Yilmaz, G., Demirli Caylan, N., and Karacan, C. D. 2015. "An intervention to preschool children for reducing screen time: a randomized controlled trial." *Child: Care, Health & Development*, 41(3), 443–9.

## CHAPTER 3

# CARING FOR CHILDREN WITH NEUROLOGICAL CONDITIONS

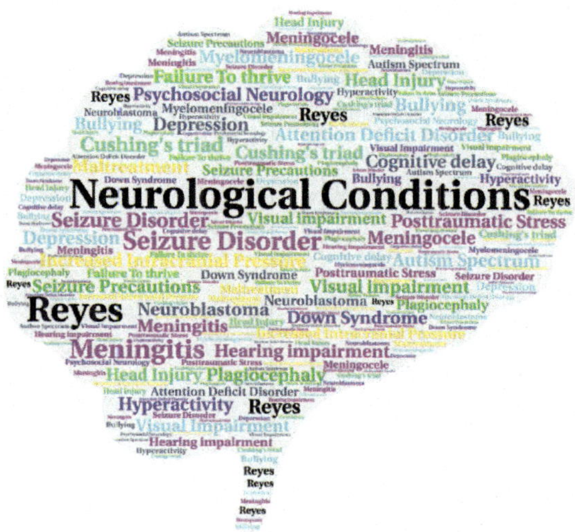


Modified from Shutterstock. Original image © johavel/ Shutterstock.com

## LEARNING OUTCOMES

1. Describe the anatomy and physiology of the neurological system.
2. Utilize the nursing process to provide safe, comprehensive health care to children with neurologic conditions.
3. Construct a comprehensive "family-centered" teaching plan for children with a neurological condition.
4. Differentiate between the assessment and interventions for bacterial vs. viral meningitis.
5. Describe the plan of care for a child with Reye's syndrome.
4. Differentiate among seizures, epilepsy, and status epilepticus.
5. Distinguish between mild and severe traumatic brain injuries.
6. Describe a plan of care for a child with Down's syndrome.
7. Create a nursing plan for a child with cerebral palsy.
8. Use the nursing process to plan care for children with meningocele, myelomeningocele, and hydrocephalus.
9. Create a holistic plan of care for a child with ADHD.
10. Describe a plan of care for a child with autism spectrum disorder.
12. Create a plan of care for a substance-exposed infant and mother.
13. Teaching/learning principles in providing anticipatory guidance in the prevention and treatment of children with neurologic conditions.

## KEY TERMS

Absence seizure
Alpha-fetoprotein
Ankle-foot orthoses
Atonic or akinetic seizure
Baclofen
Botulinum toxin a
Brain herniation
Brudzinski sign
Burr holes
Caregiver role strain
Cerebral perfusion pressure (CPP)
Cerebral spinal fluid (CSF)
Concussion
Contusion
Craniotomy
Cushing's triad
Developmental delay
Diazepam
Diazepam (Diastat)
Diplopia
Electroencephalogram (EEG)
Epicanthal folds
Epidural hematomas
Emla cream
Extension
Flexion
Gluconeogenesis
Glycogenolysis
Infantile spasms
Intracranial pressure (ICP)
Kernig's sign
Ketogenic diet
Lumbar puncture
Latex allergy
Magnetic resonance imaging (MRI)
Meningocele
Methadone
Methylphenidate
Mini-osteoplastic craniotomy
Myelomeningocele
Myoclonic seizure
NADS
Neural crests
Neural plate
Neural tube
Neural tube defects
Nuchal rigidity
Partial seizures
Phenobarbital
Phenytoin
Posturing
Pulmonary hygiene
Purpuric-type rash
Seizure precautions
Selective serotonin reuptake inhibitors (SSRI)
Status epilepticus
Stimming
Subdural hematoma
Substance withdrawal
Thimerosal
Transfontanel percutaneous aspiration
Traumatic brain injury (TBI)
Trisomy 21
Vagal nerve stimulator
Valproic acid
Ventriculoperitoneal shunt
Ventricles
Xerostomia

## THE NEUROLOGICAL SYSTEM

The brain is the most complex organ in the body (see Fig 3-1) Scientists still do not understand the brain in its entirety. However, brain development in an embryo follows a predictable trajectory. By the third week after conception, the back of the embryo begins to develop and forms a **neural plate**. By the fourth week of development, the plate folds into itself and creates a primitive spine or neural tube. This tube is complete by 18 weeks and creates the central nervous system; the brain and the spinal cord. Three layers of specialized tissue called the meninges cover the brain and spinal cord. There is **cerebral spinal fluid (CSF)** that flows through the **ventricles** of the brain, around the brain, and through the spinal cord. **Neural crests** are projections that grow from the neural tube that creates the nerves of the peripheral nervous system. Because the neural system is the earliest organ system to develop, **neural tube defects** such as spina bifida or CNS malformations can impact a child's development. Neurological disorders often produce **developmental delay** due to the pathology of the brain. The average brain grows until 20 years of age (Dowling 2004).

The brain manages many tasks for the body including cognition, motor ability, sensory interpretation, emotions and regulation of all bodily functions. Each part of the brain controls a different function in the body. Neurological disorders can include infectious diseases, trauma, concussions, and seizures (or the misfiring of the electrical system of the brain). Children respond to neurological disorders differently than adults due to differences in their anatomy. The pediatric patient has a weaker immune system, and developing head and neck when compared to an adult (Stephenson, J. P. B., & King, M. (Eds.). 2009).

The pediatric brain is susceptible to acute and chronic neurological disorders. Meningitis and Reye's syndrome are two of these disorders and can have similar manifestations. Diagnostic testing can differentiate the two disorders.

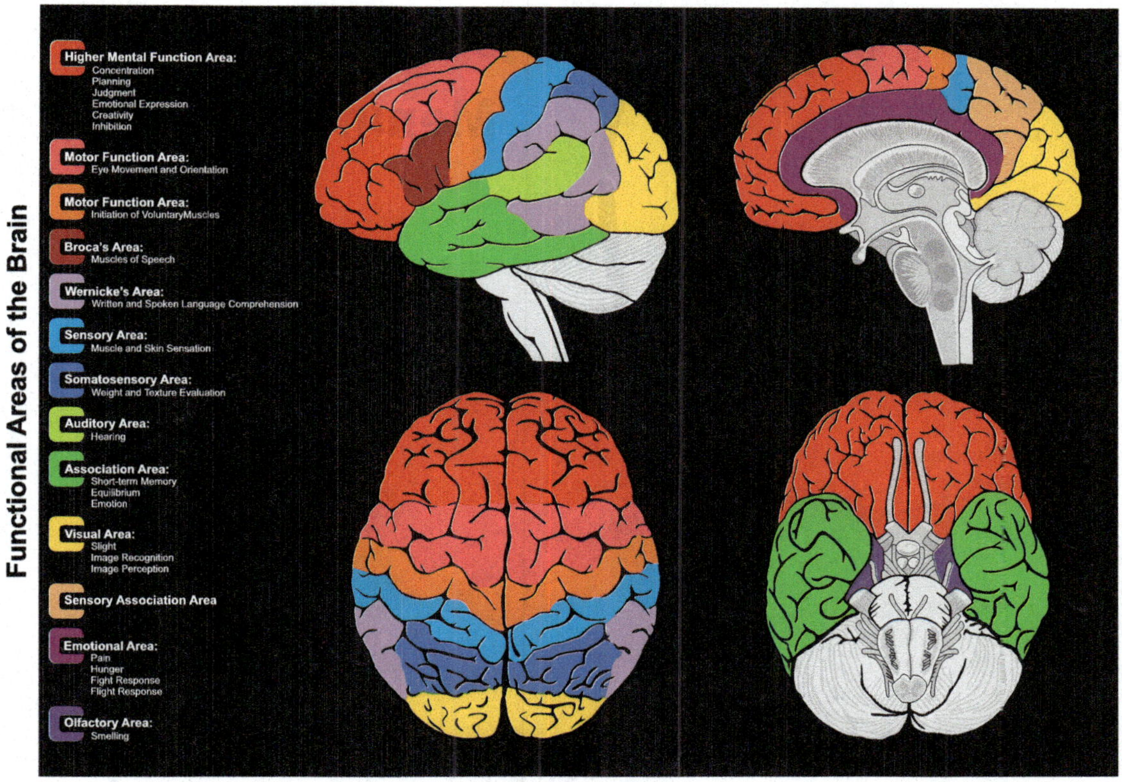



**Fig 3-1** Each region of the brain controls a different function

## QSEN Application

### Teamwork and collaboration

Neurological diseases are complex and require a multidisciplinary approach. Desirable outcomes originate from proactive teams that collaborate well with other teams. Teamwork and collaboration call for nurses to "[f]unction effectively within nursing and inter-professional teams, fostering open communication, mutual respect, and shared decision-making to achieve quality patient care. Nurses can "respect the unique attributes that members bring to a team, including variation in professional orientations, competencies, and accountabilities [and] respect the centrality of the patient/family as core members of any health care team." Children need nurses who can effectively coordinate the health care team.

From Quality and Safety Education for Nurses http://qsen.org/competencies/pre-licensure-ksas/

# ACUTE NEUROLOGICAL DISORDERS

## Meningitis

Meningitis is an infection and inflammation of the coverings of the brain and spinal cord or the meninges. Children are susceptible to infection because the blood–brain barrier has not fully developed. Meningitis infections are mostly viral, but a bacterial, amoebic, parasitic, or fungal origin is also possible (Meningitis, 2017). A foreign agent finds its way into the CSF and multiplies causing the CSF to become cloudy and produces symptoms associated with increased intracranial pressure (see Fig 3-2). (Meningitis, 2017).

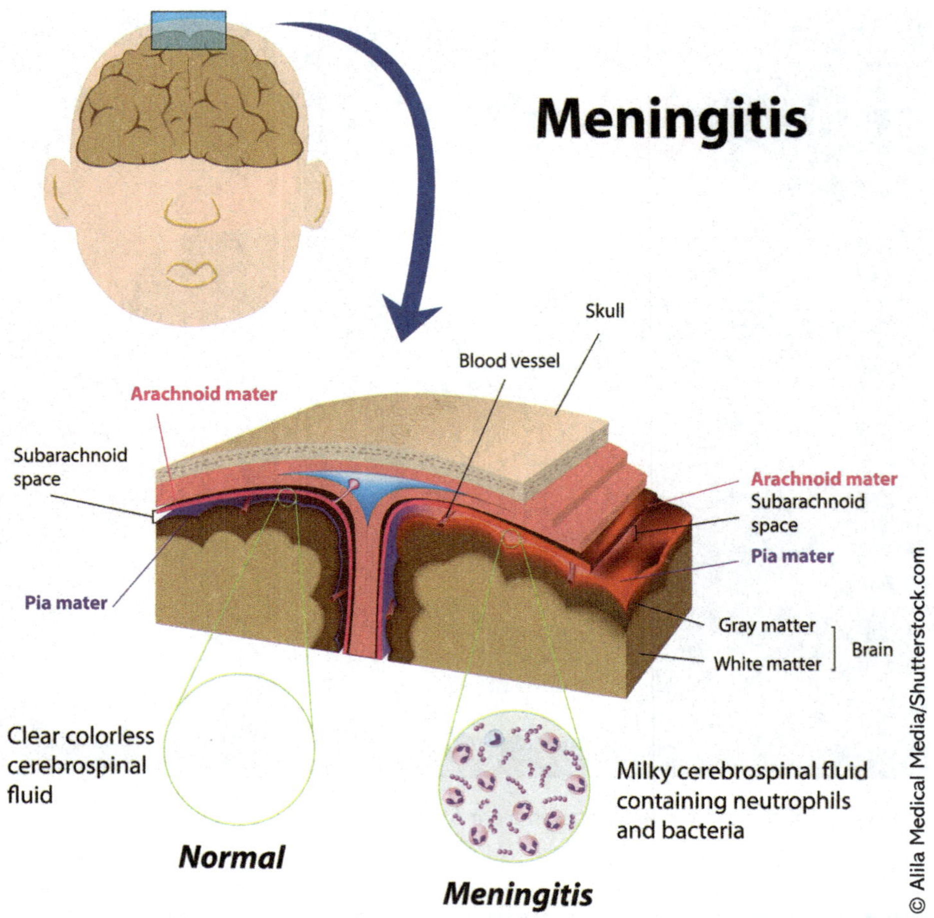


**Fig 3-2** Normal assessment findings vs. meningitis assessment findings

Children may contract meningitis through a head injury or contact with an infected person. Viral infectious agents may include enterovirus, herpes simplex, mumps and measles, and flavivirus' such as West Nile, dengue virus or Zika virus. Bacterial infectious agents may include *Neisseria meningitidis* (meningococcal), *Streptococcus pneumoniae* (pneumococcal), *Haemophilus influenzae type B* (Hib), and *Escherichia coli* (Meningitis, 2017).

## Assessment

Assessment findings will change based on the age of the child and the closure of the fontanels on the infant's head. However, the assessment is similar for viral, bacterial, fungal amoebic, or parasitic meningitis (ATI Testing 2016).

Children from 2 years of age through adolescence often present with seizures as the first presenting sign. They also present with **nuchal rigidity**, a positive **Brudzinski sign**, and a positive Kernig sign. Brudzinski's sign occurs when the knees and hips flex in response to passive flexion of the neck, due to irritation around roots of the lumbar region (Anatomy and Physiology 2016). **Kernig's sign** produces severe stiffness in the hamstring muscle, and an inability to straighten the leg when the hip flexes to 90 degrees and the failure to straighten the leg greater than 135 degrees without pain (Anatomy and Physiology 2016).

Other signs and symptoms include fever, headache, vomiting, irritability, and restlessness. There may be an altered level of consciousness from confusion to delirium, stupor, and finally, coma. There may also be petechiae or a **purpuric-type rash** if the infectious agent was meningococcal (see Fig 3-3). This hallmark sign requires immediate medical attention. There can be pain in muscles or joints with meningococcal and Hib infectious agents. (ATI Testing 2016).

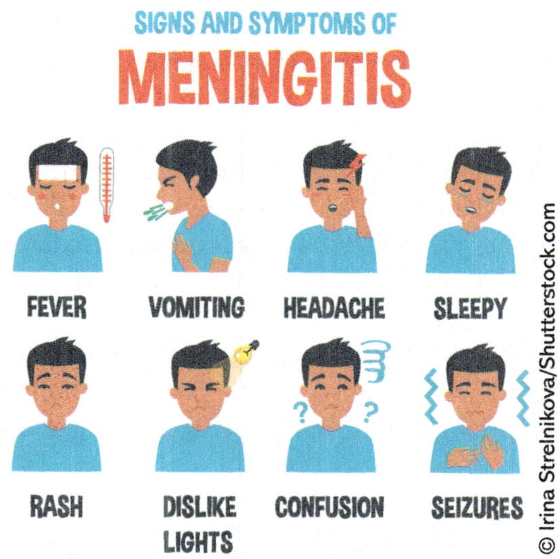


**Fig 3-3** Findings in meningitis

Newborns show few signs of meningitis infection because of their immature immune systems. They do not respond with an apparent immune response like older children. The assessment findings may include a weak cry, poor or uncoordinated suck, poor muscle tone, vomiting, or diarrhea. Newborns can develop a fever but not always. Lack of a fever does not rule out meningitis in infants. Newborns do not show nuchal rigidity; their neck assessment may appear normal (ATI Testing 2016).

Children up to 2 years of age may present with fever and irritability, bulging fontanels, poor feeding, vomiting, a high-pitched cry, and, potentially, seizures. Children this age will not display the classic Brudzinski and Kernig signs (ATI Testing 2016).

Meningitis can cause increased **Intracranial Pressure (ICP)** and decreased **Cerebral Perfusion Pressure (CPP)** due to the inflammation of the meninges. Early signs and symptoms may include an altered level of consciousness, stable vital signs, headache, blurred vision, and muscle weakness. Late symptoms include a further decrease in consciousness towards coma, a headache with increased pain, flaccid, decorticate or decerebrate posturing. **Cushing's triad** (increased systolic BP with widening pulse pressure, bradycardia, altered respirations) and elevated temperature, and projectile vomiting without nausea are ominous signs (see Fig 3-12). Newborns and infants display bulging fontanels, increased head circumference, high-pitched cry, irritability, bradycardia, and respiratory changes. Children demonstrate increased irritability, delirium, headache, nausea, vomiting, **diplopia** (double vision), seizures, bradycardia, and respiratory changes. Increased ICP is a medical emergency that can result in brain herniation if not treated immediately (ATI Testing 2016).

## Diagnostic Tests

Diagnostic tests are necessary to determine the origin of the infectious agent and subsequently the plan of care. The provider collects CSF via **lumbar puncture** and yields definitive results for meningitis. A spinal needle inserted between L3 and L4, or L4 and L5, lumbar vertebral spaces allows the collection of CSF. The pressure of the CSF is measured, and the sample is sent to the laboratory for testing to identify ICP and the specific pathogen (ATI Testing 2016).

The nurse prepares the child for this procedure with lots of reassurance and psychosocial support. The nurse ensures the child has voided before the procedure. A topical anesthetic (**EMLA cream**) is applied 45 minutes to 1 hour before the procedure. The nurse positions the child in a left side-lying position with the head flexed and knees drawn up toward the chest. The nurse holds the child and offers psychosocial support as necessary. Sedation with fentanyl and midazolam calms the child and provides pain relief. The provider cleans the skin and injects a local anesthetic. The doctor or nurse practitioner inserts the collection needle as they take a pressure reading and collects tubes of CSF. A pressure dressing that uses an elastic bandage for compression prevents further leaking of CSF from the puncture site. The nurse labels specimens and sends them to the laboratory. The nurse keeps the child flat to prevent leakage and a spinal headache. The nurse must also monitor the site for hemmorrhage, hematoma, or infection every assessment and report any abnormal findings to the provider (ATI Testing 2016).

The CSF analysis indicative of meningitis will reveal certain characteristics. Bacterial meningitis will appear cloudy, contain an elevated WBC count and have a high protein content. The sample will have a decreased glucose content as this is the source of energy for bacteria. The fluid will also have a positive Gram stain indicative of the gram positive bacteria. CSF from viral meningitis appears colorless, contains a slightly elevated WBC count, and has a normal or slightly elevated protein content; the glucose content remains normal as viruses consume host cells for energy and reproduction. Viral meningitis will have a negative gram stain (ATI Testing 2016).

A CT scan or MRI will indicate ICP or an abscess. The nurse positions the child, provides sedation and psychosocial support. (see Fig 3-4). Blood cultures may reveal a pathogen even when the CSF does not (ATI Testing 2016).

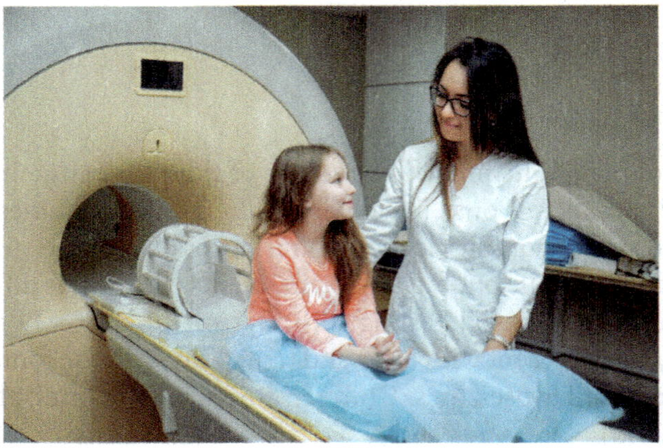


**Fig 3-4** A child about to undergo magnetic resonance imaging

## Interventions

Viral meningitis occurs as a self-limiting pathology. Parents can treat children at home. However, parents must isolate their child from the other family members, and refrain from sharing eating utensils or cups. Bacterial meningitis creates more deleterious sequelae, or harmful consequences, than viral meningitis. The nurse's priority intervention for bacterial meningitis requires isolation of suspected meningitis cases and the initiation of droplet precautions (respiratory precautions). Droplet precautions require a private room. However, patients may share a room with clients who have the same infectious disease. (March, P. P., & Schub, T. B. 2016).

A child with bacterial meningitis requires providers and visitors wear masks. The nurse initiates respiratory isolation for a minimum of 24 hours after the start of antibiotic therapy. The nurse ensures safety by keeping the bed in a low position and implementing seizure precautions. The nurse evaluates vital signs, neurologic status, urine output, and pain level after every assessment. For newborns and infants, the nurse assesses head circumference and fontanels for the size or changes in bulging. The nurse provides IV hydration and then restricts fluids until ICP normalizes, and electrolyte levels are within normal range (Wallace, D. C., & Cartwright, C. C. 2007).

The child requires an NPO status. As the child's consciousness improves, the nurse can advance the diet to clear liquids and then a diet the child can tolerate. All neurological patients require environmental management to reduce brain stimuli. Therefore, a quiet environment without bright light benefits the child. Comfort measures including a cool room and proper positioning are required. Position the child without a pillow, and slightly elevate the head of the bed 30 degrees. The child can also be placed side-lying to reduce neck discomfort. Other interventions to reduce ICP include the avoidance of coughing and straining. Finally, provide psychosocial support to child and family and keep the family updated on the child's condition (Furay, C., & Howell, T. 2010).

### Medications

Bacterial meningitis treatment includes IV antibiotics for 10 days. A broad-spectrum antibiotic covers typical pathogens until lab results accurately identify the pathogen. The provider can then change the antibiotic to match the pathogen. A corticosteroid such as dexamethasone decreases the inflammation in the initial phase of increased ICP, especially in Hib infections. The child's respiratory status requires careful monitoring if acetaminophen with codeine is administered (ATI Testing 2016).

### Teaching

Families should learn that good handwashing, a healthy diet, and immunizations can prevent infectious diseases. They should understand early, and complete treatment is necessary for upper respiratory infections as this may prevent meningitis. Children should receive the Hib and PCV vaccines at 2, 4, and 6 months of age, then again between 12 and 15 months of age (ATI Testing 2016).

## Reye's Syndrome

Reye's syndrome is an uncommon but serious condition that affects the brain and the liver causing cerebral edema and liver dysfunction. It progresses through five stages as the liver and brain fail, ending in coma and respiratory arrest. The administration of aspirin following a viral infection can induce Reye's syndrome. The reasons for the syndrome are still unknown. This syndrome affects children and adolescents who have recently had a viral infection such as influenza, gastroenteritis or varicella. The peak incidence coincides with the peak influenza season from January through March. Three to five days after a viral infection Reye's syndrome can begin. In the circulatory system, a child's blood sugar usually drops probably from the lack of eating and because the liver becomes fatty (dysfunctional) and cannot export stored glucose into the system (**glycogenolysis**) or create glucose from amino acids and other compounds (**gluconeogenesis**) (see Fig 3-6). Meanwhile, ammonia levels increase, and metabolic acidosis appears. Reye's syndrome shares many signs and symptoms with other disorders such as encephalitis, meningitis, poisoning, sudden infant death syndrome (SIDS), diabetes mellitus, and psychiatric illness. The best prognosis comes with early identification and treatment (ATI Testing 2016).

### Assessment

The first symptoms of Reye's syndrome include constant vomiting, tachypnea, and dry heaving that may appear as a symptom of the initial viral infection. The level of consciousness declines from irritability to confusion, followed by delirium or combativeness finally resulting in coma. Seizures can occur as cerebral edema increases (ATI Testing 2016) (see Fig 3-5).

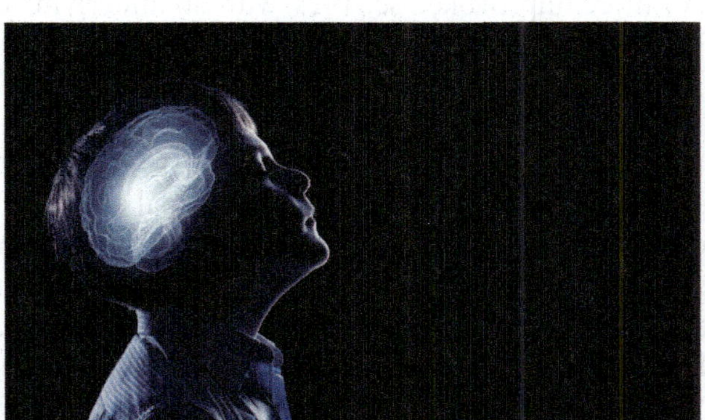



**Fig 3-5** A child with cerebral edema

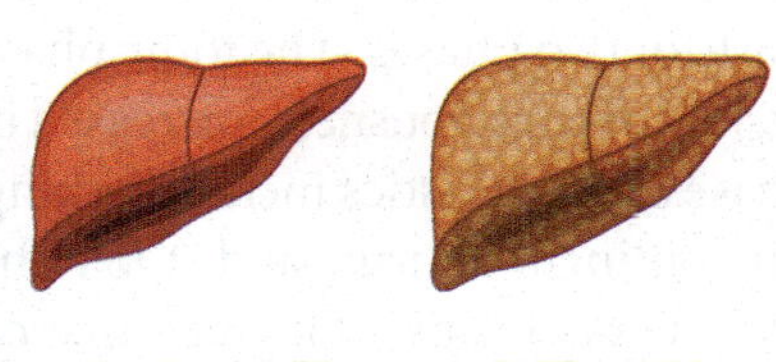




**Fig 3-6** Fatty liver from Reye's syndrome

### Diagnostic Tests

Reye's syndrome has no definitive, diagnostic test, but liver enzymes alanine aminotransferase (ALT) and aspartate aminotransferase (AST) elevate. Serum ammonia levels also elevate. A liver biopsy reveals fatty patches and confirms fatty liver degeneration. A Complete Blood Count and a Comprehensive Metabolic Panel detect dehydration and electrolyte imbalances. Extended coagulation times (PT) and blood sugars fall out of the normal range (ATI Testing 2016).

### Interventions

The nurse implements seizure precautions and initiates IV hydration. However, rapid fluid administration can exacerbate cerebral edema. The insertion of a Foley catheter allows strict intake and output measurements. The nurse positions the child to keep the child's head in a midline neutral position with the head of the bed elevated 30°. A coagulation panel may reveal a potential hemorrhage from unexplained or prolonged bleeding. The nurse should apply pressure after procedures that cause bleeding. Pain or a response to painful stimuli may require pain medications. Some patients may need a ventilator if the drive to breathe diminishes, or for the treatment of metabolic acidosis. The nurse should provide the family with psychosocial support and privacy if the child is terminal (ATI Testing 2016).

### Medications

Mannitol, an osmotic diuretic, causes a decrease in cerebral swelling relieving increased ICP, and vitamin K promotes the formation of blood clotting factors in the liver. Subcutaneous administration is the preferred route. Teach the child about dietary intake of vitamin K. IV glucose is given, and small amounts of insulin may be needed as the liver cannot store glucose so an excess can move into the body cells (ATI Testing 2016).

### Teaching

The nurse should ensure parents understand the importance of avoiding salicylates in aspirin and over the counter medications such as Pepto-Bismol. Parents should know that most children recover full liver function, but may have neurological deficits (ATI Testing 2016).

## Seizures

Seizures are disorganized electrical discharges of neurons caused by pathology. Several types of seizures exist in children. Seizure classification depends on type and etiology. A diagnosis of epilepsy, is a rule-out diagnosis where all other causes are eliminated before the condition is assumed to be seizure disorder. A chronic and recurring seizure disorder diagnosis occurs after two or more unprovoked seizures, with no underlying cause (Stephenson, J. P. B., & King, M. (Eds.). 2009). (see Fig 3-8).

### Assessment for Generalized Seizures

The generalized seizure is a type of seizure known as tonic-clonic, and previously a grand mal seizure. These seizures consists of two phases. The tonic phase causes a stiffening of the body. There may be increased salivation, flushing, loss of consciousness, increased blood pressure and heart rate, and apnea that can lead to cyanosis. The clonic phase characteristics include jerking movements of the body, followed by periods of relaxation. The child can be incontinent of urine and stool. There will be a gradual slowing of the movements until they cease. Then the child enters the postictal phase that can last for at least 30 minutes. The child remains semi-conscious and arouses with difficulty. There is possible weakness, confusion, headache, visual, or speech disturbance. The child will then sleep for several hours. The child won't recall the episode. (Kutscher, M. L. 2006)

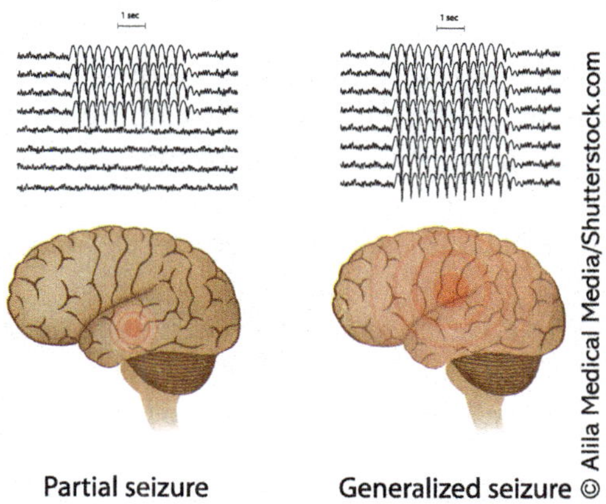


**Fig 3-7** Partial vs. generalized seizure

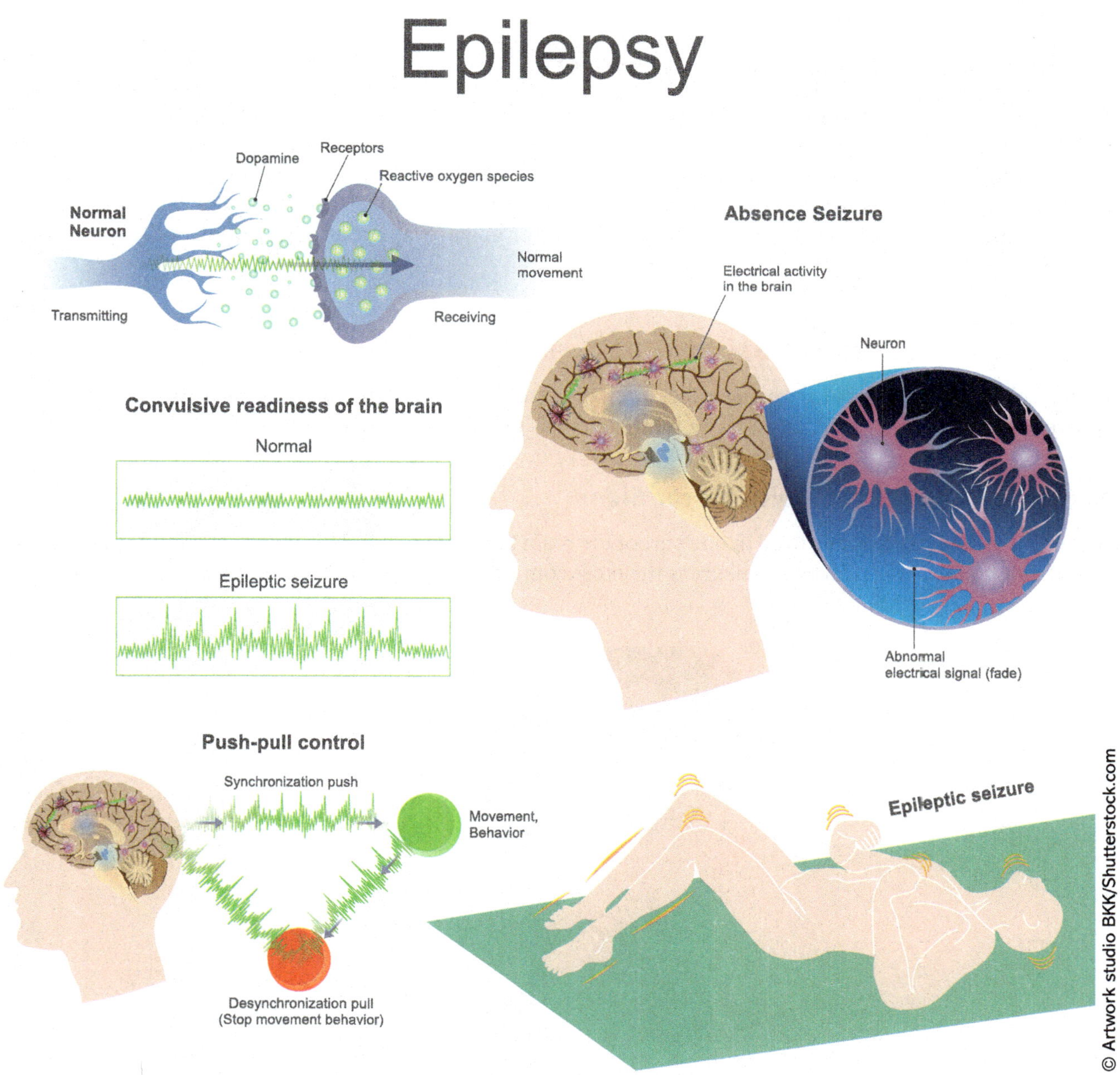


**Fig 3-8** Epileptic seizure

The **absence seizure**, or previously petit mal seizure, presents differently than the tonic-clonic seizure. The loss of consciousness presents subtly only lasting 5–10 seconds with minimal or no change in behavior. The behavior of the child may be confused with daydreaming or inattentiveness (see Fig 3-9). The child cannot hold on to objects and does not fall to the ground like a tonic-clonic seizure. There may be lip-smacking, twitching of eyelids or face, or eye fluttering. Like the tonic-clonic seizure, the child does not recall episodes but can be momentarily confused. However, the child can resume normal activity after the seizure (Kutscher, M. L. 2006).

The **myoclonic seizure** occurs in a variety of seizure occurrences. These seizures are brief startle like jerks of a muscle or muscle groups. The seizure can present symmetrically or asymmetrically, and may only involve the face or trunk or an extremity. The postictal state does not occur in a myoclonic seizure, and the child maintains consciousness.

An **atonic or akinetic seizure** creates a loss of muscle tone for a few seconds, or drop attacks. Children experience a loss of muscle tone that can result in falls and injuries. Children should wear helmets to prevent head injuries (ATI Testing 2016).

## West's Syndrome (Infantile Spasms)

West's syndrome seizure disorder usually affects young infants. Its peak onset is between 3 and 7 months of age. West's syndrome rarely occurs after 24 months of age and occurs twice as often in boys than in girls. Subtle, sudden, brief, symmetric muscle contractions signal a seizure. An infant displays a sudden, symmetric contractions (flexor spasms or flexion-extensor spasms) of muscles of the neck, trunk, and extremities. A loss of consciousness, flushing, pallor or cyanosis, and a cry or giggle may occur before or after the spasm (ATI Testing 2016).

## Assessment of Partial Seizures (Focal or Local)

Partial seizures are different than generalized seizures (see Fig 3-7). Generalized seizures affect both hemispheres of the brain. Focal seizures have a localized focus on one side of the brain.

### Simple Partial Seizures with Motor Signs

A simple partial seizure is localized in one part of the brain but may spread. This type of seizure does not cause loss of consciousness. An aversive seizure is the most common simple, partial motor seizure. During aversive

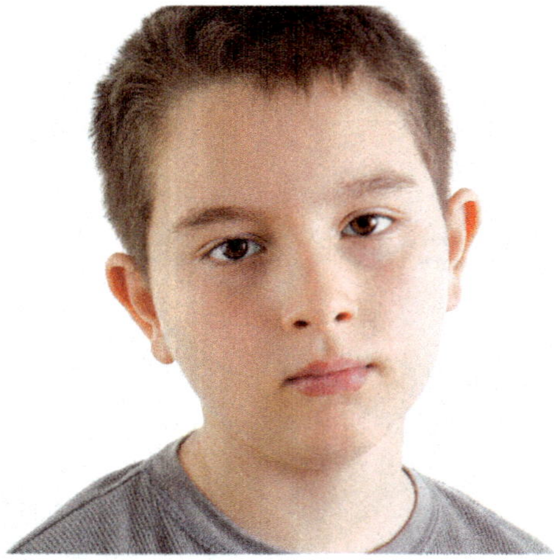



**Fig 3-9** An absence seizure can look like daydreaming.

seizures the child's eyes and head turn away from the side of focus. These seizures occur with or without loss of consciousness. A Rolandic (Sylvan) seizure is the most common seizure during sleep. The child makes tonic-clonic movements involving the face, hypersalivation, and disrupts sleep (ATI Testing 2016).

## Simple Partial Seizure with Sensory Signs

Simple, partial seizures with sensory signs create seizures that affect the senses. These seizures may present with tingling, numbness or pain, heat, or flashing lights. Children may display, hypertonia or posturing as a result (Shorvon, S. D. 2010).

## Complex Partial Seizures (Psychomotor Seizures)

Complex partial seizures come from the temporal lobe and can manifest as altered behavior, lack of response to the environment, impaired consciousness, confusion and inability to recall the event. These seizures produce a sensory aura that can manifest as feeling that starts in the stomach and rises into the throat, auditory or visual hallucinations, feelings of fear, or a distorted sense of time and self (ATI Testing 2016).

## Diagnostic Tests and Procedures

Diagnostic tests may include serum lead level, white blood cell count, blood glucose, serum electrolytes (metabolic panel), chromosomal analysis, and a toxicology screen (ATI Testing 2016).

Several diagnostic procedures can diagnose the origin of the seizures. An **electroencephalogram (EEG)** records electrical activity and can identify the source of seizure activity (see Fig 3-10). An EEG monitors the child during sleep, when awake, and with stimulation and hyperventilation. The EEG can last from 1 hour to multiple periods. The provider can monitor through video monitoring. The child must refrain from coffee for several hours prior to the procedure. The nurse should wash the child's hair before and after the procedure and not use oils or sprays afterward. The nurse prepares the child to take deep breaths during the procedure and to expect flashes of light during the procedure. Reassure the child that the test will not be painful. (Kutscher, M. L. 2006)

## Interventions

The nurse ensures safety through seizure precautions. **Seizure precautions** include padded side rails of the bed, crib, and wheelchair, placing the bed in the lowest position, removing objects in the bed that could cause injury, suction and oxygen equipment ready for use, and monitored bathing (Caple, C. M., & Schub, E. B. 2017).

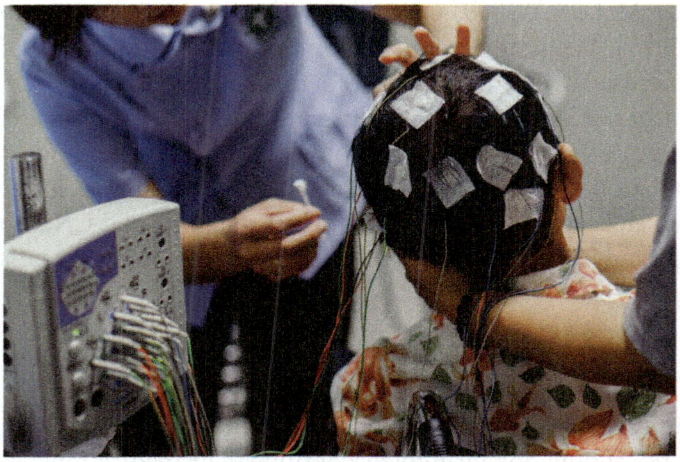



**Fig 3-10** A child having an EEG

When a child has a seizure, clear the area to protect them from injury. The nurse must also continuously monitor the airway for patency and and suctions the child when needed. The nurse should position the child in a side-lying position to minimize the risk of aspiration, loosen any restrictive clothing, and remove glasses or other devices that could cause injury. No one should ever attempt to restrain the child, open the jaw or insert an airway, or place anything in the child's mouth during seizure activity. If the child is cyanotic, the nurse administers oxygen. The nurse should document onset, time, and features of seizure (Caple, C. M., & Schub, E. B. 2017).

After a child has a seizure, the nurse should maintain the child in a side-lying position to decrease the risk for aspiration and to facilitate drainage of oral secretions. An assessment that includes vital signs, neurologic checks, and monitoring the postictal stage. The child cannot have foods or liquids until completely awake and the gag reflex has returned. Allow the child time to describe the period before, during, and after the seizure activity, and allow the child to describe any auras experienced before the seizure, aura, which can indicate the origin of seizure in the brain. If a child stops breathing, has a seizure that lasts more than 5 minutes, or if pupils are not equal after the seizure, notify the provider. In addition, if a child vomits within 30 minutes of the seizure, the seizure occurs in water, the child has status epilepticus (a seizure that lasts for 30 minutes or more), or it's the first seizure for the child also notify the provider immediately (ATI Testing 2016).

**Status epilepticus** is prolonged seizure activity in a child that lasts longer than 30 minutes or continuous seizure activity that does not end in a postictal phase. This acute condition is a medical emergency and requires immediate treatment to prevent permanent brain damage. (Caple, C. M., & Schub, E. B. 2017).

The nurse must maintain an airway, administer oxygen, establish IV access, perform ECG monitoring, and monitor pulse oximetry and other vital signs, and ABG results. Typically, the nurse administers a loading dose of diazepam or lorazepam. If seizures persist after the loading dose is given, the nurse may administer fosphenytoin and phenobarbital. (Caple, C. M., & Schub, E. B. 2017).

## Medications

Medications and possibly a **ketogenic diet** (high-fat, very-low-carbohydrate, and adequate protein) maintain wellness for children with seizure disorder. Antiepileptic drugs (AEDs) include **diazepam**, rectal **diazepam (Diastat), phenytoin**, **valproic acid**, topiramate. fosphenytoin sodium, lamotrigine, carbamazepine, clonazepam. Phenytoin needs to be kept in a narrow therapeutic index, and the administration of the drug is through a slow IV push so low blood pressure and dysrhythmias do not occur. Typically, the provider begins with a single medication at a low dosage and gradually increases the dosage until seizure activity subsides. Second-line medications, in addition to the first-line medication, treat more severe conditions. The nurse monitors the therapeutic serum medication levels for required medications (Stephenson, J. P. B., & King, M. (Eds.). 2009).

The administration of seizure medications are scheduled to enhance effectiveness, in addition to medication, adverse effects, and food interactions that are unique to each medication. Blood cell counts, liver function tests, and urinalysis tests are monitored at regular intervals to determine the adverse impact on the organ (Stephenson, J. P. B., & King, M. (Eds.). 2009).

Some children respond to a **Vagal nerve stimulator**, an implanted device surgically placed into the left chest wall under general anesthesia. The device connects to an electrode on the left vagus nerve. The device administers intermittent vagal nerve stimulation at a rate specific to the client's needs. In addition to routine stimulation, the client can create vagal nerve stimulation using a magnet held over the device once a seizure begins. This electrical stimulation will either abort the seizure or lessen its severity. The vagal nerve stimulator works similarly to a pacemaker, keeping the brain organized through regular CNS stimulation. Candidates for the device are 12 years of age and older with partial onset seizures, which are unmanageable with antiepileptic medications (ATI Testing 2016).

## Teaching

Educate the client and family about the importance of periodic laboratory testing to monitor medication concentration levels. Children should not abruptly discontinue their medications. Female adolescents should understand oral contraceptives decrease the effectiveness of seizure medications (ATI Testing 2016).

Parents should encourage the child to wear a medical alert bracelet or necklace at all times. Parents should also evaluate driving privileges for the adolescent with a seizure disorder based on the driving laws in the child's community. Parents encourage safety with each child to wear safety devices, such as helmets, while participating in activities. The family cannot ever leave the child unattended in water. Older children should shower, rather than take a tub bath, and leave the bathroom door unlocked while showering. Ask the family to try to identify triggers such as emotional stress, sleep deprivation, fatigue, and physical abuse. The nurse and family should work together to promote optimal development, make appropriate referrals and provide support for the household (ATI Testing 2016).

## Head Injury

There are several different categories of head injury concussions, contusions, lacerations, hematomas, and skull fractures. A **concussion** is a traumatic injury to the brain that interrupts brain functions. A **contusion** is bruising of the brain tissue from blunt trauma. A laceration tears the brain tissue. Hematomas can develop into the epidural space or the subdural space. **Epidural hematomas** result from arterial bleeding in between the dura mater and the skull. Because epidural hematomas originate from arterial bleeding, these hematomas develop quickly. A **subdural hematoma** consists of venous bleeding between the dura mater and the arachnoid membrane. These hematomas have a slower onset than an epidural hematoma, due to the lower pressure in the venous circulation. Subdural hematoma outcomes include higher mortality rates than epidural hematomas. Subdural hematomas can become chronic. Each hematoma can increase ICP by filling the free space in the cranium. Skull fractures can be linear, depressed, comminuted, basilar, open, or growing. A concussion, or a **traumatic brain injury (TBI)**, is the leading cause of death among children. (ATI Testing 2016). Diffuse Axonal Injuries are the most severe TBI's related to an acceleration-deceleration injury sometimes referred to as a closed-head trauma see Fig 3-11 (Whitfield, P. C. 2009).

TBI's can result from unexpected trauma, nonaccidental injuries such as shaken baby syndrome, or childhood activities such as bicycling, soccer, football, or hockey. Injuries can cause long-term effects such as epilepsy, cognitive deficits, and behavioral, learning or emotional challenges. Brain injuries can be primary or secondary. Primary injuries occur with the initial injury). Secondary injuries come from the inevitable cerebral edema that increases ICP and if not well controlled could result in brain herniation. **Brain herniation** results when the pressure in the brain causes a downward shift through the foramen magnum causing sudden death (ATI Testing 2016).

### Assessment

With all head injuries, the length of the period of unconsciousness defines the severity of the injury. Minor injuries occur with minimal or no loss of consciousness, vomiting, irritability, lethargy, and drowsiness. As a head injury progresses the vital signs decline with an altered mental state, increased agitation, and focal neurological deficits. A severe injury includes increased ICP, **posturing** (flexion and extension), alterations in pupillary response, optic disc swelling, bradycardia, Cheyne-Stokes respirations, decreased response to painful stimuli, decreased motor response, decreased consciousness, and coma. **Flexion**, also known as decorticate posturing, indicates severe dysfunction of the cerebral cortex. The child postures with the arms, wrists, elbows, and fingers flex and bent inward toward the heart with the legs extended and rotated internally. **Extension** indicates severe dysfunction at the level of the midbrain. The child postures with a backward arching of the legs and arms, flexed wrists and fingers, extended neck, clenched jaw, and possibly an arched back. Because young children possess fontanels, they can more easily compensate for increased ICP. Assessment findings will be different based on the age of the child (ATI Testing 2016).

Infants display bulging fontanels, separation of cranial sutures, irritability, restlessness, increased sleeping, high-pitched cry, poor feeding, setting-sun sign, and distended scalp veins (see Fig 3-12). Older children present with nausea, headache, forceful vomiting, blurred vision, increased sleeping, inability to follow simple commands, a decline in school performance, and seizures. Monitor vital signs for Cushing's triad pupils, the level of consciousness, motor activity, sensory perception, and verbal responses at regular intervals.

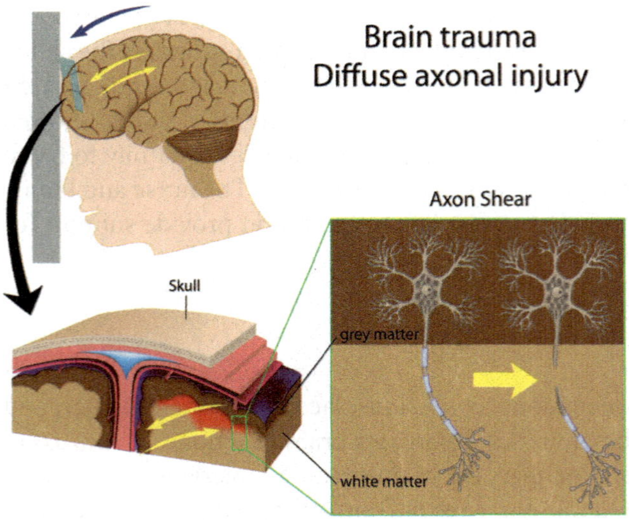




**Fig 3-11** Primary injuries cause axon shearing

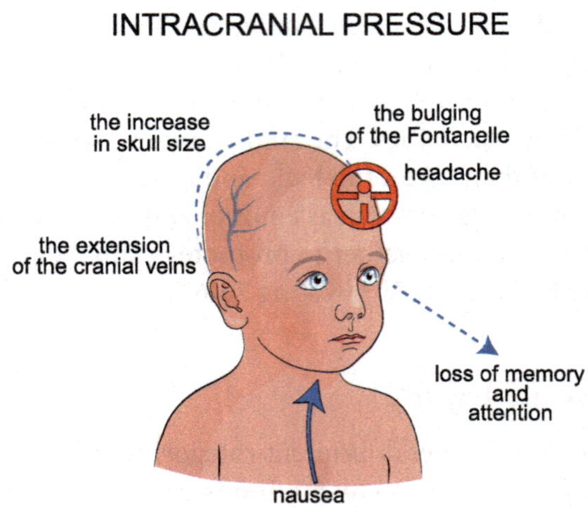




**Fig 3-12** Children younger than 18 months of age expand them their head circumference in response to increased ICP

Use the Glasgow Coma Scale as indicated (see Fig 3-13) The nurse assesses the child for clear fluid drainage from ears or nose for CSF. If so, the nurse reports this finding to the provider. The nurse also assesses the child for bleeding from the ear or bruising behind the ear as that indicates a basal skull fracture and is reported to the provider (ATI Testing 2016).

Epidural and subdural hematomas are complications that develop as a result of a head injury. An epidural hematoma presents with a brief loss of consciousness followed by a period of a couple of hours where the child will assess as normal. However, after this period the child appears lethargic and may become comatose due to the rapid accumulation of blood in the epidural space. Birth injury, falls or violent shaking (shaken baby syndrome) can cause a subdural hematoma (ATI Testing 2016).

The result of sustained, increased ICP is brain herniation. The impending signs include loss of blinking, loss of gag reflex, pupils failing to react to light, with systemic hypertension, bradycardia, coma, respiratory arrest, and death (ATI Testing 2016).

| Behaviour | Response |
|---|---|
| Eye Opening Response | 4. Spontaneously<br>3. To speech<br>2. To pain<br>1. No response |
| Verbal Response | 5. Oriented to time, person and place<br>4. Confused<br>3. Inappropriate words<br>2. Incomprehensible sounds<br>1. No response |
| Motor Response | 6. Obeys command<br>5. Moves to localised pain<br>4. Flex to withdraw from pain<br>3. Abnormal flexion<br>2. Abnormal extension<br>1. No response |



**Fig 3-13** Glasgow coma scale

## Diagnostic Procedures and Tests

A cervical spine x-ray is necessary to rule out cervical spine injury. In addition, computerized tomography and magnetic resonance imaging of head and neck might be performed with and without contrast if indicated.

Children may need an ICP monitor to keep ICP between 1 and 10 mm Hg. A level greater than 20 mm Hg is dangerous. Woten, M. B., & Mennella, H. A. (2017).

## Interventions

The nurse should promote safety, so the child does not further injure themselves. Thus, the nurse must stabilize the spine until a spinal cord injury is ruled out. Seizure precautions include padded bed rails that protect children with agitation from harm. The nurse must also maintain a patent airway with oxygen saturation levels greater than 95%. The health-care team can provide mechanical ventilation as indicated. The nurse promotes the child's safety by leaving the side rails up, padding the side rails, and keeping the call light within reach. The nurse must position the child to prevent elevation in ICP including positioning the child's head midline and neutral with the bed elevated to 30°, to promote venous drainage and avoid extreme flexion, extension, or rotation of the head. The nurse aligns the child's body to prevent hip flexion or extension. The child may have a footboard or splints to help with positioning. The nurse will minimize oral suctioning and refrain from contraindicated interventions such as nasal suctioning. The child cannot cough, blow their nose, or strain (Valsalva maneuver) while defecating because these activities increase ICP in the brain. To make sure the positioning does not cause problems with skin breakdown the nurse repositions the child every 2 hours. The nurse controls the environment to create a calm, restful environment without too many visitors or loud noises. Nurses must also cluster their nursing tasks to maximize rest periods and conserve energy for the child (ATI Testing 2016).

The nurse places an indwelling urinary catheter for strict output measurements and to regulate fluid and electrolyte values and osmolarity for changes in sodium regulation, the onset of diabetes insipidus, or severe hypovolemia. The nurse administers adequate IV fluids to maintain cerebral perfusion. However, any fluid volume might increase ICP. Nutritional support is necessary and may include total parenteral nutrition or enteral nutrition (ATI Testing 2016).

The nurse should also support the family through psychosocial interventions that include ongoing communication with the client and family. It also may include instruction on how to communicate with their child through touching, cuddling, talking, and assisting with care as appropriate (ATI Testing 2016).

## Medications

Medications that treat increased ICP, balance electrolytes, and prevent seizures are required to manage head injuries. Mannitol, an osmotic diuretic, treats cerebral edema and improves consciousness, vomiting, and behavioral or personality changes. The high incidence rate of electrolyte imbalances and metabolic acidosis during the treatment necessitate close monitoring. Antiepileptics prevent or treat seizures that might occur. In brain injuries with CSF leakage, lacerations, or penetrating injuries antibiotics treat infections. Analgesics (acetaminophen) treat headaches and pain. Proper management of pain will keep ICP from increasing (ATI Testing 2016).

## Surgical Procedures

**Transfontanel percutaneous aspiration** removes excess fluid through the infant's fontanel. If continuous drainage benefits the child, a subdural drain or **burr holes** with or without a subdural drain maintains appropriate CSF levels. A traditional **craniotomy** removes a flap of skull and then replaces the bone once the swelling has subsided. However, the use of a **mini-osteoplastic craniotomy** may be more therapeutic than using burr holes (Klimo, J., Matthews, A., Lew, S. M., Zwienenberg-Lee, M., and Kaufman, B. A. 2011).

# COGNITIVE AND SENSORY IMPAIRMENTS

Congenital cognitive impairments include Down's syndrome, cerebral palsy, neural tube defects or spina bifida, and the resulting hydrocephalus. Down's syndrome (**Trisomy 21**) is a common chromosomal abnormality that affects the child's growth and development and results in cognitive and sensory impairments. Neural tube defects occur around the fourth week of gestation because the spine does not completely develop, neurologic deficits may occur.

Hydrocephalus occurs when there is too much production and too little reabsorption of CSF that typically causes increased ICP. Cerebral palsy (CP) is a neuromuscular disorder that occurs while the brain is developing. CP affects muscle control and coordination, muscle tone, reflexes, posture and balance, fine motor skills, gross motor skills and oral motor functioning and swallowing (ATI Testing 2016).

Sensory impairments in children most commonly impact the eyes and ears. Vision and hearing are necessary to allow the normal growth and development of a child to progress. Therefore, early identification is essential to supporting a child's development (ATI Testing 2016).

## Down's Syndrome

Down's syndrome is a condition where there are three chromosomes at chromosome 21 in every cell of the body. Many medical conditions accompany Down's syndrome including congenital heart malformation, hypotonicity, dysfunction of the immune system, thyroid dysfunction, and leukemia (ATI Testing 2016).

### Assessment

Children with Down's syndrome can present with some or all of the following assessment findings. Infants may have an enlarged anterior fontanel, and a flattened forehead. They have a characteristic upward, and outward slant to their eyes (see Fig 3-14). They have a small nose with depressed nasal bridge (saddle nose). The ears are small ears with short pinna. The eyes have **epicanthal folds** (a fold of the upper eyelid, covering the inner corner or medial canthus of the eye). Their mouths contain a high-arched narrow palate with a protruding tongue. The neck is short and broad. The ribcage is shorter than typical children. Congenital heart disease affects about 40%–45% of children. The abdomen naturally protrudes. They may have an incurved fifth finger (clinodactyly). The feet are broad, with short feet and stubby toes. There is a large space between the big and second toes, with a plantar crease on the sole. The hands are short with stubby fingers. The hands have a transverse palmar crease. Children with Down's syndrome often have dry skin that cracks easily. They

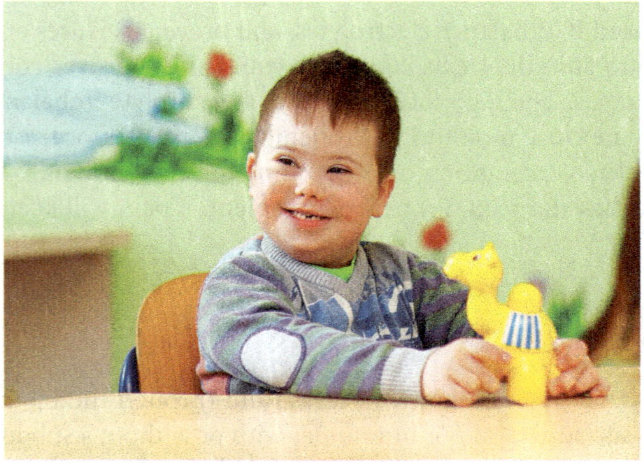



**Fig 3-14** A child with Down's syndrome

are hyperflexible, may have muscle weakness and hypotonia. Children with Down's syndrome have a short stature. They also can have congenital or acquired hypothyroidism and must be continually assessed for these issues. Children will have varying degrees of intellectual disability. Development can be 2–3 years behind their chronological age. Other possibilities include bone anomalies such as hip subluxation and patella dislocation, and gastrointestinal conditions such as duodenal atresia, tracheoesophageal fistula, and Hirschsprung's disease. Children with Down's syndrome may have sensory deficits. Some children have ocular problems that include strabismus, nystagmus, astigmatism, myopia, hyperopia, head tilt, excessive tearing, and cataracts. Many have hearing loss, frequent otitis media, narrow canals, and impacted cerumen. Both height and weight are slower in children with Down's syndrome. Early weight gain without growth in height and can result in excessive weight by 36 months. Sexual development of male and female genitalia can be underdeveloped and delayed (ATI Testing 2016).

## Diagnostic Tests

Pregnant mothers receive screenings for **alpha-fetoprotein** (AFP) in maternal serum. An elevation in AFP suggests a congenital disability, further diagnostic testing is necessary. As a newborn, chromosome analysis and echocardiography are used to determine how the extra chromosomal material manifests in each child, and to determine if there are congenital heart defects (ATI Testing 2016).

### Clinical Pearl

There are two important ways to support the family of a child with Down's syndrome at the time of diagnosis. The first communication to the family should include "congratulations" as the family welcomes a new member of the family. Mothers may still be in shock from the birth experience, and have earned congratulations for their hard work. Also, nurses can make sure they have materials to connect parents to organizations for Down's syndrome. Materials from the National Association for Down's syndrome are available. **NADS** are available to support children and families with Down's syndrome. http://www.nads.org/

## Interventions

Surgical interventions vary according to the individual, associated congenital anomalies. These can range from cardiac anomalies to strabismus. The nurse provides standard postoperative care with an emphasis on wound care, respiratory care, pain management, post-operative teaching, and home-care management. Children with Down's syndrome may have difficulty feeding due to their protruding tongue and low muscle tone. The nurse should help swaddle the infant to prevent heat loss due to limp, extended body position. Support family with feeding difficulties, and monitor the newborn's dietary intake. The child's skin must be kept clean, dry and moisturized. Assist the parents to hold and bond with their child. Listen to the concerns of the parents and discuss ethical dilemmas regarding treatment for physical defects. Make appropriate referrals for social work, home health, school early intervention, genetic counseling, speech therapy, physical therapy, and occupational therapy (ATI Testing 2016).

## Teaching

Teach the family to reposition an infant frequently to minimize skin breakdown, prevent respiratory infection and promote growth and development. The child assumes responsibility for care as they are able, and are taught how to aspirate nasal secretions and use cool mist humidifiers in the room to assist in moistening

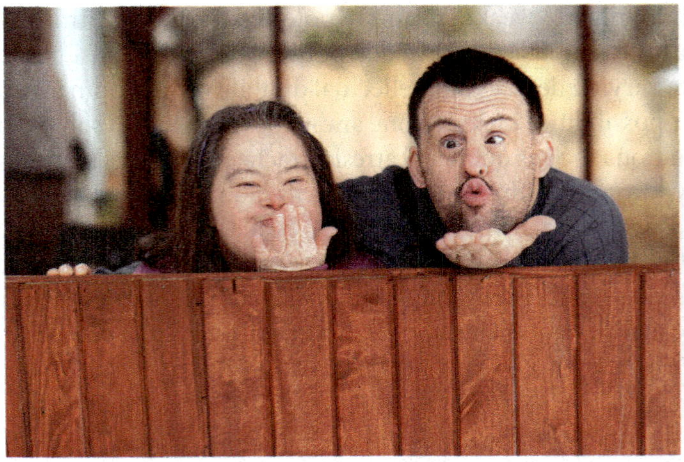


**Fig 3-15** A couple with Down's syndrome

secretions. Parents must rinse the child's mouth after feedings. Children with Down's syndrome experience tooth decay and respiratory infections caused by **xerostomia** (dry mouth) related to mouth breathing because of a small nose. Parents should reposition infants frequently and moisturize skin to prevent rashes and skin breakdown associated with hypotonia or muscle weakness. The family must take extra time for feeding to accommodate the child's protruding tongue. The wellness of these children depends on a healthy diet, exercise, and infection control. Nurses and families must promote a diet high in unprocessed food to increase fiber and extra unsweetened fluids to prevent constipation. Parents should track children's high-quality food choices and calorie intake. Children also need exercise and should be encouraged to be active most days of the week to prevent obesity. Wellness appointments are essential for children with Down's syndrome. These visits can troubleshoot any acute problems, keep children up to date with vaccinations, and monitor the child for growth and development milestones. Eyesight and hearing screenings, rule out these issues that can create developmental delays. Wellness visits reinforce the need for routine immunizations. (Schub, T. B., & Boling, B. C. 2016).

Down Syndrome manifests in many ways and can be mild or severe. It is important not to limit expectations for children with Down Syndrome. Children with Down Syndrome can grow into adults with jobs, become athletes and have healthy adult relationships like typical adults (see Fig 3-15).

# CHRONIC NEUROMUSCULOSKELETAL DISORDERS

Neuromuscular disorders can affect voluntary muscles, nerves, or neuromuscular junctions that originate from the brain's cortex to the neuromuscular junction. Two common neuromuscular pathologies are cerebral palsy and spina bifida (ATI Testing 2016).

## Cerebral Palsy

Cerebral palsy (CP) is a nonprogressive disorder of movement, muscle tone, coordination, and posture (see Fig 3-16). CP can cause altered perception and sensation with visual, hearing, and speech impairments, seizures, and cognitive disabilities. Standard visual impairments in children with CP include myopia, hyperopia, astigmatism, anisometropia, amblyopia, strabismus, cataracts, and glaucoma. Visual disturbance can come from the inability to focus on one object at the same time. Children with CP may have hearing problems. hear. Speech impairments come from the child's inability to control the muscles in their mouths. Cognitive disabilities vary with individuals who have CP; some have intellectual disabilities and others do not. All injuries occur during the development of the brain, often before birth. The exact cause of CP is not known. The associated risk factors

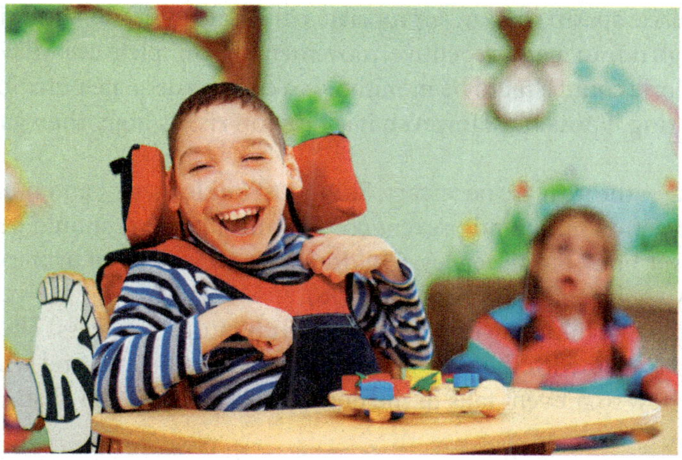



**Fig 3-16** A child with cerebral palsy

of CP may present in the prenatal, perinatal, and postnatal periods. Brian anomalies, cerebral infections, head trauma (shaken baby syndrome), or anoxia to the brain can all cause CP. Maternal infection such as chorioamnionitis, placental abnormalities, or kernicterus can also cause CP (Stephenson, J. P. B., & King, M. (Eds.). 2009).

### Assessment

There are different types of CP with different assessment findings. Children may have spastic CP, dyskinetic CP, and ataxic CP. Children with CP will not meet their developmental milestones and retain their primitive infant reflexes such as the Moro or the tonic neck reflex and display hyperreflexia. Children will have a weak suck reflex and have feeding difficulties such as tongue thrusting, gagging, choking, and have poor head control. Children with CP assume a rigid posture and extremities with an abnormal posture. Vision, speech, or hearing impairments and seizures are common (ATI Testing 2016).

## Spastic CP (Pyramidal)

Spastic CP characteristics include hypertonicity, muscle tightness or spasticity; increased deep tendon reflexes; clonus; and poor control of fine and gross motor skills that affect motion, balance, and posture. Hypertonicity can manifest in all four extremities (tetraplegia), in the lower extremities (diplegia), in three limbs (triplegia), in one limb (monoplegia), or one side of the body (hemiplegia). Children with spastic CP have a modified gait. They appear crouched with a scissoring motion of the legs with feet plantar flexed (ATI Testing 2016).

Dyskinetic CP (nonspastic, extrapyramidal) Dyskinetic CP may be athetoid or dystonic. Athetoid CP characteristics include involuntary jerking movements that appear slow, writhing, and wormlike. These actions involve the extremities, trunk, neck, face, and tongue. Dystonic CP characteristics include slow, twisting movements that affect the trunk or extremities with abnormal posturing from muscle contractions. Drooling and speech impairment results from the involvement of the muscles of the pharynx, larynx, and oral regions (ATI Testing 2016).

## Ataxic CP (Nonspastic, Extrapyramidal)

Ataxic CP forces the child to assume a wide-based gait and creates difficulty with coordination. Children struggle to perform repetitive movements. Children with ataxic CP have no coordination to complete purposeful movements such as reaching for a toy or other routine tasks (Stephenson, J. P. B., & King, M. (Eds.). 2009).

Nursing care includes maintaining a patent airway by elevating the head of the bed to promote the draining of oral secretions and ventilation and suctioning as needed. The nurse must monitor for aspiration while the child eats or drinks. **Pulmonary hygiene** techniques such as chest physiotherapy and suctioning are helpful.

Evaluate pain related to muscle spasm with an appropriate pain scale tool, and administer medication if necessary. Nutrition needs are high due to many, repetitive, movements to complete everyday tasks (ATI Testing 2016).

Height, weight, and calorie count should be monitored to ensure adequate nutrition. Familiar foods should be given in the hospital setting if possible. However, if aspiration risk is high, then gavage feedings are appropriate (ATI Testing 2016).

Interventions to maintain the skin are necessary. Skin must be clean, dry, and moisturized. Splints, braces, and **ankle-foot orthoses** position limbs and prevent contractures. Patients should be turned every 2 hours to prevent skin breakdown over bony prominences. Children with CP will need urinary straight catheterization administered by the family or the child (ATI Testing 2016).

Rest periods are essential for children with CP and help with muscle soreness. These children are placed on fall precautions while hospitalized with the bed rails raised, padded side rails and wheelchair arms to prevent falls. Parents should learn how to prevent falls in the home environment (ATI Testing 2016).

### Medications

**Baclofen** is an antispasmodic, centrally acting skeletal muscle relaxant that decreases muscle spasm and severe spasticity. Baclofen may be taken orally or intrathecally (into the spinal cord) for CP. It is most effective when used in a pump to deliver medication into the spinal cord. Baclofen causes muscle weakness, increased fatigue, and different adverse effects such as diaphoresis and constipation. A balanced diet with plenty of water and fiber prevents constipation (ATI Testing 2016).

### Diazepam and Antiepileptics

**Diazepam** is a skeletal muscle relaxant used to decrease muscle spasms and severe spasticity, in addition to seizures in older children and adolescents. The nurse and family must monitor for drowsiness, fatigue, and signs of overdose from these medications (ATI Testing 2016).

### Botulinum Toxin A

**Botulinum toxin A** reduces spasticity in particular muscle groups in the lower extremities essentially paralyzes muscles; therefore, temporary muscle weakness will occur, the nurse must monitor for safety issues such as falls. The onset of the medication is 24–72 hours, with a peak of 2 weeks, lasting for 3–6 months (ATI Testing 2016).

A multidisciplinary approach is best for this chronic disease that has no cure. Speech, physical, occupational therapists will coordinate care to maintain function and development in children with CP. The nurse integrates education specialists and medical specialists into the plan of care. Referrals for specialized equipment that can assist with coordination, speaking, mobility, and an increased level of independence. Some children may need a voice-activated wheelchair. If contractures occur, then surgeons can release tendons and muscles correct the contractures or other spastic deformities. The nurse should identify all resources, including respite care support groups, and CPR training for children with CP and their families (ATI Testing 2016).

## Spina Bifida

Spina bifida is a condition where the bony processes of the spine fail to close; these defects are called neural tube defects (NTDs) (see Fig 3-17). These defects are present at birth and affect the CNS and spine (ATI Testing 2016).

Spina bifida occulta usually affects the lumbosacral area, but the protrusion is covered by skin making it hidden. Spina bifida occulta is the least severe defect. Spina bifida cystica is a visible protrusion outside of the spine and comes in two types (see Fig 3-18). A **meningocele** is a protrusion of the meningeal sac that contains spinal fluid and meninges. A **myelomeningocele** is a protrusion that contains the meningeal sac, spinal fluid, meninges, and nerves. Maternal malnutrition, exposure to teratogens, and especially a lack of folic acid can cause NTDs (ATI Testing 2016).

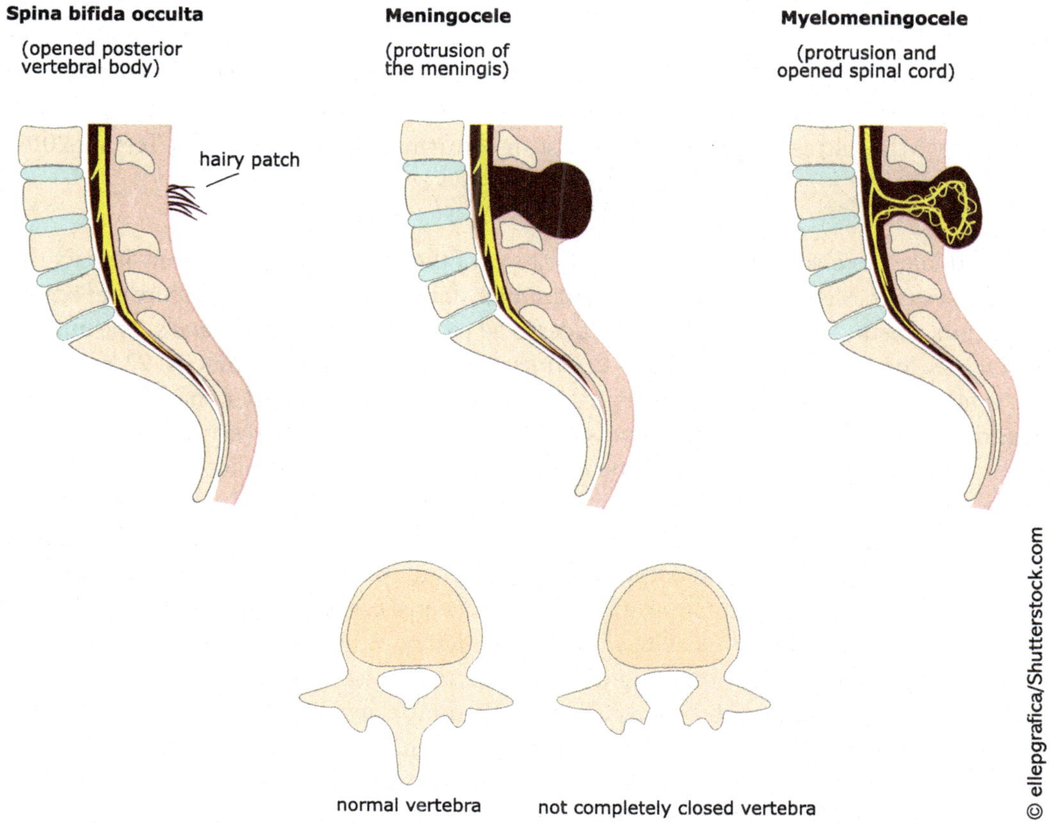


**Fig 3-17** Neural tube defect

## Assessment

There will be a protruding sac midline of the osseous spine (cystica). In the occulta type findings include dimpling in the lumbosacral area, a port wine angioma, dark hair tufts in the sacral area, or a subcutaneous lipoma. Laboratory testing includes a serum alpha-fetoprotein between 16 and 18 weeks of gestation indicate possible NTD in pregnant mothers, and blood cultures on the infant determine causative pathogen if the defect has become infected (ATI Testing 2016).

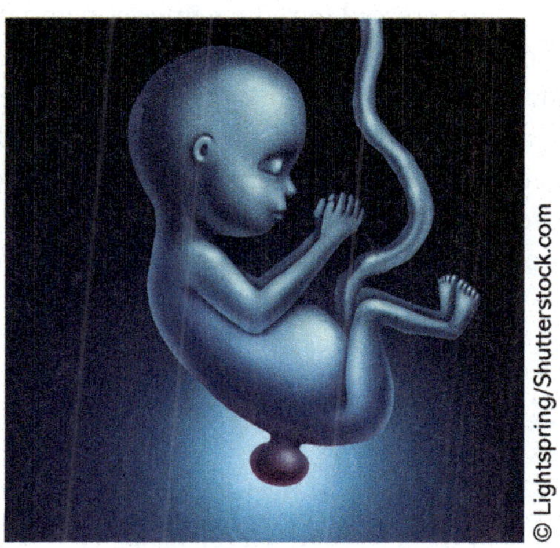


**Fig 3-18** NTD in utero

### Diagnostic Testing

A prenatal assessment ultrasound can show visual deficits. A chorionic villus sampling or amniocentesis follows an elevated alpha-fetoprotein level to detect anencephaly or myelomeningocele. Imaging of the neonatal brain and spine by MRI, ultrasonography, and CT scan confirms the diagnosis (ATI Testing 2016).

### Interventions and Teaching

The level of neurologic involvement related to the location of the sac, and may negatively impact the respiratory, bowel or bladder systems. Meticulous skin care can minimize skin breakdown from pressure and bowel and bladder output. In addition, a neurological assessment includes head circumference and fontanels. The nurse must prepare the child and family for surgery to close the defect. Surgery will occur within the first 24–72 hours after birth. The priority intervention is to protect the sac from injury and infection. A sterile, moist, nonadherent dressing with 0.9% sodium chloride on the sac can achieve this. Dressing changes to the sac occur every 2 hours along with an assessment of the sac for leaks, irritation, abrasions, and signs of infection (fever, irritability, and lethargy). The neonate is placed in the prone position with hips flexed, legs abducted. Nurses administer IV antibiotics as prescribed. Rectal temperatures are contraindicated, as well as cuddling or putting pressure on the sac. After the surgical procedure, the nurse monitors vital signs, input and output, CSF leakage, and pain status. The nurse will care for the surgical incision with dressing changes. The nurse positions the neonate in a prone position until the provider orders additional positions. The nurse then restarts feedings and provides Range of Motion (ROM) exercises (ATI Testing 2016).

This chronic disorder requires ongoing assessments that include head circumference, skin integrity. Cognitive development, bladder and bowel functioning, motor development, infections, body image concerns, and allergy assessments for urticaria or wheezing, which can progress to anaphylaxis. A **latex allergy** often occurs with other allergies to certain foods such as bananas, avocados, kiwi, and chestnuts. The nurse can provide the family with a list of household items that can contain latex balloons, bandages, and pacifiers storage bags, to make sure the family prevents exposure to the child (ATI Testing 2016).

The nurse helps secure medical equipment to supports the child in the home environment. The nurse must emotionally support the child and family and promote independence for the child throughout the child's lifespan (ATI Testing 2016).

Children may be at risk for increased intracranial pressure. A **Ventriculoperitoneal shunt** may be placed to drain the excess CSF into the abdomen (see Fig 3-19). Shunts can malfunction and show signs of occlusion of infection that include headaches, vomiting, lethargy, irritability, swelling or redness around the shunt, periods of confusion, seizure, or decreased school performance. Infants display a high-pitched cry, lethargy, vomiting, bulging fontanels, widening cranial suture lines, increased head circumference. Children exhibit a headache, lethargy, nausea, vomiting, double vision, decreased school performance of learned tasks, decreased the level of consciousness, seizures. Parents must notify the health-care provider if any of these signs are noted (ATI Testing 2016).

Children with bladder involvement (spasms or flaccidity) require monitoring for blood or infection in the urine. A vesicostomy (a temporary stoma created to reduce infection and damage to the kidneys). Orthopedic problems may include clubfoot, scoliosis, and other malformations of the feet and legs (ATI Testing 2016).

New developments in fetal surgery address the myelomeningocele defect. Surgeons can now operate on the fetus in utero to avoid the damage to the neural sac from the labor and birth process (Adzick, N. S. 2012).

A child with spina bifida benefits from a multidisciplinary approach that includes neurosurgery neurology, urology, orthopedics, pediatrics, physical therapy, occupational therapy, and social services. The closure of a meningocele or a myelomeningocele is done as quickly as possible to minimize complications of injury or infection (ATI Testing 2016).

# SENSORY DEFICITS

## Visual Impairment

Visual disturbances can manifest in several ways. Myopia (nearsightedness), occurs when objects are clear close-up, but not in the distance, headaches and vertigo, eye tearing, difficulty reading, poor school performance,

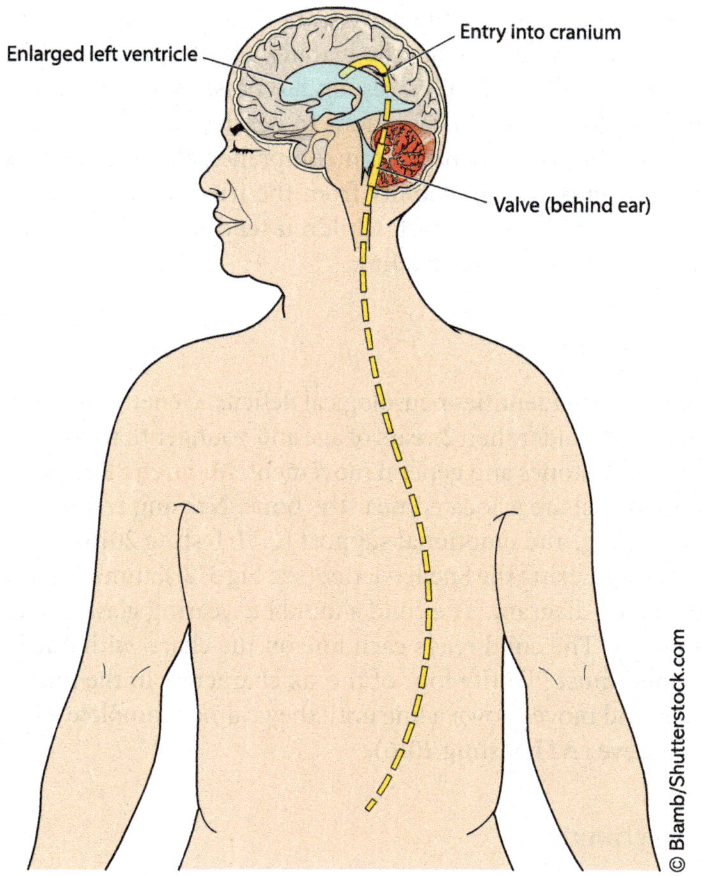


**Fig 3-19** Ventroperitoneal shunt in an adolescent

and, clumsiness. Hyperopia (farsightedness) allows for distant objects to appear clearly, but not objects that are close. However, because a farsighted eye requires more accommodation than a nearsighted eye, this is not usually detected until 7 years of age when children can accommodate. Astigmatism produces uneven vision in the eye, so only parts of letters on a page are visible. A child may move his or her head to view all words. Anisometropia causes different refractive strength in each eye and may cause a headache and vertigo, excessive eye rubbing, and poor school performance (ATI 2016). Amblyopia (lazy eye) occurs when there is reduced visual acuity in one eye. Strabismus can manifest as esotropia (inward deviation of the eye) or exotropia (outward deviation of the eye) (ATI Testing 2016).

Children will possess an abnormal corneal light reflex or cover test and have misaligned eyes. They may frown or squint, have difficulty seeing print clearly, close one eye to enable better vision, tilt their head to one side, and may present with a headache, dizziness, diplopia, photophobia, and crossed eyes (ATI Testing 2016).

Cataracts cause a decreased ability to see clearly with a possible loss of peripheral vision; These children will not have a red reflex (ATI Testing 2016).

Glaucoma produces corneal haziness, the perception of halos around objects, red eyes, photophobia, enlargement of the eyeball (buphthalmos), excessive tearing (epiphora), spasmodic winking (blepharospasm), and potential pain. (ATI Testing 2016).

Children may present with a partial visual impairment. Impairments include visual acuity such as a from a visual acuity of 20/70 to 20/200, legal blindness with a visual acuity of 20/200 or worse, or a visual field of 20 degrees or less in the child's stronger eye (ATI Testing 2016).

Children with hearing loss may experience conductive losses that causes the ear to not recognize sounds. Which can result from otitis media, external ear infection, foreign bodies, or excessive ear wax. They may experience sensorineural losses that involve interference of the transmission along the nerve pathways, which can result from congenital disabilities, or secondary to acquired infection, the use of ototoxic medication, and exposure to constant noise from a Neonatal Intensive Care Unit. Children may experience central auditory imperception that includes aphasia, and agnosia (the inability to interpret sounds).

Infants do not show a startle reflex and fail to respond to noise or spoken words. They will not vocalize 7 months of age. Older children show several adaptations to hearing deficits. They employ the use of gestures instead of talking after 15 months and may have an incomprehensible speech pattern by 24 months of age. Children may yell to express themselves, irritability from the frustration of not being able to communicate thoughts, and may seem withdrawn or shy affect. Children tend to speak in a monotone voice and require repetition to understand language (ATI Testing 2016).

## Diagnostic Procedures

A complete neurological assessment identifies neurological deficits. Genetic and metabolic testing is conducted to determine anomalies. Children, older than 2 years of age and younger than 5 years of age undergo screenings for growth and development milestones and general movement. **Magnetic Resonance Imaging (MRI)** is used to evaluate structures or abnormal areas located near the bone. Nursing responsibilities for those diagnostic tests include sedation, positioning, and emotional support (ATI Testing 2016).

Visual screening is completed using the Snellen letter (see Fig 3-21), tumbling E, or picture chart. The child is placed 10 feet from the Snellen diagram. The child should be wearing glasses, if appropriate, and keep both eyes open during the screening. The child reads each line on the chart, with one eye covered, starting at the bottom of the chart. The child must identify four of the six characters in the line correctly to pass. The child begins at the top of the chart and moves down a line until they cannot complete a line. The practitioner repeats the procedure with the other eye (ATI Testing 2016).

## Interventions and Teaching

Care must be customized to each child as each child will have a different manifestation of the disorder. Therefore, he or she will need growth and development screenings, hearing, and speech evaluations on a yearly basis. Therapies, modified household devices such as a flashing light when the doorbell or phone rings, telecommunication devices, closed captioning on the television, lip reading, and use of cued speech (hand gestures with verbal communication) promote independence. A sign language or an interpreter may be used if appropriate when working with a child who has hearing loss. The nurse should always talk to the child, not the interpreter. In addition, eye surgery, eye laser surgery, and patching can support children's visual deficits. Nurses must help parents and the child to promote maximum independence with self-care activities. Personal freedom allows the child to create and maintain a positive self-image and a high level of self-esteem. Families

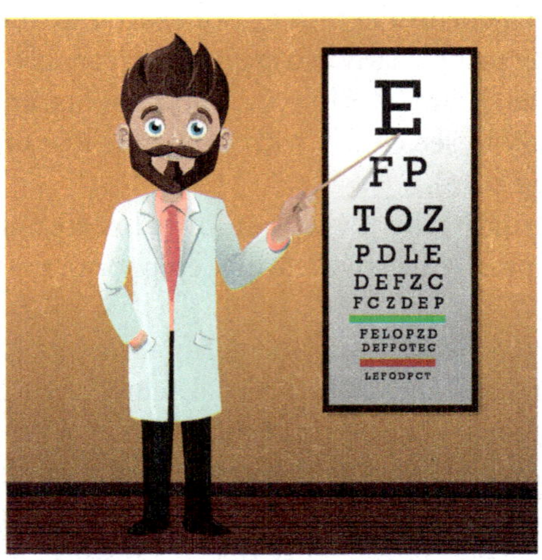




**Fig 3-20** A Snellen eye chart

need a proactive framework to develop coping skills, resilience, and minimize **caregiver role strain**. Once these parameters are defined, interventions and communications are appropriately determined based on the child's developmental level, rather than chronological age. The nurse must communicate with the child directly, through augmented communication such as electronic devices for speech and other types of communication tools, but include parents when necessary. Parents should have care taught and reinforced by the nurse during hospitalization. Encourage the family to provide routine care in the inpatient setting, so they will be competent to perform these tasks at home (ATI Testing 2016).

# NEUROLOGICAL PSYCHOSOCIAL ISSUES OF INFANTS, CHILDREN AND ADOLESCENTS

## Attention-Deficit/Hyperactivity Disorder

Attention-deficit/hyperactivity disorder characteristics include inattentiveness, hyperactivity, and impulsiveness. There are differences in the brain of a child with ADD/ADHD when compared with typical children (see Fig 3-21). These symptoms are usually revealed before age 7, and can persist into adulthood. Symptoms present between the ages of 4 and 18 years, and present in more than one setting. These symptoms impair social or academic development. A diagnosis includes six or more findings from a category. There is a genetic component or a history of toxin or medicine exposure (ATI Testing 2016).

### Assessment

Inattention in a child occurs when the child fails to pay close attention to detail or make careless mistakes. Children with ADHD, fail to interpret incoming stimuli and have a general difficulty sustaining attention. They appear not to listen, and fail to follow through on instructions. They have trouble organizing activities, and they avoid or dislikes activities that require mental effort for a long period of time, such as reading, or writing. They can lose things, because they are easily distracted, and forgetful. These symptoms must occur for at least 6 month to obtain a diagnosis (Thompson, R. (Ed.). 2012).

Hyperactivity in the child manifests as fidgeting, failure to remain seated, inappropriate running, difficulty engaging in quiet play, and a sense of being "busy" all the time, and excessive talking (ATI Testing 2016).

Impulsivity symptoms include blurting out responses inappropriately, difficulty with waiting to take a turn, striking out, biting, and shouting (ATI Testing 2016). Children with ADHD are easily labelled by society as "problem children". Health care providers should help parents process any negative social pressures by assuring them the symptoms are a disease that has treatment options (see Fig 3-23).

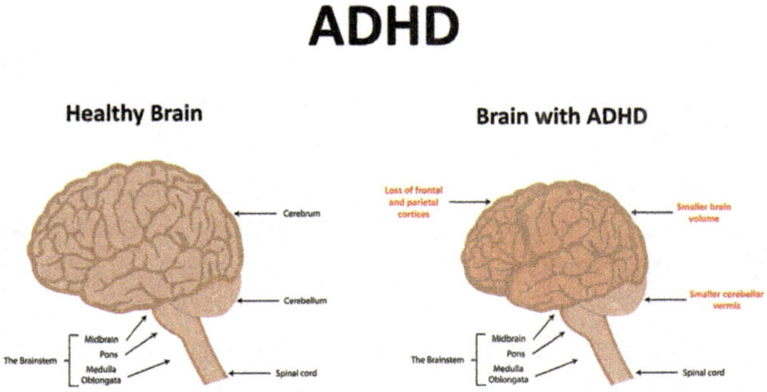


© joshya/Shutterstock.com

Fig 3-21 Typical brain vs. ADHD brain

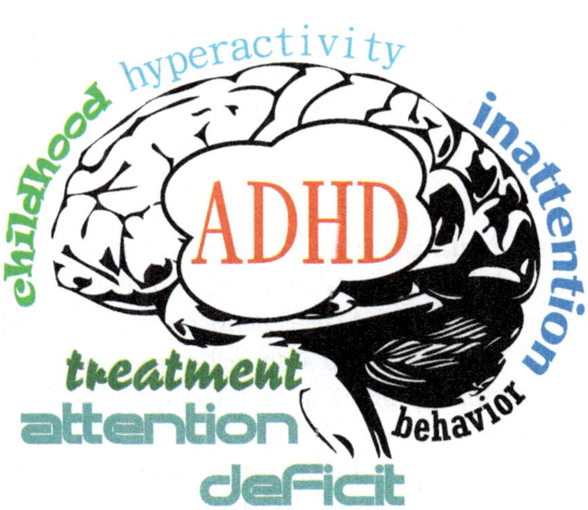


© Oxlock/Shutterstock.com

Fig 3-22 Symptoms of ADHD

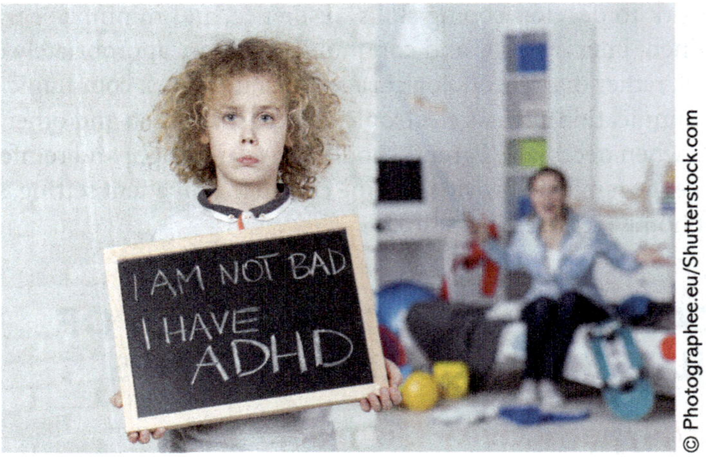
I AM NOT BAD
I HAVE
ADHD
© Photographee.eu/Shutterstock.com

**Fig 3-23** ADHD can be mistaken for bad behavior

## Interventions and Teaching

All children benefit from art therapy, play therapy, and Cognitive Behavioral Therapy (CBT). Children complete a medical, developmental, or behavioral assessment to guide interventions. All children need a safe environment and a calm, firm, respectful approach because children imitate these social cues. The nurse must obtain the child's attention before giving directions, and provide short and clear explanations. The nurse must be sure to have the child's attention before giving concise and clear instructions and illustrations. Children complete tasks better when adults set clear limits and consequences. Physical activities help the child expend energy and supports general focus. It is important to concentrate on the strengths of the child and family and not just the chronic problems. Adults should provide specific positive feedback when a child meets a goal. The nurse can help the family support their child by identifying issues that create power struggles, and ideas to manage such matters. The parents and the nurse can develop coping strategies for the child to handle the stress of the pathology. The child and family need therapy to manage behavioral issues that arise with expected growth and development milestones. The nurse must also help the family identify age-appropriate consequences from behavioral issues to address in therapy (ATI Testing 2016).

The priority intervention for children with ADHD is to provide a structured environment with a steady routine. A predictable day supports the growth and development of all children and will especially help children with ADHD, charts, and stickers can help children stay organized for the day. Chores can be broken down into steps to help children complete tasks. Studying must also be consistent and routine, occurring in the same space and at the same time if possible. A therapeutic environment is necessary for a child's school environment that includes scheduled breaks, verbal and visual instruction, and extra time for testing. It is best to complete academic tasks early in the morning with small class sizes to support learning (ATI Testing 2016).

## Medications

**Methylphenidate** or dextroamphetamine are psychostimulants that increase dopamine and norepinephrine levels. Medications are given 30 minutes before a meal. The last dose should be administered before 1800 to prevent disturbed sleep or insomnia, and caffeine is avoided. A tricyclic antidepressant can treat insomnia. Adverse effects include insomnia, anorexia, nervousness, hyper/hypotension, tachycardia, and anemia. Medications should be stored safely as this drug has the potential for abuse by people who do not have ADHD (ATI Testing 2016).

Atomoxetine is a selective norepinephrine reuptake inhibitor that increases concentrations of norepinephrine and epinephrine. It requires a gradual increase in dose to reach therapeutic results. This drug has less potential for abuse. The nurse must monitor for adverse effects such as suicidal ideation (ATI Testing 2016).

## Autism Spectrum Disorder

Autism Spectrum Disorder is a neurodevelopmental disorder with spectrum of behaviors that impact an individual's ability to communicate and create relationships with others in a social setting (see Fig 3-24). There is a potential genetic component to the disorder, but the exact cause is unknown (ATI Testing 2016).

**Thimerosal**, a vaccine preservative, was thought to precipitate autism in the MMR vaccine. However, autism has no definitive cause. The use of Thimerosal has stopped since 1999 in vaccines as a reassurance to the public (Ball L. K., Ball R., Pratt R. 2001).

### Assessment

Autism spectrum disorder creates developmental delays in at least of one of the following measures including social interaction, social communication, or imaginative play before 3 years of age. Children may show unusual distress when routines change; they may create unusual attachments to objects and lack the ability for free-flowing conversation. Children may use gestures instead of words, have delayed or absent language skills, or exhibit humming or grunting in place of words. Children with Autism may also have an inability to adjust their gaze to look at something new, referring to themselves using incorrect grammar, or become withdrawn or exhibit a labile mood, lack of empathy, and a decreased response to pain. Children often prefer time spent alone rather than with others, avoid eye contact, possess heightened or lowered senses. Children with Autism are not interested in imitating the actions of others or engaging in pretend play. They have a short attention span, intense temper tantrums, aggression, repetitive movements (**stimming**), and an IQ score less than 70 (ATI Testing 2016).

### Diagnostic Tools

The nurse may assist with screening tools or refer the family to specialist practitioners, such as the Denver II Developmental Screening Test, the Checklist for Autism in Toddlers (CHAT) or the Pervasive Developmental Disorders Screening Test (ATI Testing 2016).

### Interventions and Teaching

Early identification produces the best prognosis for children with Autism. A referral to early intervention, physical therapy, occupational therapy, and speech and language therapy benefits the child. Behavior modification is essential to promote positive reinforcement, increase social awareness, develop verbal communication, decrease or manage unacceptable behaviors, set realistic goals, create a structure to support small successes, set clear rules. In addition, children with Autism need reduced environmental stimulation, good nutritional,

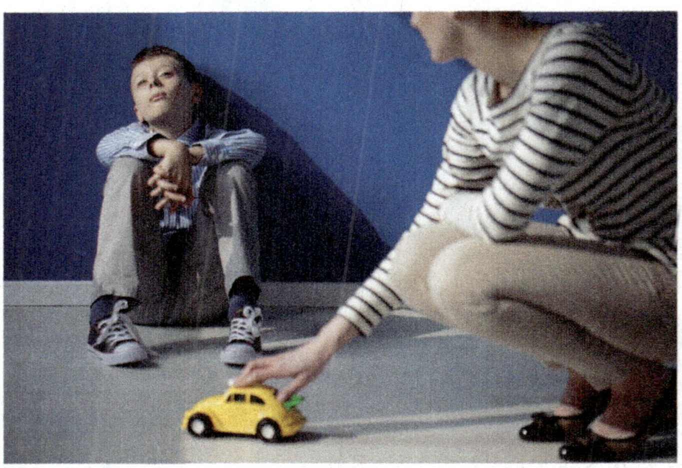

© Photographee.eu/Shutterstock.com

**Fig 3-24** A mother tries to engage her son with autism

and methodical way to introduce new situations. They need developmentally appropriate play to engage their attention. Communication must also be developmentally appropriate. The nurse must provide emotional support and resources for caregiver role strain such as support groups or therapy (ATI Testing 2016).

### Medications

Medications aim to control communication difficulties, social challenges, and stimming behaviors. Drugs aim to treat aggression, anxiety, hyperactivity, irritability, mood swings, compulsions, and attention problems. **Selective Serotonin Reuptake Inhibitors (SSRI)** are used to decrease aggression Antipsychotics, and melatonin can help with insomnia (ATI Testing 2016).

Practitioners order medications for use "off-label" to treat Autism. Therefore, more research is necessary to develop medications specifically for this pathology (ATI Testing 2016).

## Substance-Exposed Infants

Maternal substance ingestion during pregnancy consists of any use of alcohol or drugs. Intrauterine drug exposure can cause congenital anomalies, neurobehavioral changes, and evidence of withdrawal in the neonate. These changes are related to the particular drug or the combination of medicines used, the dosage, the route of administration, or metabolism and excretion by the mother and her fetus. In addition, the timing of exposure and length of exposure predicts severity. **Substance withdrawal** in the neonate happens when the serum concentration of the substance troughs causing withdrawal symptoms. These infants are cared for in the Neonatal Intensive Care Unit (NICU) (see Fig 3-25). These substances include heroin, opiates, alcohol, tobacco, methadone, and prescription medications (ATI Testing 2016).

Mothers who ingest alcohol may develop Fetal alcohol spectrum disorder (FASD), formerly referred to as fetal alcohol syndrome (FAS). Neonates with FASD develop the disease from the chronic or periodic use of alcohol during pregnancy. FASD is term used to describe a range of clinical effects. FAS refers to children who exhibit a triad of characteristic facial anomalies and growth delays with a confirmed history of maternal alcohol consumption. Neonates who have FAS are at risk for specific congenital physical defects, along with long-term complications (Nelson, M. M. 2013).

### Assessment

The neonatal abstinence scoring system directs the comprehensive assessment for substance-exposed infants. Neurological symptoms scored include increased wakefulness, a high-pitched, shrill cry, inconsolable

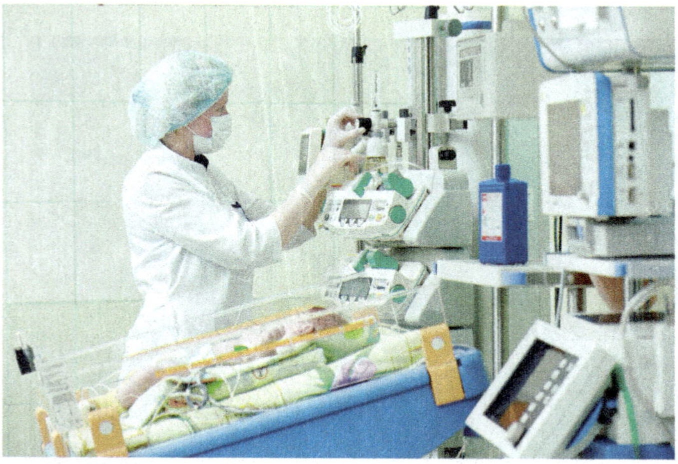



**Fig 3-25** Substance exposed infants are monitored in the nursery or Neonatal Intensive Care Unit (NICU) for withdrawal symptoms

crying, irritability, tremors, hyperactive responses to stimuli including an increased Moro reflex, increased deep-tendon reflexes, increased muscle tone, abrasions and excoriations on the face and knees, and seizures (ATI Testing 2016).

Newborns have metabolic, circulatory, and respiratory symptoms that include nasal congestion with flaring, frequent yawning, skin mottling, tachypnea greater than 60/minute, and sweating.

Infants respond to withdrawal in characteristic ways to certain substances (ATI Testing 2016).

## Heroin Withdrawal

Neonatal abstinence syndrome symptoms comprise of a low-birth weight and small for gestational age (SGA), decreased Moro reflexes (when typically increased), jittery, hyperactive, and hypothermia or hyperthermia. The infant has a shrill persistent cry (ATI Testing 2016).

## Methadone Withdrawal

Neonatal abstinence syndrome symptoms comprise of an increased incidence of seizures, sleep pattern disturbances, higher birth weights, and greater risk of sudden infant death syndrome (SIDS) (ATI Testing 2016).

## Cocaine Exposure

These babies can appear normal or exhibit neurologic problems at birth. Newborns can show neurobehavioral depression or excitability. High-pitched cry, abnormal sleep patterns, excessive sucking, hypertonicity, tremors, irritability, inability to console, and a reduced tolerance to changes in routine (ATI Testing 2016).

## Methamphetamine Withdrawal

Infants exposed to methamphetamine includes a small head circumference, SGA, agitation, vomiting, rapid respiratory rate, bradycardia or tachycardia, jitteriness, sleep pattern disturbances, emotional disturbances, and delayed growth and development (ATI Testing 2016).

## Fetal Alcohol Syndrome

Children with Fetal Alcohol Syndrome (FAS) display distinguishing craniofacial features such as microcephaly, small eyes with epicanthal folds, and short palpebral fissures, thin upper lip, flat midface and an ill-defined philtrum (Avital, O. M. 2017).

Children with FAS lack stranger-anxiety, and appropriate judgment skills. They may have many organ abnormalities, such as limb defect and heart defects, including ventricular septal defects. Children with FAS may experience prenatal and postnatal growth restriction, developmental delays and neurologic abnormalities, an IQ deficit, and diminished fine motor skills, and Attention Deficit Disorder (ATI Testing 2016).

## Tobacco Exposure

Children exposed to tobacco smoke often experience prematurity, low birth weight, an increased risk for SIDS, an increased risk for bronchitis, pneumonia, and developmental delays. Nurses will elicit neurological reflexes, assess for fluids and electrolytes imbalances, monitor for dehydration with skin turgor, mucous membranes, fontanels, input, and output status (ATI Testing 2016).

## Diagnostic Tests

Blood tests differentiate between neonatal drug withdrawal and central nervous system irritability. These tests include a CBC, blood glucose levels, calcium, electrolytes, and a drug screening of urine or meconium to identify any substances. (ATI Testing 2016).

A Complete Metabolic Panel may show electrolyte imbalances. A chest x-ray for children with FAS rules out congenital heart defects (ATI Testing 2016).

## Interventions

Interventions for maternal substance use and neonatal effects or withdrawal result from the continuous evaluation of the neonatal abstinence scoring system assessment. The nurse clusters nursing care (provides all nursing care at once) for newborns to minimize stimulation and decrease environmental stimuli. Children have difficulty feeding and digesting and must be given small, frequent, high-calorie meals with adequate fluid intake. The newborn may require **gavage feedings** (nasogastric feeding). Elevate the infant's head during and following feedings, and burp the newborn to reduce vomiting and aspiration. Specialized nipples may help babies with a weak suck reflex to feed. The nurse must have suction equipment available if the infant aspirates. Children receive IV hydration and electrolytes. The nurse should swaddle the newborn to reduce self-stimulation and protect the skin from abrasions (ATI Testing 2016).

For newborns addicted to cocaine, adults should avoid eye contact as it overstimulates the child. The use of vertical rocking and a pacifier may help.

A lactation consultation to evaluate whether breastfeeding is desired or contraindicated to avoid passing narcotics in breast milk. Infection prevention promotes the infant's growth and development. The nurse must initiate a consult with child protective services (ATI Testing 2016).

## Medications

### *Phenobarbital*

Phenobarbital works as an anticonvulsant. It decreases CNS irritability and controls seizures.

### *Morphine and Clonidine*

Morphine and clonidine decrease central nervous system irritability.

### *Methadone*

Infants and mothers receive **methadone** for heroin or methadone addiction. There are no contraindications for methadone during breastfeeding (ATI Testing 2016).

## Teaching

The mother needs a referral to a drug and alcohol treatment center. If the mother used or now uses methadone, then explain the importance of increased SIDS rates in infants of mothers who used methadone during pregnancy (ATI Testing 2016).

# CHAPTER HIGHLIGHTS

- The neurological system is a complex network of nerves and supportive cells that relay messages back and forth from the brain to the body.
- Bacterial meningitis is potentially life-threatening and can cause long-term effects. There may be cognitive, behavioral, or hearing deficits.

- Reye's syndrome is a rare encephalopathy that can result in death. The syndrome manifests with a combination of aspirin and a viral illness like influenza or chickenpox.
- Prolonged, generalized seizures are known as status epilepticus and are medical emergencies. Airway management, supplemental oxygen, and benzodiazepines treat these seizures.
- Traumatic brain injury is the leading cause of death for children. Trauma from falls, motor vehicle accidents, and non-accidental injury are the primary reasons.
- Concussions are head injuries that may precipitate a loss of consciousness. They are mild diffuse axonal injuries that occur from the stretching, shearing, or compression of axons during an impact to the head. They result in dizziness, headache, unsteady gait, or amnesia.
- Down's syndrome encompasses a broad range of congenital anomalies related to a genetic disorder. This disorder originates from the abnormal division of chromosome cells at chromosome 21.
- Cerebral palsy results from damage to the cerebrum, or the region of the brain that controls motor function. The disorder affects muscle tone, coordination, and posture.
- Spina bifida is an incomplete closure of the spine and spinal cord that causes a herniation of the meninges and possibly, the spinal nerves. Spina bifida may present as meningocele, myelomeningocele, and spina bifida occulta. Folic acid prevents spina bifida.
- Hydrocephalus results from the accumulation of CSF in the brain. The CSF does not circulate, obstructed by blockages or the inability of the cerebral ventricles to absorb CSF. Hydrocephalus can occur related to congenital anomalies or infections, hemorrhages, or tumors that increase intracranial pressure.
- Although the pathophysiology of ADHD still eludes scientists, it is thought to create deficits in the neurotransmitters catecholamine, dopamine, and norepinephrine. Stimulants create a paradoxical effect on the neuropathways in children with ADHD.
- Autism spectrum disorder is a disorder that creates a developmental delay. It impairs social interactions and communication skills.
- Children exposed to illicit drugs in utero can develop Neonatal Abstinence Syndrome and experience withdrawal symptoms. A multidisciplinary approach allows for the detoxification of the infant and treatment for the mother.

## REFERENCES


Adzick, N. S. 2012. "Fetal Surgery for Myelomeningocele: Trials and Tribulations." *Journal of Pediatric Surgery*, 47(2), 273–81. http://doi.org/10.1016/j.jpedsurg.2011.11.021.

Anatomy and Physiology II Laboratory Manual, 3rd Ed. 2016. [Bookshelf Online]. Retrieved from https://online.vitalsource.com/#/books/9781465292582/.

ATI Testing. 2016. Nursing Care of Children. Retrieved from http://www.atitesting.com/ati_next_gen/DisplayResources.aspx?Name=rm_rn_ncc_2016_ebook_20170417.pdf.

Avital, O. M. (2017). Fetal Alcohol Syndrome. CINAHL Nursing Guide.

Ball L. K , Ball R , Pratt R. D. 2001. An assessment of Thimerosal use in childhood vaccines. *Pediatrics*, 1147–1154.

Caple, C. M., & Schub, E. B. (2017). Seizure Precautions for Children: Initiating and Maintaining. CINAHL Nursing Guide.

Caple, C. M., & Schub, T. B. (2016). Lumbar Puncture. CINAHL Nursing Guide.

Dowling, J. 2004. *The great brain debate nature or nurture?* Washington, D.C.: Joseph Henry Press.

Furay, C., & Howell, T. (2010). Paediatric neuroanaesthesia. Continuing Education In Anaesthesia, Critical Care & Pain, 10(6), 172–176.

Immunization Schedules. (2017, February 06). Retrieved September 01, 2017, from https://www.cdc.gov/vaccines/schedules/hcp/imz/child-adolescent.html.

Jaffe, S. A. (2016). Reye's Syndrome. CINAHL Nursing Guide.

Kabir, S., Rajaraman, C., Rittey, C., Zaki, H., Kemeny, A., & McMullan, J. (2009). Vagus nerve stimulation in children with intractable epilepsy: indications, complications and outcome. Child's Nervous System, 25(9), 1097. doi:10.1007/s00381-009-0849-z

Klimo, J. R., Matthews, A., Lew, S. M., Zwienenberg-Lee, M., and Kaufman, B. A. 2011. Minicraniotomy versus bur holes for evacuation of chronic subdural collections in infants-a preliminary single-institution experience. Retrieved July 13, 2017, from https://www.ncbi.nlm.nih.gov/pubmed/22044363.

Kutscher, M. L. (2006). Children with seizures : a guide for parents, teachers, and other professionals. Retrieved from https://ebookcentral-proquest-com.chamberlainuniversity.idm.oclc.org

March, P. P., & Schub, T. B. (2017). Autism Spectrum Disorder. CINAHL Nursing Guide.

Meningitis. 2017. Retrieved July 09, 2017, from https://www.cdc.gov/meningitis/index.html.

Nelson, M. M. (2013). Neonatal Abstinence Syndrome: The Nurse's Role. International Journal Of Childbirth Education, 28(1), 38–42.

(Rana, M., Upadhyay, J., Rana, A., Durgapal, S., & Jantwal, A. (2017). A Systematic Review on Etiology, Epidemiology, and Treatment of Cerebral Palsy. International Journal Of Nutrition, Pharmacology, Neurological Diseases, 7(4), 76–83. doi:10.4103/ijnpnd.ijnpnd_26_17

Reynolds, C. R. ,Vannest, K. J & Fletcher-Janzen, E. (Eds.) (2013). Ketogenic diet. Encyclopedia of special education: a reference for the education of children, adolescents, and adults with disabilities and other exceptional individuals (4th ed.). Hoboken, NJ: Wiley. Retrieved from https://chamberlainuniversity.idm.oclc.org/login?url=http://search.credoreference.com/content/entry/wileyse/ketogenic_diet/0?institutionId=8802

Schub, T. B., & Boling, B. C. (2016). Down Syndrome. CINAHL Nursing Guide.

Shorvon, S. D. (2010). Handbook of epilepsy treatment. Retrieved from https://ebookcentral-proquest-com.chamberlainuniversity.idm.oclc.org

Stephenson, J. P. B., & King, M. (Eds.). (2009). Handbook of neurological investigations in children. Retrieved from http://ebookcentral.proquest.com.chamberlainuniversity.idm.oclc.org

Teddy, S., Latief, A., and Madiyono, B. 2016. "Profile of children with increased intracranial pressure on mannitol treatment." *Paediatrica Indonesiana*, 44(4), 148–152. doi: http://dx.doi.org/10.14238/pi44.4.2004.148–52.

Thompson, R. (Ed.). (2012). Adhd : cognitive symptoms, genetics and treatment outcomes. Retrieved from https://ebookcentral-proquest-com.chamberlainuniversity.idm.oclc.org

Wallace, D. C., & Cartwright, C. C. (2007). Nursing Care of the Pediatric Neurosurgery Patient. Berlin: Springer.

Whitfield, P. C. (2009). Head Injury : A Multidisciplinary Approach. Cambridge: Cambridge University Press.

Wolfe, P. 2010. Brain Matters: Translating Research into Classroom Practice (2). Alexandria, US: ASCD. Retrieved from http://www.ebrary.com.proxy.chamberlain.edu:8080.

Woten, M. B., & Mennella, H. A. (2017). Intracranial Pressure Monitoring: Performing in the Pediatric Patient. CINAHL Nursing Guide.

CHAPTER 4

# CARING FOR CHILDREN WITH RESPIRATORY CONDITIONS

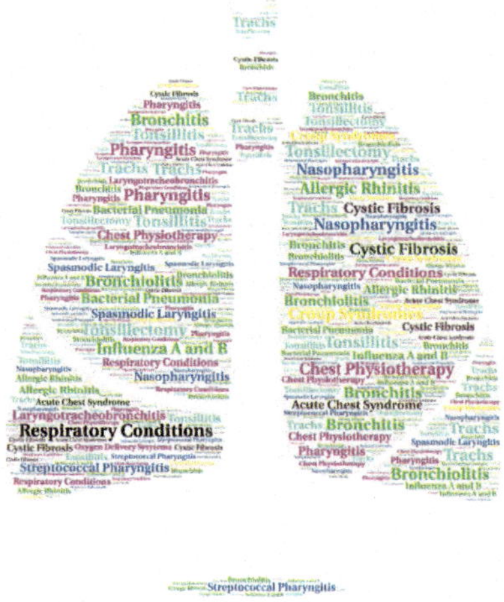


Modified from Shutterstock. Original image © Pikovit/Shutterstock.com

## LEARNING OUTCOMES

1. Describe the anatomical differences between children and adults, and integrate care for children with respiratory conditions.
2. Recognize different respiratory conditions that cause impaired breathing and respiratory distress in children.
3. Synthesize data from evidence-based practice, physical assessment, developmental milestones, and the family members to create a plan of care for children with respiratory conditions.
4. Plan nursing interventions and evaluate outcomes for children with chronic respiratory conditions in the home setting.
5. Utilize the nursing process to provide safe and comprehensive health care to children with respiratory conditions.
6. Teaching/learning principles in providing anticipatory guidance in the prevention and treatment of health problems in maternal and medical/surgical settings.

## KEY TERMS

Adenoids
Antihistamines
Antipyretic
Beta-adrenergic
Beta lactam antibiotic
Cephalosporins
Corticosteroids
Decongestants
Dry powder inhalers
Dysphonia
Eustachian tube
Group a beta-hemolytic streptococcal infections (GABHS)
Hemoptysis
Immunoglobin E (IgE)
Inspiratory stridor
Ipratropium
Leukotriene modifiers
Macrolide
Mast cell stabilizers
Metered dose inhalers
Nasal smear
Nebulized racemic epinephrine
Pharyngeal tonsils

The respiratory system is the most critical organ system to be assessed in children, because it is the most often affected. The respiratory system is particularly vulnerable, because it is one of the last systems to develop in the human body. Thus, it is more susceptible to acute and chronic illness until the lungs and the immune system mature.

An infant's lungs do not begin to work until the first breath occurs at birth. However, by 3–6 months of age, the immune system loses the benefit of maternal antibodies that create resistance to infection. Infants, who do not breastfeed, do not receive immune system support during the first several months. Viral infections peak in the preschool and toddler years, and decrease after 5 years of age as the immune system strengthens. Therefore, viral agents that cause serious illness in infancy may only cause mild illness in older children (ATI Testing 2016).

The anatomy of a child's respiratory system makes him or her more vulnerable than adults. Children have a short, narrow airway that causes airway resistance, easily occludes with mucus or edema, and subsequently causes infections (see Fig 4-1) (ATI Testing 2016). Children also have weak intercostals that are not effective until after 6 years of age (ATI Testing 2016). Children also consume more oxygen than adults do, and have higher oxygen requirements during respiratory distress (see Fig 4-3) (ATI Testing 2016). An infant's airway may be no larger than a diameter of a straw, or 4 mm. A child's middle finger can roughly estimate the diameter of the airway (Adewale, L. 2009).

Infections quickly travel to the lower airways and the middle ear. Pathogens enter the middle ear through a short **Eustachian tube** (ATI Testing 2016). The severity of these issues increases if the child has decreased resistance related to poor nutrition, anemia, a compromised immune system, or breathing second-hand smoke. Prevention includes frequent hand washing, isolation from others with the infection, and a healthy diet high in nutrients such as Vitamin D and zinc (Allan, G. M. and Arroll, B. 2014; Bhutta, Z.A., 2017).

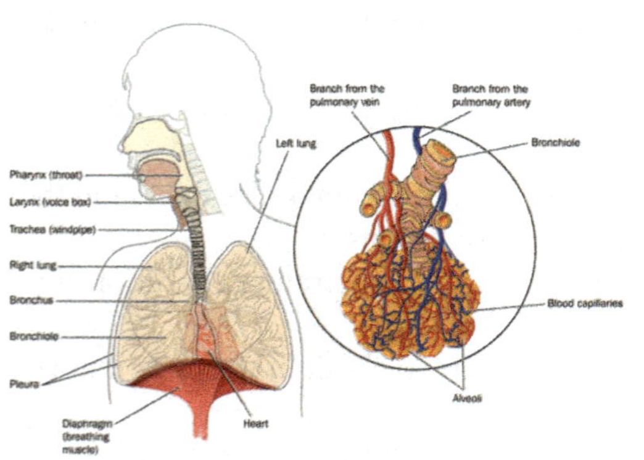


Fig 4-1 Respiratory system anatomy

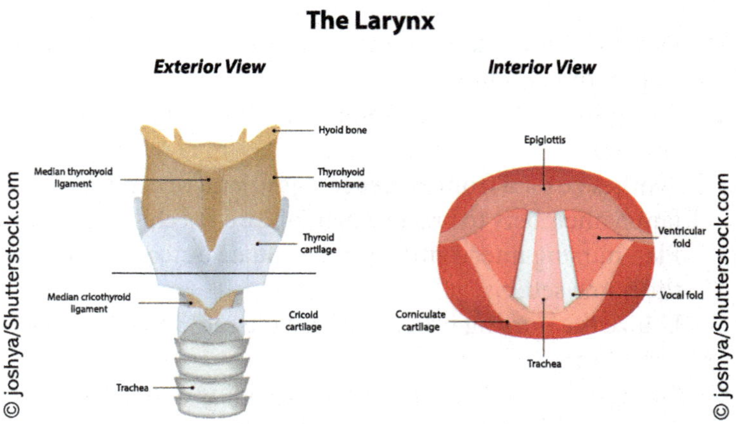


Fig 4-2 Anatomy of the larynx

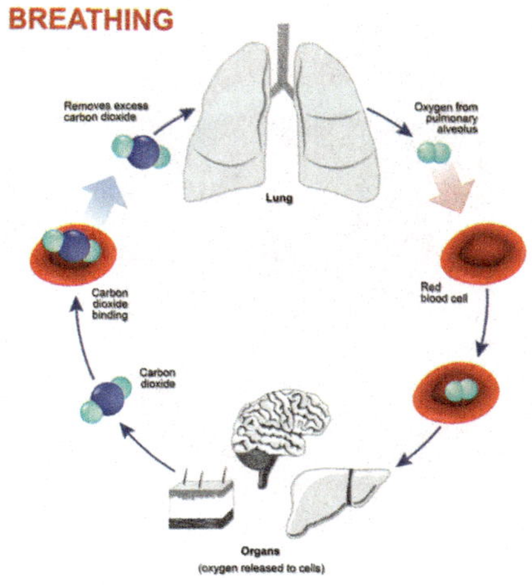




**Fig 4-3** Oxygen circulation

When the weather gets cold, children experience respiratory infections such as Respiratory Syncytial Virus (RSV) and Mycoplasma pneumoniae, probably as a result of close contact with other human beings as a consequence of the cold weather. Children with chronic respiratory diseases, such as Asthma or Cystic Fibrosis, have a greater incidence of respiratory infections.

Acute and infectious respiratory illnesses often present with a sore throat in children. A sore throat can become allergic rhinitis, nasopharyngitis, pharyngitis, tonsillitis, bacterial epiglottis, croup, bronchitis, bronchiolitis, pneumonia, or Influenza A and B. Illnesses affect the upper (oronasopharynx, pharynx, larynx, and upper part of the trachea) and/or lower (bronchi, bronchioles, and alveoli) respiratory tracts (ATI Testing 2016).

# ACUTE RESPIRATORY CONDITIONS

## Respiratory Assessment

The nursing assessment starts with the history of the illness that includes recent infections, medications taken, immunization status, and family coping. Assessment findings may include a sore throat, decreased activity level, chest pain, fatigue, difficulty breathing, shortness of breath, cough, and decreased appetite. Viral infections present as red and swollen throat infections. Bacterial infections may duplicate the viral presentation with potential additional symptoms such as a swollen uvula, white spots, and a gray furry tongue (see Fig 4-4). Viral infections generally need supportive care and bacterial infections require antibiotic therapy (ATI Testing 2016).

## Allergic Rhinitis

Allergic rhinitis creates a seasonal reaction to allergens, typically in the fall or spring. Symptoms include watery **rhinorrhea** (a runny nose), stuffy nose, irritation and itching of the eyes, nose, pharynx, snoring, fatigue, malaise, headache, and poor performance in school (ATI testing 2016).

### Assessment

Children may present with a high fever, tachypnea, or a pale color that progresses to cyanosis. Children can show irritability, restlessness, and lethargy. Symptoms of chest pain, dullness upon percussion with adventitious breath sounds (rhonchi, fine crackles), a productive or a nonproductive cough, retractions, nasal flaring can occur. Children can experience abdominal pain, diarrhea, lack of appetite, and vomiting (ATI Testing 2016).

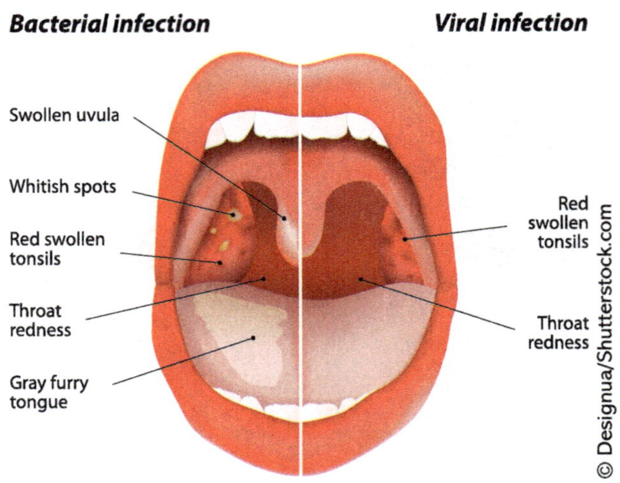


**Fig 4-4** Viral versus bacterial sore throats

### Diagnostic Tests

A **nasal smear** collected from nasal secretions measures the number of eosinophils and level of IgE antibodies. IgE antibody mediates the body's response to allergens. Eosinophils signify inflammation. Blood samples also reveal increased total **Immunoglobin (IgE)** and eosinophils and confirm allergic rhinitis. Both IgE and eosinophil levels increase with allergic rhinitis. Children may also need skin tests or various challenge tests to determine the offending allergen (ATI Testing 2016).

### Interventions, Medication, and Teaching

The nurses and parents administer medications such as **corticosteroids, antihistamines, beta-adrenergic decongestants, mast cell stabilizers, leukotriene modifiers,** and **ipratropium**. Parents should receive instruction about the specific allergen and ways to avoid exposure. Parents must also learn how to administer corticosteroids, antihistamines, beta-adrenergic decongestants, mast cell stabilizers, leukotriene modifiers, and ipratropium, as ordered by the doctor or nurse practitioner. New interventions for seasonal allergic rhinitis include injection immunotherapy (New therapies with (Doyle, M. J. 2017; Calderon MA, Alves B, Jacobson M, Hurwitz B, Sheikh A, Durham S. 2007).

## Nasopharyngitis

Nasopharyngitis is the common cold (see Fig 4-5). It is a self-limiting virus that lasts for 4–10 days (ATI Testing 2016).

### Assessment

Children present with a fever, decreased appetite and restlessness, sneezing, irritability, difficulty sleeping, decreased appetite and dryness and irritation of nasal and pharynx passages (see Fig 4-6) (ATI Testing 2016).

### Interventions and Teaching

Children recover at home with the help of their parents. Parents administer an **antipyretic** for fevers. Although fevers are a therapeutic response to pathogens, children have an immature immune system and should receive ibuprofen; it is more effective than acetaminophen (Allan, G M., and Arroll, B. 2014). Parents may give decongestants for children older than 6 years of age, and cough suppressants using care to not over sedate the child. The child needs rest and vaporized air (cool mist).

Children do not need antihistamines or antibiotics (ATI Testing 2016).

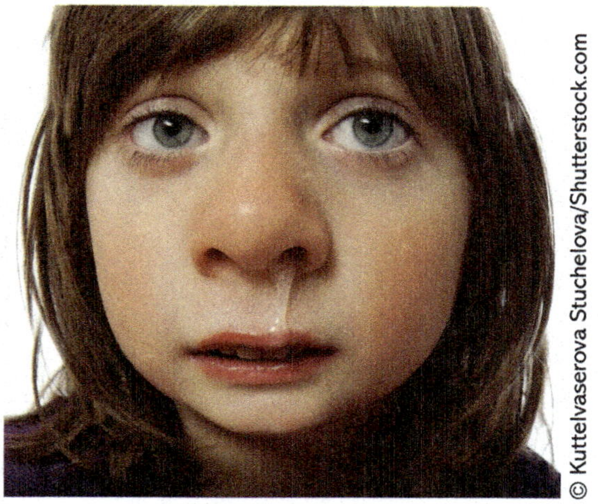


Fig 4-5 Child with a common cold

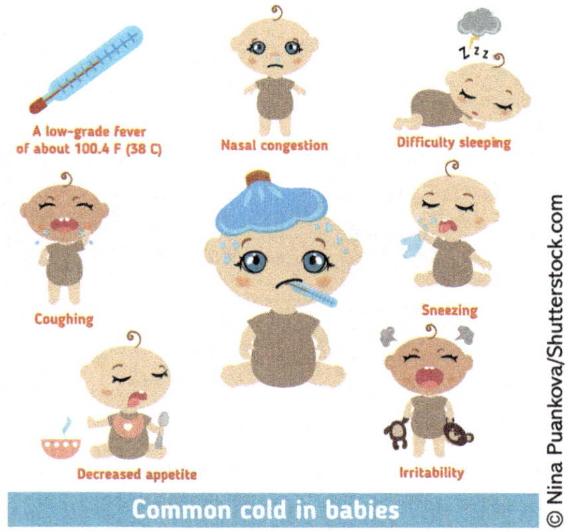


Fig 4-6 Symptoms of the common cold

## Acute Streptococcal Pharyngitis (Strep Throat)

**Group A beta-hemolytic streptococcal infections (GABHS)** is an infection of the upper airway (ATI Testing 2016).

### Assessment

GABHS infections present with an abrupt onset characterized by pharyngitis, headache, fever and abdominal pain. The tonsils and pharynx reveal inflammation and a coating of exudate that usually appears by the second day of illness (ATI Testing 2016).

### Diagnostic Tests

A throat culture or rapid antigen testing diagnoses GABHS infection (ATI Testing 2016).

### Interventions, Medications, and Teaching

Parents will administer antipyretics for fever. The child receives a **beta-lactam antibiotic** (penicillin or amoxicillin) or a **macrolide** (erythromycin) antibiotic. Parents give oral penicillin or amoxicillin for at least 10 days, or the provider can administer IM penicillin G benzathine. For penicillin allergies oral erythromycin, clarithromycin, azithromycin, clindamycin, and oral **cephalosporins** are effective to treat GABHS. Parents must complete the entire course of antibiotics (ATI Testing 2016).

## Tonsillitis and Tonsillectomy

Tonsils are mounds of lymph-type tissue found in the pharynx (see Fig 4-7). Tonsils fight respiratory and gastrointestinal infections. They filter pathogenic organisms by producing B cells that secrete antibodies. Acute tonsillitis occurs when the tonsils become inflamed and reddened. Acute tonsillitis can become chronic (ATI Testing 2016).

Chronic throat infection (more than 7 in a year) or sleep disordered breathing (a sleep related breathing abnormality) are indications for tonsillectomy (Clinical Practice Guideline 2011).

In some instances, enlarged tonsils can block the nose and throat (see Fig 4-8). Blockages interfere with normal breathing, sinus drainage, sleeping, swallowing, and speaking. They may also affect the function of the Eustachian tube, leading to otitis media or hearing deficits. **Pharyngeal tonsils** referred to as the **adenoids** may

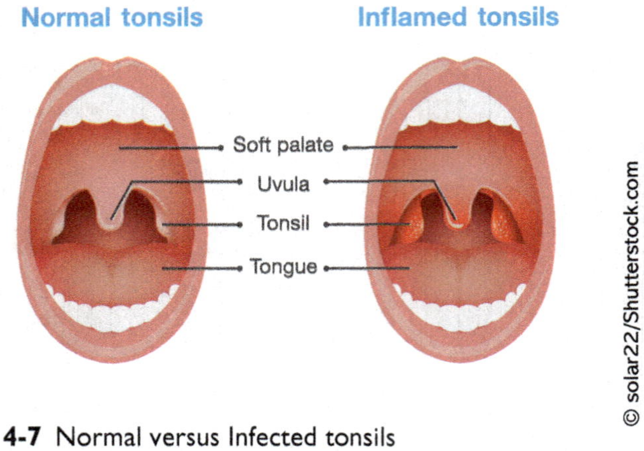


**Fig 4-7** Normal versus Infected tonsils

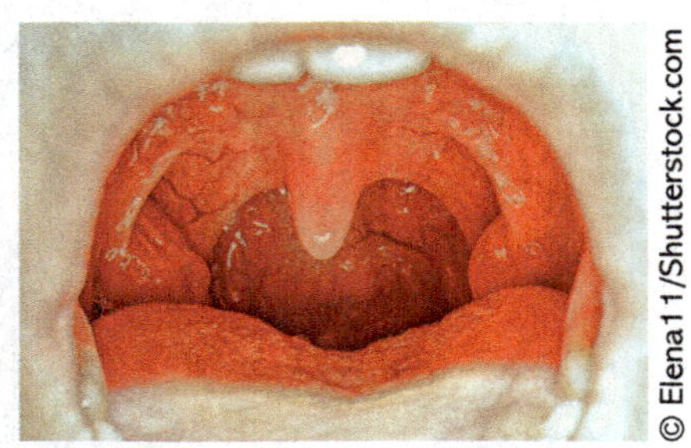


**Fig 4-8** Tonsillitis

need removal during a surgical procedure called an adenoidectomy. Chronically infected tonsils with GABHS can threaten the heart or kidney via rheumatic fever or glomerulonephritis (ATI Testing 2016).

## Assessment

Children complain of a sore throat with difficulty swallowing with a history of respiratory infection, otitis media, or hearing problems. Children present with tonsil inflammation, fever, mouth breathing, mouth odor, snoring, and a nasal quality to their voice (ATI Testing 2016).

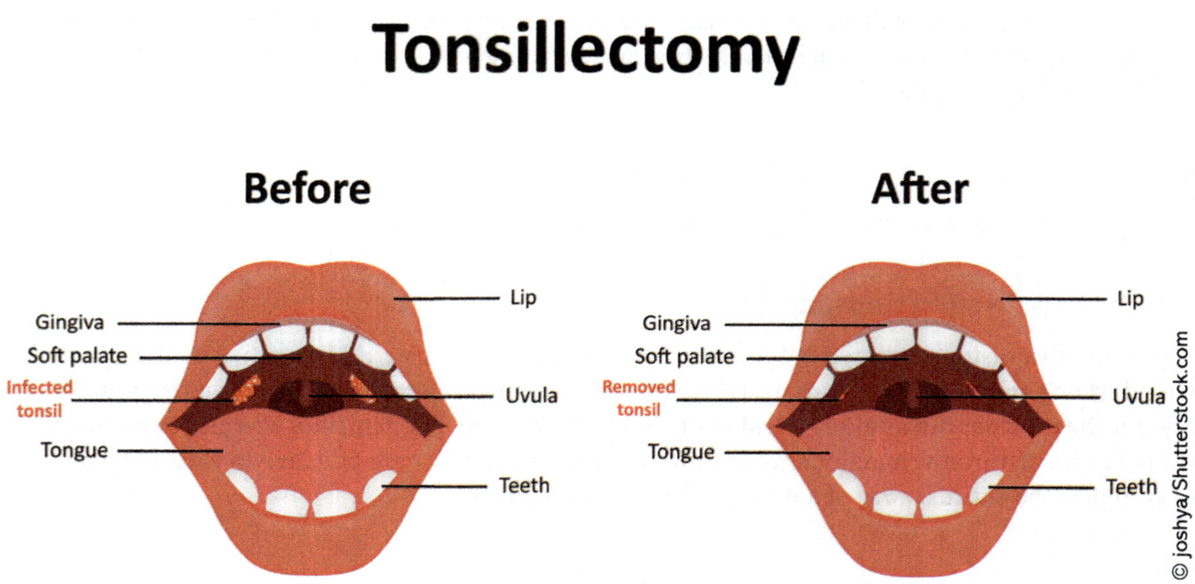


**Fig 4-9** Tonsillectomy

## Tonsillectomy Hemorrhage Assessment

Assess the child for a patent airway related to secretions, edema or difficulty breathing, and vital signs. Signs of bleeding include frequent swallowing, clearing the throat, restlessness, bright red emesis, tachycardia, and/or pallor. The nurse assesses for signs of bleeding tachycardia, repeated swallowing and clearing of the throat, and **hemoptysis** (blood-tinged sputum). Hypotension manifests as a late sign of shock and demands an urgent call to the provider. The nurse should report the tachycardia to the provider as an early sign of shock. (ATI Testing 2016).

### Diagnostic Tests

A throat culture for group A beta-hemolytic streptococci (GABHS) evaluates the pathogen causing the inflammation (ATI Testing 2016).

### Interventions for Tonsillectomy (see Fig 4-9)

Dehydration requires IV fluid administration and strict Input and Output (I&O) monitoring. Supportive care that includes rest, warm fluids, warm salt-water gargles are appropriate for viral tonsillitis. However, bacterial tonsillitis requires an antibiotic prescription (ATI Testing 2016).

The child needs comfort measures including using liquid analgesics or tetracaine lollipops on a regular schedule as prescribed, and use of an ice collar, ice chips or sips of water.

The child's diet needs modification to include clear liquids and fluids after a return of the gag reflex, avoidance of red-colored fluids so that identification of blood is possible. Children refrain from citrus juice, and milk-based foods. The nurse advances the diet to soft and bland foods. The child should not clear the throat, cough, use straws, or blow the nose to protect the surgical site (ATI Testing 2016).

Parents should understand that there can be clots or blood-tinged mucus in the vomitus. However, they should notify the nurse or provider, if bright red bleeding occurs, the child has excessive swallowing, experiences difficulty in breathing, has difficulty with oral intake, has an increase in pain, or any indications of infection.

Parents must ensure objects stay out of the child's mouth. The child and family should temporarily limit activity to decrease the potential for bleeding. A full recovery can take approximately 14 days (ATI Testing 2016).

### Medications

Children receive antipyretics/analgesics to reduce fever and pain (acetaminophen or ibuprofen), and hydrocodone, if the child cannot drink fluids. Parents must learn appropriate weight-based dosages for their particular child, to prevent overdosing in the home setting. Parents must administer the entire prescription to the child for an effective outcome (ATI Testing 2016).

## Bacterial Epiglottitis (Acute Supraglottitis)

Bacterial epiglottitis creates a swelling of the epiglottis that occludes the airway and is a medical emergency usually caused by *Haemophilus influenza* (ATI Testing 2016).

### Assessment

There are predictive signs associated with epiglottitis, including the absence of a cough, excessive drooling, and agitation. Children characteristically assume the tripod position, where they sit upright with the chin pointing out, mouth opened, with the tongue protruding. Children have **dysphonia** or a muffled, froglike, croaking voice. Children have dysphagia (difficulty swallowing) of their own secretions that cause drooling. An **inspiratory stridor** (noisy inspirations) presents with suprasternal and substernal retractions. Children have a sore throat, high fever, and are unsettled (ATI Testing 2016).

### Diagnostic Test

A lateral neck radiograph of the soft tissues confirms the swelling of the epiglottis (ATI Testing 2016).

### Interventions, Medications, and Teaching

The nurse must protect the airway by avoiding a throat culture or using a tongue blade. The nurse prepares for intubation. The nurse implements droplet isolation precautions for the first 24 hours after IV antibiotics begin. Humidified oxygen and continuous pulse oximetry keep oxygen saturation within normal limits. The nurse initiates IV hydration, corticosteroids, and IV antibiotic therapy. The parents complete a 10-day course of oral antibiotics as prescribed. Parents must understand the rationale for completing the entire course of antibiotics (ATI Testing 2016).

## Acute Laryngotracheobronchitis (ALTB) or Croup

Acute Laryngotracheobronchitis occurs when RSV, influenza A and B, Mycoplasma pneumonia, or Parainfluenza types 1, 2, and 3 create a distinctive cough known as croup (ATI Testing 2016).

### Assessment

Children present with a low-grade fever, restlessness, hoarseness, a barky cough, dyspnea, inspiratory stridor, and retractions. In addition, infants may display nasal flaring, intercostal retractions, tachypnea, and continuous stridor (see Fig 4-10) (ATI Testing 2016).

### Interventions, Medications, and Teaching

Oxygen administered with a cool mist maintains oxygen saturation within normal limits. IV fluids or oral intake maintain hydration that prevents dehydration and thins mucus secretions. The nurse or a respiratory therapist gives **nebulized racemic epinephrine**, corticosteroids: oral or IM (dexamethasone), or nebulized (budesonide) as prescribed. Medications are given through a nebulizer transform liquid medications into a fine mist dispersed through a mask and into the respiratory tract. These droplets create a fine spray, with smaller drops than those created by inhalers. Parents can use cool or warm humidity to subside a croup attack at home, but they should bring the child in for evaluation, if the child had difficulty breathing (ATI Testing 2016).

A best practices recommendation for any child with mild, moderate, or severe croup symptoms is to receive one dose of corticosteroids in the Emergency Department (Cincinnati Children's Hospital Medical Center 2011).

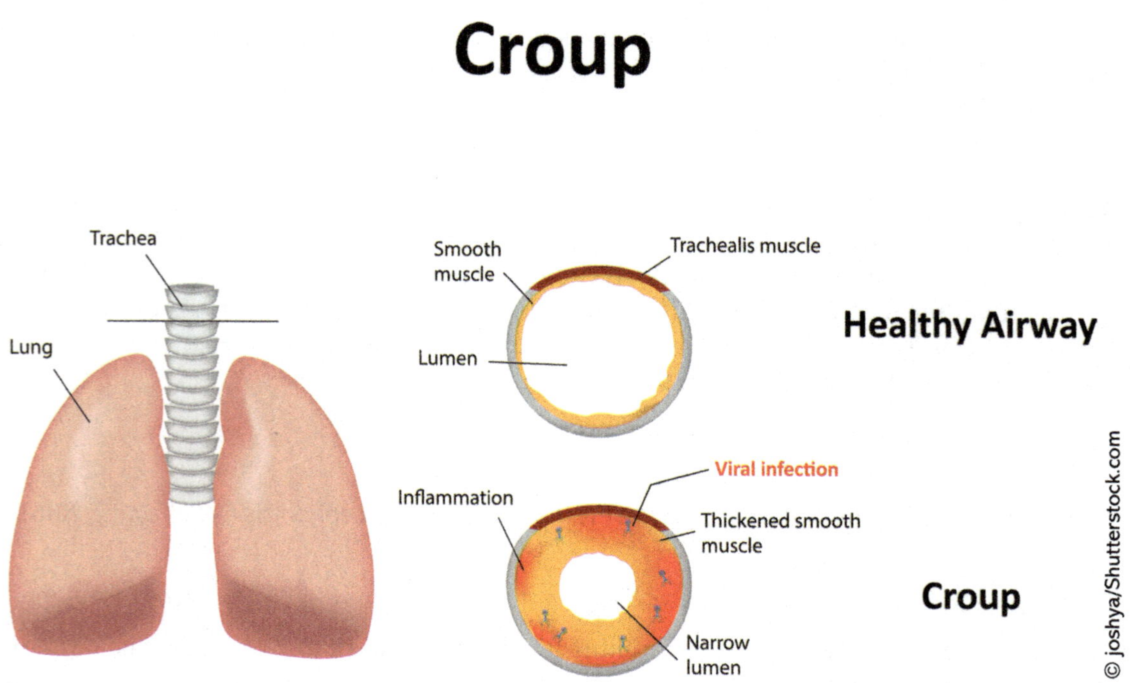


**Fig 4-10** Croup causes the child's airway lumen to narrow

# Bronchitis

Bronchitis consists of a self-limiting upper respiratory infection and inflammation of the large airways (see Fig 4-11) (ATI Testing 2016).

## Assessment

Children present with a persistent dry, hacking cough as a related to inflammation of the bronchial tubes that usually resolves in 5–10 days (ATI Testing 2016).

## Diagnostic Test

The nurse sends nasopharyngeal secretions to the lab for evaluation (ATI Testing 2016).

## Interventions, Medications, and Teaching

Parents care for children in the home setting. Parents are taught to administer an antipyretic agent and a cough suppressant. They should humidify the air with a cool mist vaporizer (ATI Testing 2016).

# Bronchiolitis

Bronchiolitis causes inflammation in the smaller airway passages or bronchioles (see Fig 4-12). RSV (Respiratory Syncytial Virus) commonly causes inflammation of the bronchioles. Preterm children are most susceptible (ATI Testing 2016).

## Assessment

The initial presentation includes rhinorrhea, intermittent fever, pharyngitis, coughing, sneezing, wheezing, and possible ear or eye infection.

As the pathology progresses children display increased coughing and sneezing, fever, tachypnea and retractions, refusal to nurse or bottle feed, and copious secretions. Once the disease becomes severe, tachypnea (greater than 70/min), listlessness, apneic spells, poor air exchange, poor breath sounds, cyanosis characterize the disease (ATI Testing 2016).

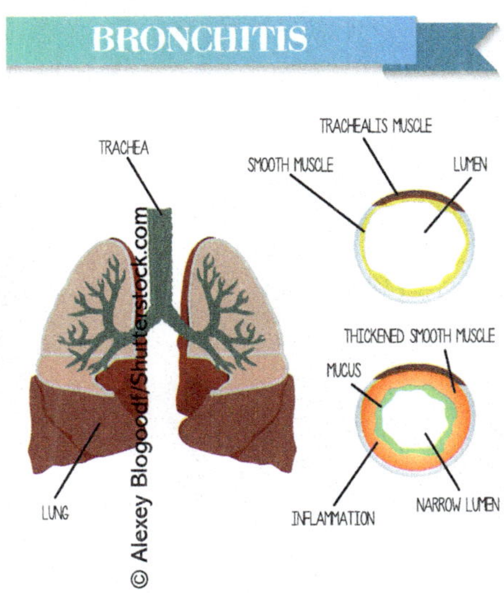


**Fig 4-11** Inflammation in Bronchitis (tracheobronchitis)

## Diagnostic Tests

The nurse collects nasopharyngeal secretions. The lab uses either rapid immunofluorescent antibody-direct fluorescent antibody staining or enzyme-linked immunosorbent assay techniques for RSV antigen detection (see Fig 4-12) (ATI Testing 2016).

## Interventions

The nurse's priorities are the child's airway and supplemental oxygen to maintain an oxygen saturation equal to or greater than 90%. The child should be breastfed or given oral intake. If the child cannot, IV fluids meet fluid needs until the acute phase has passed. The nurse may use nasopharyngeal or nasal suctioning as needed.

Medications may include antibiotics if a coexisting bacterial infection presents; however, corticosteroids and bronchodilators produce ineffective results. The nurse should also refrain from chest physiotherapy (ATI Testing 2016).

### Clinical Pearl

For more than 50 years, uncuffed tracheal tubes were used for endotracheal intubation. The standard has been to use these uncuffed tubes in children under 8 years of age because the pediatric larynx (see Fig 4-2) was assumed to be funnel-shaped and the concern that the cuff will cause damage to the airway mucosa, creating subglottic stenosis. According to Motoyama, this assumption is incorrect (Motoyama, E. K. 2014). Regardless of this difference there are known issues with uncuffed tracheal tubes including ventilation leaks around the tube. These leaks yield false readings of end-tidal carbon dioxide monitoring and increased costs of inhaled anesthetics, increased pollution of the environment, and an increased risk of aspiration. Randomized Controlled Trials (RCTs) and prospective cohort studies reveal new cuffed endotracheal tubes reduce the need for tracheal tube exchanges and do not increase the risk for post-extubation stridor compared with uncuffed ETTs (Shi, F., Xiao, Y., Xiong, W., Zhou, Q., and Huang, X. 2016).

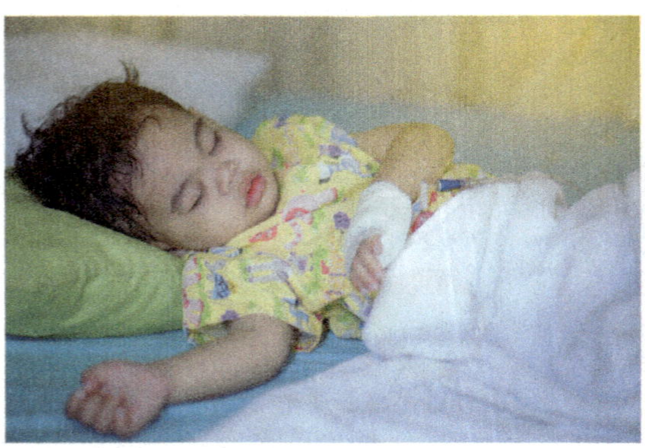



**Fig 4-12** Infant with RSV resting

Respiratory Syncytial Virus

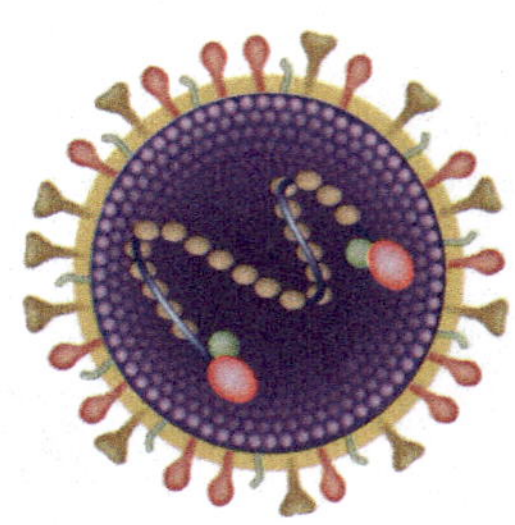



**Fig 4-12** RSV is the most common pathogen that causes bronchiolitis

## QSEN Application

According to QSEN, Evidence-Based Practice (EBP) requires nurses to "integrate best current evidence with clinical expertise and patient/family preferences and values for delivery of optimal health care and use health research methods and processes, alone or in partnership with scientists, to generate new knowledge for practice".

The best practice guidelines come from randomized, controlled trials. Nurses should seek out these types of studies when implementing EBP (From Quality and Safety Education for Nurses http://qsen.org/competencies/pre-licensure-ksas/)

Children with severe manifestations may need mechanical ventilation and a possible tracheotomy. A tracheotomy creates a secure, artificial airway into the trachea. Artificial airways are placed orotracheally, nasotracheally, or through a tracheostomy that connects to a ventilator (ATI Testing 2016).

Pediatric tracheostomy tubes have a more acute angle than adult tubes. They become malleable with body temperature and curve with the shape of the child's trachea. Pediatric tubes have no inner cannula because the plastic or silastic material prevents the collection of dried secretions. Nursing considerations include oxygenation, ventilation (respiratory rate, effort, oxygen saturation, and hourly vital signs. The nurse should not suction routinely, but only as often as necessary to maintain patency of the tube, audible/noisy secretions, crackles, restlessness, tachypnea, tachycardia, and mucus in the airway (ATI Testing 2016). Coarse crackles are low pitched sounds that sound like bubbling; fine crackles are high pitched sounds that sound like a fire crackling.

Excessive suctioning can cause mucosal damage, bleeding, bronchospasm, and increase infection risk. The nurse uses a surgical aseptic technique during suctioning to prevent infection. The nurse should provide tracheostomy care every 8 hours and change disposable tracheostomy tubes every 6–8 weeks or as per protocol. The nurse should reposition the child every 2 hours to prevent atelectasis, pneumonia, and skin breakdown. The nurse will keep an emergency tracheostomy tube (one size smaller) at the bedside in case of decannulation. The nurse monitors the tracheostomy site for drainage or breakdown. The nurse cleans the stoma with soap and water. If there is an event of accidental decannulation during the first 72 hours after surgery is an emergency. The tracheostomy has not healed and replacement requires a smaller tube. The nurse should change or replace a tracheostomy tube with another RN for safety reasons. Parents caring for the tube at home must have a second tube and scissors to cut the old strings in the event of decannulation (ATI Testing 2016).

### Teaching

Children can receive the medication, palivizumab, once per month during the RSV season (From November through April). Parents must understand the commitment to prevent future cases of bronchiolitis (Bollani, L. et al. 2015).

## Viral and Bacterial Pneumonia

Bacterial Pneumonia manifests from a Streptococcus pneumoniae, Group A streptococci, Staphylococcus aureus, Mycoplasma catarrhalis, or Mycoplasma pneumoniae infection (see Fig 4-14) (ATI Testing 2016).

### Assessment

Children present with a high fever, tachypnea, retractions and nasal flaring, and a cough that can be unproductive or productive with white sputum. Children experience chest pain, dullness with percussion, adventitious breath sounds (rhonchi, fine crackles), and a pale appearance that advances to cyanosis (ATI Teaching 2016).

Children can appear irritable, restless, or lethargic. They may also have abdominal pain, diarrhea, lack of appetite, and vomiting. The nurse evaluates input and output for dehydration status. Pneumonia can cause a pneumothorax or a collection of air in the pleural space (see Fig 4-13). Pneumonia can also cause a plural effusion or an accumulation of fluid in the pleural space. Pneumothorax or plural effusion symptoms include dyspnea, decreased oxygen saturations, tachycardia, chest pain, back pain, and decreased air movement on the affected side (see Fig 4-15) (ATI Testing 2016).

### Diagnostic Tests

Chest X-rays detect the location of infiltrates while nasopharyngeal specimens, blood cultures, and possible sputum cultures evaluate and guide medication therapy. If a streptococcal infection is suspected, an anti-streptolysin titer confirms this diagnosis (ATI Testing 2016).

### Interventions

Viral infections require supportive care including oxygen with a cool mist and continuous pulse oximetry. The nurse gives antipyretics for fever. Chest physiotherapy therapy and postural drainage help break up and remove secretions (ATI Testing 2016).

Chest physiotherapy is a set of interventions that include manual or mechanical percussion, vibration, cough, forceful expiration (or huffing), and breathing exercises. The nurse positions the child to use gravity to move secretions into the central airways, where coughing or suctioning removes excess secretions. In addition to these interventions, children with bacterial pneumonia require IV antibiotics (ATI Testing 2016).

Nursing responsibilities for complications such as a pneumothorax or pleural effusion are similar. They include the preparation of the child for an emergent needle aspiration to pull out the air in the pleural space with an insertion of a chest tube to closed drainage. The nurse will also maintain the chest tube, and administer oxygen (ATI Testing 2016).

## Influenza A and B

Influenza A and B cause a seasonal epidemic every year in the United States. It may present as mild, moderate, or severe (see Fig 4-16) (ATI Testing 2016).

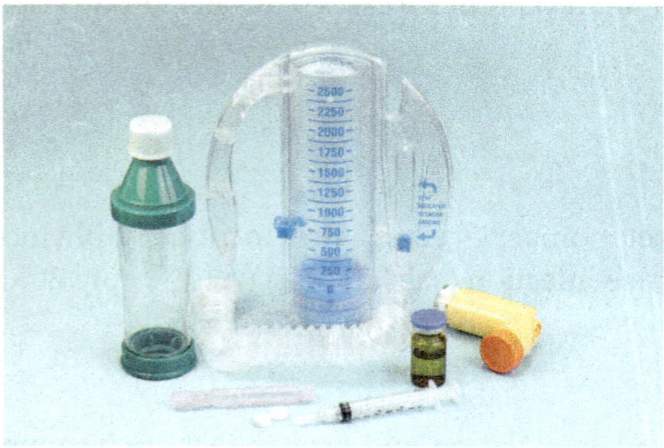



**Fig 4-13** An incentive spirometer prevents atelectasis and pneumothorax

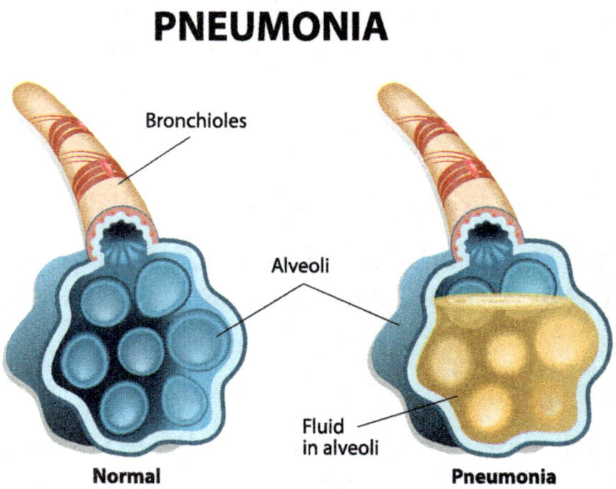




**Fig 4-14** Pneumonia infected alveoli

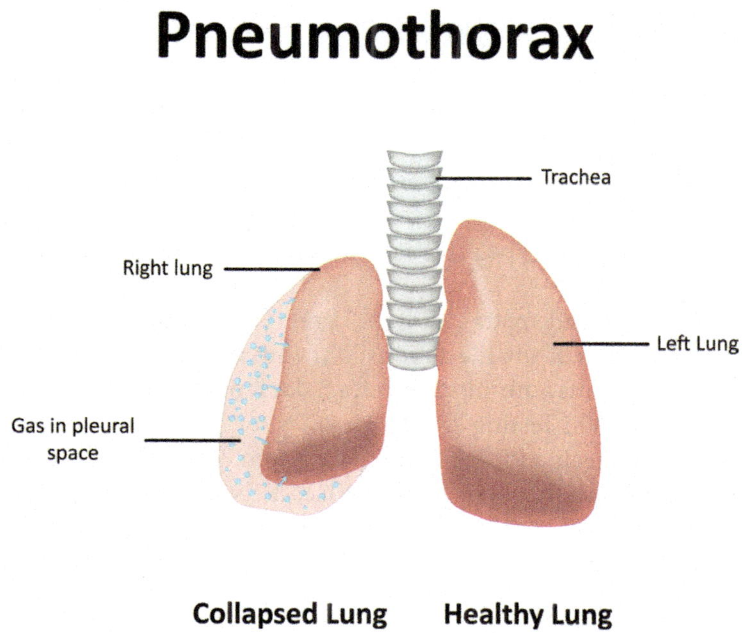




**Fig 4-15** Pneumothorax in left lung

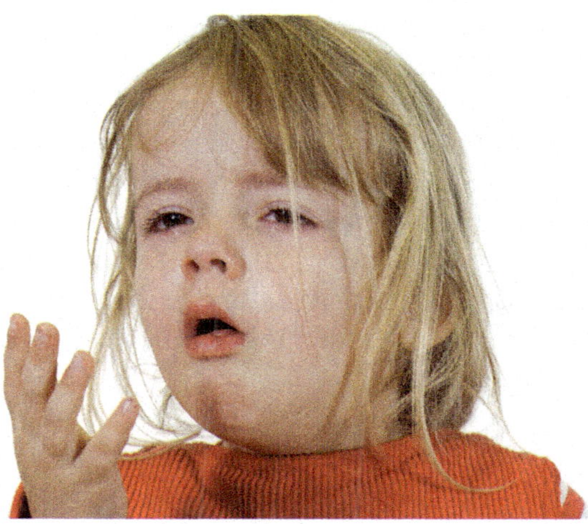



**Fig 4-16** A child with the flu

## Assessment

Children present with a sudden onset of fever and chills, a dry throat, cough and nasal mucosa, a flushed face, myalgia, and fatigue (ATI Testing, 2016).

## Diagnostic Tests

The nurse collects nasopharyngeal secretions for viral culture or rapid detection testing. The lab identifies Influenza A and B by fluorescent antibody and indirect immunofluorescent antibody staining (ATI Testing 2016).

### Interventions, Medication, and Teaching

Parents can manage the symptoms of Influenza A or B in the home environment. A parent should offer fluids regularly and allow the child to take as much as tolerated. Parents should use acetaminophen or ibuprofen for fever, as prescribed (ATI Testing 2016).

Medications include amantadine and rimantadine for type A. Both drugs shorten the duration of the illness when given within 24–48 hours of the onset of symptoms. However, amantadine has more adverse effects. The provider usually prescribes rimantadine (type A) orally two times per day for 7 days for children older than 1 year (ATI Testing 2016).

Zanamivir treats type A and B, and treats children 7 and older, or provides prophylaxis for children 5 and older if initiated within 48 hours of manifestations. Zanamivir is inhaled two times per day for 5 days. Oseltamivir treats type A and B. Parents administer this for 5 days for children older than 1 year of age if given within 48 hours of manifestations (ATI Testing 2016).

Parents can use the Influenza vaccine for prevention. Children 6 months or older receive the inactivated influenza vaccine. Children, who have heart or lung disease, diabetes or kidney failure, respiratory conditions, are pregnant, have a severe chicken egg allergy or have a history of Guillain-Barré syndrome should refrain from the live vaccine, but can use the attenuated type. Contrary to popular belief immunocompromised patients can receive the influenza vaccine (Zbinden, D., and Manuel, O. 2014).

# CHRONIC RESPIRATORY CONDITIONS

## Asthma

Asthma is a disease marked by chronic inflammation of the airways that causes intermittent and reversible airflow obstruction of the bronchioles. The bronchioles are obstructed by inflammation or airway hyper-responsiveness (ATI Testing 2016). Asthma diagnoses fall into one of four categories based on symptoms: intermittent, mild persistent, moderate persistent, and severe persistent (see Fig 4-17) (ATI Testing 2016, p. 99).

An asthma attack precipitates from a particular trigger. Triggers may include mold, cockroach antigen, dust, dust mites, grasses, pollen, trees, shrubs, molds, spores, air pollution, weeds, tobacco smoke, wood smoke, odors, and sprays. Environmental triggers include exercise, cold air, or changes in weather or temperature, environmental changes such as a recent move or change of school, infections/colds, animal hair or dander. Medication triggers can include aspirin, nonsteroidal anti-inflammatory drugs, antibiotics, and beta blockers. Emotional triggers can come from strong emotions like fear, anger, laughing, and crying. Other triggers can

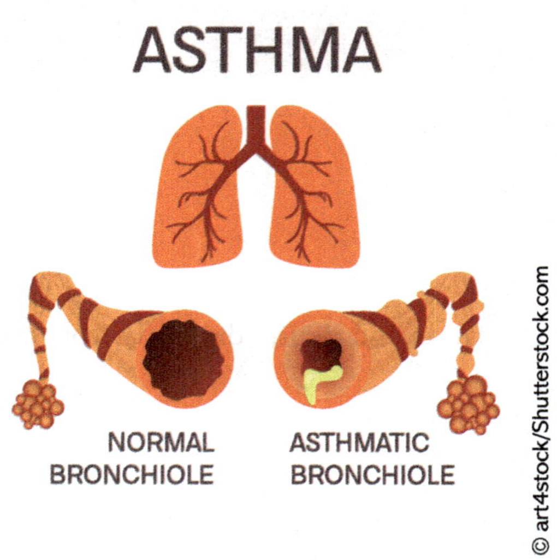


**Fig 4-17** Inflammation and obstruction in Asthma

include Gastroesophageal reflux, tracheoesophageal fistula, food allergies, or additives (sulfites). Endocrine triggers can include menses, pregnancy, and thyroid disease (ATI Testing 2016).

## Assessment

Children complain of chest tightness, shortness of breath, dyspnea, cough, an audible wheezing throughout with possible crackles, use of accessory muscles, a decreased oxygen saturation (low $SaO_2$), and mucus production. Children will appear restless, irritable, with anxiety, sweating (ATI Testing 2016).

Three categories define the pathology of asthma: Intermittent, Persistent (mild to moderate), and Severe persistent. An Intermittent diagnosis presents with an asthma attack 0–2 times/week more than twice/week, but not daily. The attacks require the use of a short-acting bronchodilator less than twice a week. Mild intermittent presents with an asthma attack more than twice a week but not daily with the use of a short-acting bronchodilator more than twice a week, but not daily. A moderate persistent diagnosis presents with a daily asthma attack and requires the use of a short acting bronchodilator (ATI Testing 2016). Severe persistent symptoms are several times a day and can interfere with sleeping and normal activities.

The nurse monitors airway patency, respiratory rate, symmetry, effort, use of accessory muscles, and breath sounds in all lung fields. The nurse monitors the work of breathing through an assessment of shortness of breath, dyspnea, and audible wheezing. If the child wheezes and ceases to wheeze, a severe constriction of the alveoli has occurred, and the child can no longer perform gas exchange. The nurse monitors the efficiency of gas exchange with a peak flow meter used at the same time each day (see Fig 4-22). The nurse ensures the marker reads zero, and the child stands up straight and has no food or gum in his or her mouth. The child closes his or her lips around the mouthpiece and blows as forcefully as possible (see Fig 4-23). The nurse reads the number on the meter and notes the color range. The nurse measures three readings and records the best result. The red zone indicates the need for an intervention; the yellow zone indicates closer monitoring for the child, and the green zone means adequate gas exchange for the child (ATI Testing 2016).

Complications of asthma include status asthmaticus and respiratory failure. Symptoms of status athmaticus include wheezing, labored breathing, nasal flaring, lack of air movement in lungs, use of accessory muscles, distended neck veins, and the risk for cardiac and respiratory arrest (ATI Testing 2016).

## Respiratory Failure

Any time a child becomes hypoxemia they may decompensate and experience respiratory failure. The nurse must monitor oxygen levels, acid–base balance, and prepare for intubation and ventilation if needed (ATI Testing 2016).

## Diagnostic Tests

Diagnostic tests include a CBC blood test and pulmonary function tests. Pulmonary function tests are diagnostic for asthma and its severity. Tests are done every 1–2 years and compared to the child's baseline (ATI Testing 2016).

The provider measures peak expiratory flow rates (PEFR) or the maximum amount of air forcefully exhaled in 1 second. After three attempts, the nurse charts the best reading. Bronchoprovocation testing includes exposure to methacholine, cold air, or histamine. An exercise challenge identifies exercise-induced asthma.

A skin prick test identifies allergens that trigger asthma. A chest x-ray shows evidence of hyperexpansion and infiltrates. The nurse will check a CBC and chest x-ray results, and Arterial Blood Gas (ABG) (ATI Testing 2016).

## Interventions

The nurse administers oxygen therapy as prescribed, and sets up endotracheal intubation equipment. IV access allows for fluids or medications if needed. The nurse positions the child with the head of the bed at 30 degrees to promote ventilation (ATI Testing 2016).

The child may receive a nebulizer treatment through the Respiratory department if he or she is an inpatient. However, home health nurses administer respiratory treatments, and they may take 10–15 minutes. The nurse determines the appropriate delivery system, either a mouthpiece, mask, or blow-by. The nurse obtains a pre-procedure baseline assessment, including vital signs and oxygen saturation. The nurse empties the medication into a small container and attaches the device to air or oxygen source. The nebulized particles absorb into the capillaries in the lungs. The nurse ensures the child to take slow, deep breaths by mouth. As the child breathes, the nurse monitors for pulmonary edema or bronchospasm (see Fig 4-18). The nurse evaluates vital signs, oxygen saturation, and lung sounds at the completion of treatment. The nurse monitors the oral mucosa for infection secondary to use of inhaled medication. The nurse also monitors long-term symptoms of oral corticosteroid use including weight gain, elevated blood pressure, electrolyte imbalance, glucose, and growth delays. The nurse should model a calm, supportive demeanor, to minimize anxiety in the child and family (ATI Testing 2016).

Vitamin D is now known to decrease the number of asthma attacks that require treatment with oral steroids and decreases the number of hospitalizations needed to control asthma attacks. Vitamin D inhibits cytokines and increases responsiveness to inhaled corticosteroids. However, the serum level for optimal effectiveness is not yet known (Martineau, A. R. et al. 2016).

Interventions for status asthmaticus include continuous cardiorespiratory monitoring, evaluation of Arterial Blood Gas (ABG) and serum electrolytes, upright positioning, humidified oxygen, IV access, and three nebulizer treatments of a beta2-agonist, 20–30 minutes apart or continuously. Additional ipratropium bromide can increase bronchodilation if added to the breathing treatment. Corticosteroid administration follows bronchodilation. Magnesium sulfate IV decreases inflammation and improves pulmonary function and peak flow rate among children who have moderate to severe asthma when treated in the emergency department

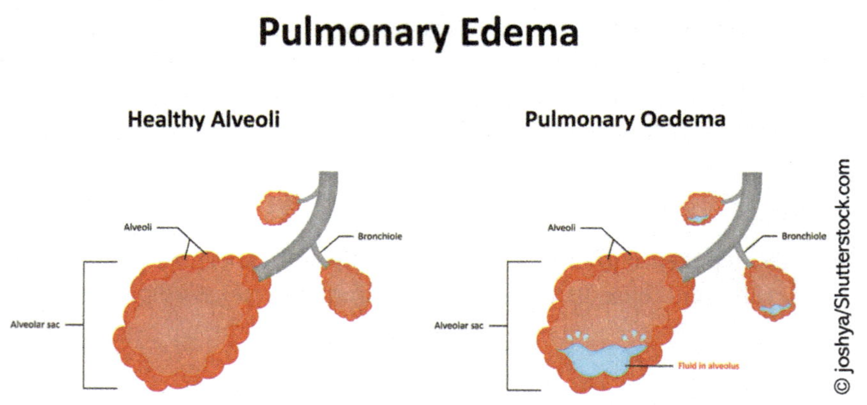


**Fig 4-18** Pulmonary edema in the alveoli

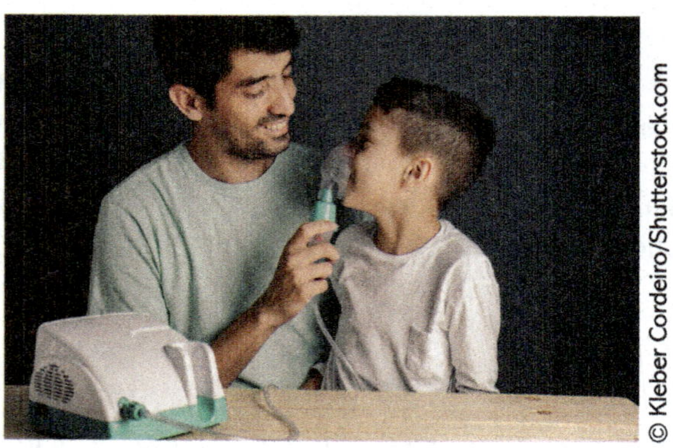


**Fig 4-19** A father administering a nebulizer treatment at home

or pediatric ICU. Finally, heliox (a mixture of helium and oxygen), administered via a nonrebreathing mask decreases airway resistance and work of breathing. If persistent hypoxia continues, respiratory failure presents and requires intubation and ventilation. Therefore, the nurse must always have equipment for emergency intubation (ATI Testing 2016).

## Medications

Children with asthma use bronchodilators (inhalers) for acute asthma attacks and use short-acting beta2 agonists (SABAs) such as albuterol, levalbuterol, or terbutaline. SABAs can prevent exercise-induced asthma. Long-acting beta2 agonists (LABAs) such as formoterol and salmeterol, prevent asthma attacks, especially at night and minimize the use of SABAs. LABAs do not treat acute asthma attacks and work with anti-inflammatory therapy. Children use an inhaler to deliver these medications (see Fig 4-20) (ATI Testing 2016).

Anticholinergic medications such as atropine and ipratropium block the parasympathetic nervous system, providing relief of acute bronchospasms. These medications use a nebulizer to deliver the medication to the child (ATI Testing 2016).

Anti-inflammatory agents minimize airway inflammation, Children with asthma use as a maintenance medication every day. Corticosteroids can be give parenterally (methylprednisolone), orally (prednisone), or by nebulizer such as budesonide (see Fig 4-19). Children can take oral systemic steroids like prednisone for short periods of 3–10 days (ATI Testing 2016). There is a small growth reduction in children up to 18 years of age in the first year of use of corticosteroids, but this effect is less evident in subsequent years (Zhang, L., Prietsch, S. O. M. and Ducharme F. M., 2014).

SABAs combined with corticosteroids improves lung function. Children may need additional medications such as anticholinergics. Children who use anticholinergics report more vomiting and tremors than children not on anticholinergics. Parents should monitor the child's response to the various medications. Children and parents must understand the importance of using the maintenance corticosteroids with the SABA's, and not just the SABAs (Griffiths, B and Ducharme, F. M. 2013).

Children may need leukotriene modifiers. Leukotriene modifiers such as zafirlukast or montelukast interrupt the action of leukotrienes. Leukotrienes impair mucociliary clearance, enhance mucus secretion, draw white blood cells to the airways, and create pulmonary vascular permeability to cause edema. Similarly, mast cell stabilizers such as cromolyn interrupt the inflammatory action of the mast cells (ATI Testing 2016).

Some children require monoclonal antibodies for adequate asthma control. Monoclonal antibodies such as omalizumab use immunotherapy to treat moderate to severe persistent allergic asthma uncontrolled by inhaled corticosteroids in children 12 years old.

The nurse teaches parents and the child how to use a **Metered Dose Inhalers** (MDIs) (see Fig 4-20) and a **Dry Powder Inhalers** (DPIs). The parent learns a methodical way to use an MDI (see Fig 4-21). Parents must

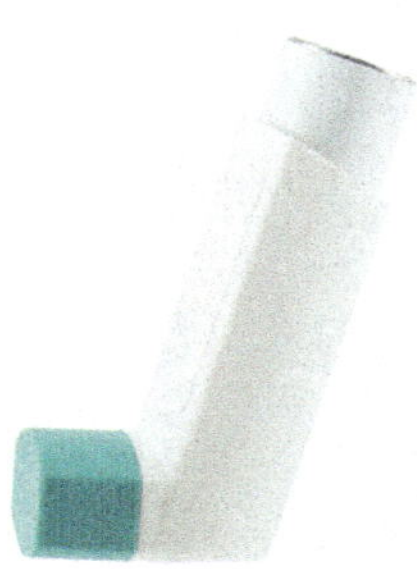

© Orawan Pattarawimonchai/ Shutterstock.com

**Fig 4-20** A metered dose inhaler

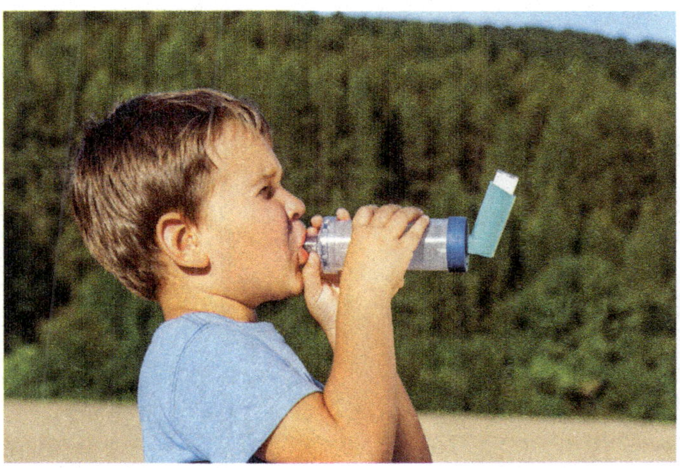

© Beneda Miroslav/Shutterstock.com

**Fig 4-21** An inhaler with a spacer

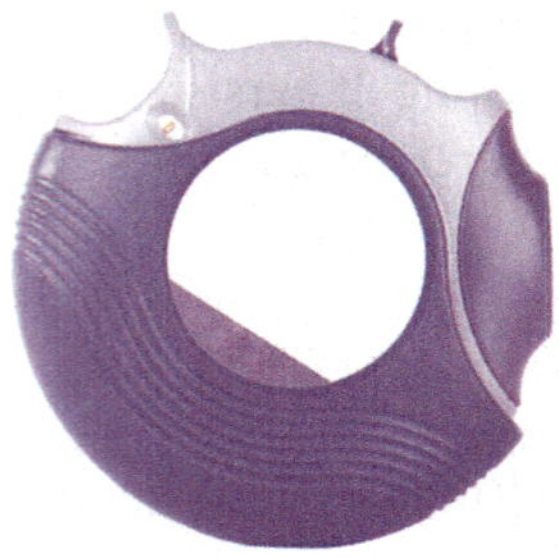


**Fig 4-22** A dry powder inhaler (DPI)

remove the cap, and shake the inhaler 5–6 times, and attach a spacer. A spacer facilitates the entire dose of medication into the lungs (see Fig 4-21). The child takes a deep breath, exhales, and tilts the head back. The child inhales a slow, deep breath for 3–5 seconds and holds the breath for 5–10 seconds to promote penetration into the air passages. An additional puff requires the child to wait 1 minute between puffs. Then the child removes the inhaler and exhales through the nose (ATI Testing 2016).

If a child needs DPI delivery system, additional teaching includes not shaking the device and following the manufacturer's directions to prepare the medication (see 4-22). The child exhales completely, places the inhaler in the mouth, and takes a deep breath through the mouth. The child holds the breath 5–10 seconds. The child removes the inhaler out of the mouth and slowly exhales through pursed lips and continues normal breathing. The parents or child should rinse the canister, inhaler, and cap once a day with warm water. The inhaler must be dried before reuse (ATI Testing 2016).

Parents and children are taught to troubleshoot the administration of medications. Medicine dosages are inaccurate if inhalation occurs rapidly, if the child has impaired coordination, or if the child forgets to hold his or her breath (ATI Testing 2016).

Parents must monitor for oral infections related to corticosteroid use, and teach the child to rinse the mouth with water after administration. If rinsing does not occur regularly a candida (yeast) infection can develop. They also must monitor any tachycardia or tremors related to albuterol (SABA) use. Children who use ipratropium can suck on hard candies to help with dry mouth. Parents must reinforce premedication before strenuous exercise (ATI Testing 2016).

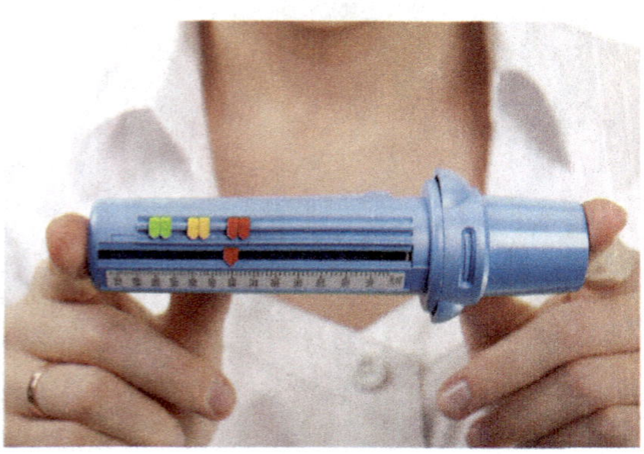


**Fig 4-22** A peak expiratory flow meter (PEFM)

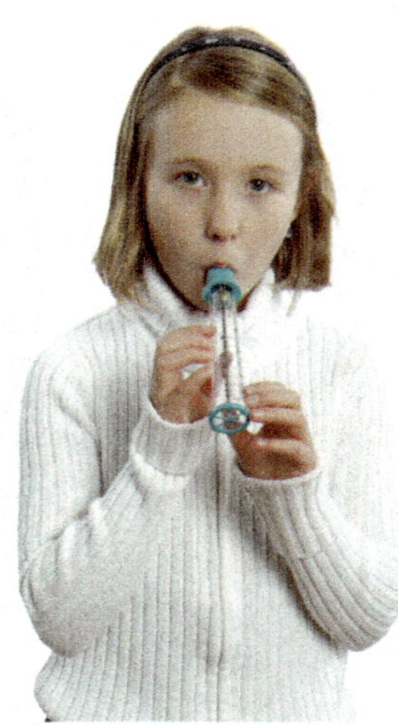


**Fig 4-23** A girl using the PEFM

The family should return home with an asthma action plan that helps direct any care needed at school. The family keeps a record of PEFR results to show the child's "best" efforts, and to provide warning signs of increased pathology (ATI Testing 2016).

The nurse reinforces the signs and symptoms of an asthma exacerbation such as decreased PEFR, greater use of SABA medications, and difficulty speaking or eating. The nurse reviews the administration and rationale of the prescribed medications (rescue medications vs. maintenance medications). The nurse ensures the family and child understands infection control and good hand-washing skills. The nurse also makes sure the family understands the impact of a diet high in nutrients and low in processed foods. Mucous producing foods like dairy should be minimized. The parents should also ensure that the child engages in physical exercise most days of the week. Parents should make a plan to reduce allergens and triggers in the environment. These interventions promote airway clearance (ATI Testing 2016).

Parents should receive education about complications of asthma such as status asthmaticus and respiratory failure. Status asthmaticus or a life-threatening episode of airway obstruction that does not respond to traditional medications requires emergency medical care, as respiratory failure does (see Assessment for status athmaticus and respiratory failure) (ATI Testing 2016).

Self-management skills are the key to improving lung function. When children are compliant they have increased feelings of self-control, decreased missed days of school, and decreased emergency room admissions. It is also more beneficial to teach children and parents to manage asthma based on peak flow readings as opposed to symptoms. Benefits are measurable 7–12 months after initial teaching is complete (Wolf, F. et al. 2002).

The nurse must address cultural concerns related to the child's asthma and exacerbations related to marginalized housing, environmental hazards, impaired social structures, and low-income neighborhoods. The nurse selects interventions in the context of the child and family's cultural lens and practices (Cincinnati Children's Hospital 2013).

## Cystic Fibrosis (CF)

Cystic fibrosis is a respiratory disorder that originates from the inheritance of a mutated gene (see Fig 4-24). Children with Cystic Fibrosis have mucous glands that secrete copious quantities of thick, tenacious mucus. This mucus causes a mechanical obstruction of organs that include the pancreas, lungs, liver, small intestine, and the reproductive system. Children also have an increase in salt and enzymes in the saliva, an increase in salt in expired sweat, and autonomic nervous system abnormalities (see Fig 4-25) (ATI Testing 2016).

### Assessment

A diagnosis of cystic fibrosis requires both biological parents to carry the recessive trait for cystic fibrosis. Cystic Fibrosis occurs mostly in children with Caucasian ethnicity. A meconium ileus may be the first sign of cystic fibrosis in the neonate. A meconium ileus presents as a distention of the abdomen, vomiting, and the inability to pass stool. Early respiratory symptoms include wheezing, rhonchi, a dry, nonproductive cough. As the disease progresses the child develops dyspnea, a paroxysmal cough (a violent cough), obstructive emphysema, and atelectasis on chest x-ray (see Fig 4-16). In its advanced stages, the symptoms include cyanosis, a barrel-shaped chest, clubbing of fingers and toes, and multiple bouts of bronchitis or bronchopneumonia (ATI Testing 2016).

The tenacious mucus also impedes the gastrointestinal system. Symptoms include large, frothy, bulky, greasy, foul-smelling stools or steatorrhea, an insatiable appetite (early), then a loss of appetite (late), failure to gain weight or weight loss, and delayed growth patterns. Children with cystic fibrosis have a distended abdomen, thin arms, and legs, a deficiency of fat-soluble vitamins and anemia. Sweat, tears, and saliva consist of a large percentage of sodium and chloride. Endocrine and reproductive symptoms include thick cervical mucus that may impede sperm motility and decreased or absent sperm production (ATI Testing 2016).

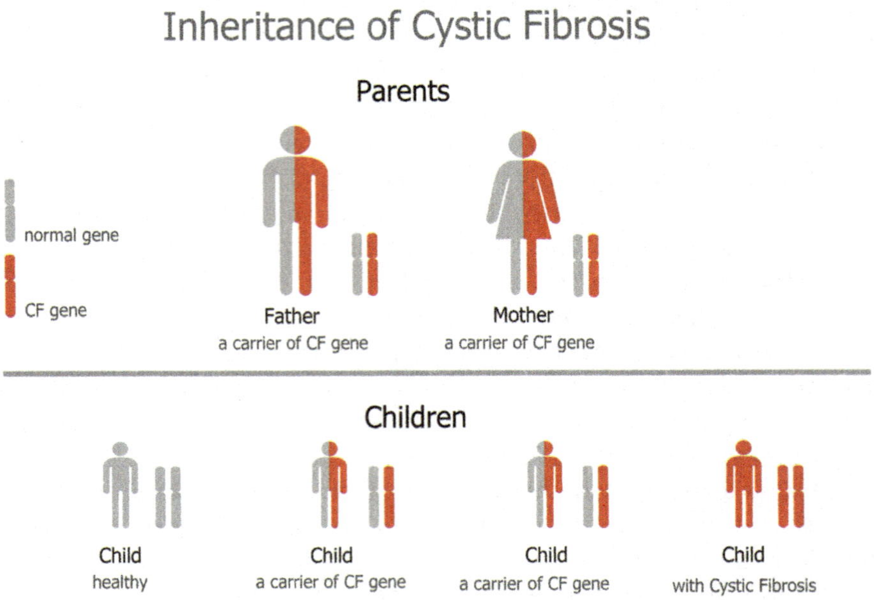




**Fig 4-24** Genetic inheritance of CF

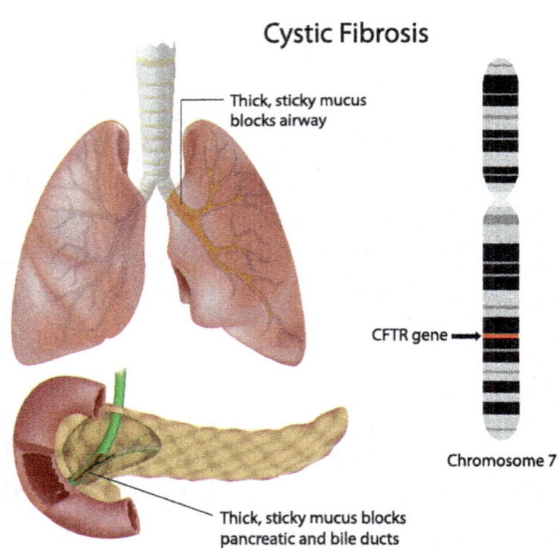




**Fig 4-25** CF affects breathing and digestion

## Diagnostic Tests

DNA testing identifies the mutation in the child with cystic fibrosis. An abdominal x-ray diagnoses a meconium ileus. The nurse supports the sweat chloride test through hydration of the child. Thus, the provider uses a device that uses an electrical current and stimulates sweat production from two different sites. The expected reference range is chloride content less than 40 mEq/L and sodium content less than 70 mEq/L. Children are diagnosed with cystic fibrosis when the chloride level exceeds 40 mEq/L for infants less than 3 months of age, and greater than 60 mEq/L for all others; and a sodium level greater than 90 mEq/L (ATI Testing 2016).

Sputum cultures can identify typical pathogens growing in the tenacious mucous such as *Pseudomonas aeruginosa, Haemophilus influenzae, Burkholderia cepacia, Staphylococcus aureus, Escherichia coli,* or *Klebsiella pneumoniae* (ATI Testing 2016).

Blood samples identify nutritional deficiencies of fat-soluble vitamins (A, D, and E) Ongoing tests include Pulmonary function tests (PFTs), chest x-rays for diffuse atelectasis and obstructive emphysema, stool analysis for the presence of fat and enzymes. A 72-hour sample with documented food intake reveals patterns of malabsorption (ATI Testing 2016).

## Interventions and Medications

The nurse must monitor respiratory status, administer oxygen, and obtain IV access. Children with cystic fibrosis usually have a peripherally inserted central catheter (PICC) that allows for home IV antibiotic therapy. Respiratory medications include SABA's such as albuterol, and cholinergic antagonists (anticholinergics) such as ipratropium bromide or fluticasone propionate/salmeterol.

Dornase alfa acts to decrease the viscosity of mucus to improve lung function (ATI Testing 2016).

Respiratory interventions include airway clearance therapy (ACT) to loosen and expectorate of pulmonary secretions. ACT occurs twice a day (morning and evening). However, ACT should not happen immediately before or after meals. Several methods of ACT are available. Children with cystic fibrosis commonly use chest physiotherapy (CPT) with postural drainage, or positive expiratory therapy (PEP). PEP uses a device, such as a flutter mucus clearance device, to support breathing with an emphasis on strong exhalations. Children may use active-cycle-of-breathing techniques, known as "huffing" or forced expiration. Nurses or parents may use autogenic drainage with an electronic chest vibrator or handheld percussor along with breathing techniques, or children may benefit from a high-frequency chest compression device combined with nebulization therapy. The nurse may administer aerosol therapy such as a bronchodilator or human deoxyribonuclease before ACT or IV, or aerosolized antibiotics. Physical exercise benefits the child's respiratory by mobilizing secretions and strengthening the cardiovascular and respiratory systems (ATI Testing 2016).

Children with cystic fibrosis are susceptible to respiratory infections. The nurse or parents should administer antibiotic via the IV or aerosol route. Common medications include tobramycin, ticarcillin, or gentamicin. Practitioners often prescribe high doses of antibiotic that require peak and trough levels to maintain a therapeutic dose for children with cystic fibrosis (ATI Testing 2016).

Gastrointestinal interventions include a well-balanced diet high in protein and calories that include three meals a day with snacks. Oral hydration promotes the thinning of mucus secretions (ATI Testing 2016).

## Interventions and Medications

Pancrelipase treats pancreatic insufficiency associated with cystic fibrosis. The nurse or parents give pancreatic enzymes within 30 minutes of eating a meal or snack. The nurse or parents should administer capsules or sprinkle capsules on food for all meals and snacks. Dosages of enzymes increase when eating high-fat foods. The nurse monitors stools for adequate dosing (1 to 2 stools/day). Vitamin supplements include a multivitamin and vitamins A, D, E, and K. The use of laxatives or stool softeners, such as a polyethylene-glycol electrolyte laxative solution, treat constipation. The nurse administers histamine-receptor antagonist and motility medications for symptoms of Gastroesophageal Reflux Disease (GERD). Endocrine interventions treat cystic fibrosis related diabetes (CFRD). Blood glucose levels may necessitate insulin administration as oral glycemic medications lack effectiveness for cystic fibrosis (ATI Testing 2016).

Children with cystic fibrosis require a multidisciplinary approach. The nurse should identify community resources and a support group in addition to information on respite care. Wellness promotion should consider the developmental stage of the child. Young children need interventions to promote growth and adolescents may need more psychosocial support for conditions such as depression. In the last stages of the disease, the family benefits from home palliative care for their family member (ATI Testing 2016).

## Artificial Airway

### Interventions and Medications

Children with tracheostomy tubes require routine safety measures, periodic airway clearance, and good skin care. The safety considerations for a tracheostomy tube include the type of tie used to secure the tube such as twill, self-fastening, or metal bead chain; and the correct tension to secure the tube without causing skin breakdown. Children need suctioning at least twice a day. The suctioning technique has several components that include a pre-measured depth of the catheter, a less than 5-second pass to clear the secretions, suctioning on the withdraw of the catheter, and maintaining the lowest amount of suction. For infants, the suction ranges from 60 to 80 mm of Hg, children need 80–100 mm of Hg, and adolescents require 80–120 mm of Hg. Children are also assessed to determine pre-oxygenation or post-oxygenation needs. The nurse should not routinely use normal saline to clear the secretions. Good skin care includes daily cleansing with soap and water, using 0.5% hydrogen peroxide for encrusted secretions. A drain sponge dressing wicks moisture from the site (Cincinnati Children's Hospital Medical Center Best Evidence Statement (BESt) 2011).

# CHAPTER HIGHLIGHTS

- The respiratory system is the most vulnerable organ system in children and is the leading cause of hospitalization for children.
- Children have major differences in their anatomy such as a shorter and narrower airway. This makes children susceptible to inflammation and obstruction.
- Early signs of respiratory distress are restlessness, tachypnea, tachycardia, diaphoresis, nasal flaring, retractions grunting, dyspnea, and wheezing.
- Late signs of respiratory distress are bradypnea, bradycardia, peripheral or central cyanosis, stupor, and coma.
- Laryngotracheobronchitis is a viral croup disorder that presents with a low-grade fever, restlessness, hoarseness, barky cough, dyspnea, inspiratory stridor, and retractions.
- Epiglottitis is caused by bacteria that makes the epiglottis to swell. This is a medical emergency that requires medical treatment and could be fatal. It is prevented by the pneumococcal vaccine. Symptoms include absence of cough, drooling, and the tripod position.
- Respiratory Syncytial Virus (RSV) is the most common pathogen responsible for bronchiolitis, an inflammation of the bronchioles. It is common in children who were born prematurely.
- Asthma is a condition that includes inflammation and excessive mucus production in the airways. An uncontrolled asthma attack that lasts for 30 minutes is called status asthmaticus.
- Cystic fibrosis is a genetic condition that causes a defective chloride ion to create tenacious mucus to impair lung, digestive, endocrine, and reproductive systems of the body.
- Tonsillectomies have fallen out of favor because tonsils support the immune system. They are still used for recurrent respiratory illness.

# REFERENCES

Adewale, L. 2009. "Anatomy and assessment of the pediatric airway." *Pediatric Anesthesia*, 191–8.

Allan, G. M. and Arroll, B. 2014. "Prevention and treatment of the common cold: making sense of the evidence." *CMAJ: Canadian Medical Association Journal*, 186(3), 190–9. http://doi.org/10.1503/cmaj.121442.

ATI Testing. 2016. "Nursing Care of Children." Retrieved from http://www.atitesting.com/ati_next_gen/DisplayResources.aspx?Name=rm_rn_ncc_2016_ebook_20170417.pdf.

Best Evidence Statement (BESt)—Cincinnati Children's ... 2013. Retrieved September 9, 2017, from https://www.bing.com/cr?IG=6FFBEA19AA294AA7ACD341862C95C6F6&CID=2EDAA07F866B69EA1380AA87876D68E6&rd=1&h=JsqOwQGHWZldpzGwbzZ1rgTeZJEo5EvpsAWSZlxolJg&v=1&r=https%3a%2f%2fwww.cincinnatichildrens.org%2f-%2fmedia%2fcincinnati%2520childrens%2fhome%2fservice

%2fj%2fanderson-center%2fevidence-based-care%2frecommendations%2ftype%2fcultura lly%2520sensitive%2520education%2520best%2520164&p=DevEx,5034.1

Bidell, T. R., & Shweder, R. A. (2009). The Child : An Encyclopedic Companion. Chicago: University of Chicago Press.

Bollani, L., Baraldi, E., Chirico, G., Dotta, A., Lanari, M., Vecchio, A. D., Romagnoli, C. et al. 2015. "Revised recommendations concerning palivizumab prophylaxis for respiratory syncytial virus (RSV)." *Italian Journal of Pediatrics*, 411. doi: 10.1186/s13052-015-0203-x.

Calderon MA, Alves B, Jacobson M, Hurwitz B, Sheikh A, Durham S. (2007). Allergen injection immunotherapy for seasonal allergic rhinitis. Cochrane Database of Systematic Reviews, Issue 1. Art. No.: CD001936. DOI: 10.1002/14651858.CD001936.pub2.

Cincinnati Children's Hospital Medical Center: Best Evidence Statement Children with Croup and Use of Steroids in the Emergency Department. 2011. Retrieved from http://www.cincinnatichildrens.org/svc/alpha/h/health-policy/best.htm, BESt 113, 1–4, 11-03-2011.

Cincinnati Children's Hospital Medical Center Best Evidence Statement (BESt). 2011. Retrieved from https://www.cincinnatichildrens.org/-/media/cincinnati%20childrens/home/service/j/anderson-center/evidence-based-care/recommendations/type/trach-care.pdf?la=en.

Clinical Practice Guideline: Tonsillectomy in Children. 2011. Retrieved July 23, 2017, from http://journals.sagepub.com/doi/abs/10.1177/0194599810389949?journalCode=otoj#article.

Doyle, M. J. (2017). ALLERGIC RHINITIS. Dermatological Nursing, 16(1), 27–31.

Griffiths, B.and Ducharme, F. M. 2013. "Combined inhaled anticholinergics and short-acting beta2-agonists for initial treatment of acute asthma in children." *Cochrane Database of Systematic Reviews*, Issue 8. Art. No.: CD000060. doi: 10.1002/14651858.CD000060.pub2.

Martineau, A. R., Cates, C. J., Urashima, M., Jensen, M., Griffiths, A. P., Nurmatov, U., Sheikh, A., and Griffiths, C. J. 2016. "Vitamin D for the management of asthma." *Cochrane Database of Systematic Reviews*. Issue 9. Art. No.: CD011511. doi: 10.1002/14651858.CD011511.pub2.

Motoyama, E. K. 2014. "The Shape of the Pediatric Larynx: Cylindrical or Funnel Shaped." Retrieved July 25, 2017 from https://www.researchgate.net/publication/24283171_The_Shape_of_the_Pediatric_Larynx_Cylindrical_or_Funnel_Shaped doi: 10.1213/ane.0b013e31819ed494.

QSEN Competencies. n.d. Retrieved June 30, 2017, from http://qsen.org/competencies/pre-licensure-ksas/.

Shi, F., Xiao, Y., Xiong, W., Zhou, Q. and Huang, X. (2016). "Cuffed versus uncuffed endotracheal tubes in children: a meta-analysis." *Journal of Anesthesia*, 30(1), 3–11. doi: 10.1007/s00540-015-2062-4.

Wolf, F., Guevara J. P., Grum, C. M., Clark, N. M., and Cates, C. J. 2002. "Educational interventions for asthma in children." *Cochrane Database of Systematic Reviews*, Issue 4. Art. No.: CD000326. doi: 10.1002/14651858.CD000326.

Zhang, L., Prietsch, S. O. M., and Ducharme, F. M. 2014. "Inhaled corticosteroids in children with persistent asthma: effects on growth." *Cochrane Database of Systematic Reviews*, Issue 7. Art. No.: CD009471. doi: 10.1002/14651858.CD009471.pub2.

Zbinden, D. and Manuel, O. 2014. Influenza vaccination in immunocompromised patients: efficacy and safety. Retrieved July 23, 2017, from https://www.ncbi.nlm.nih.gov/pubmed/24491087.

Zulfiqar A. Bhutta. 2017. "Vitamin D reduces respiratory tract infections frequency." *The Journal of Pediatrics*, 186, 209.

CHAPTER 5

# CARING FOR CHILDREN WITH INFECTIOUS DISEASES

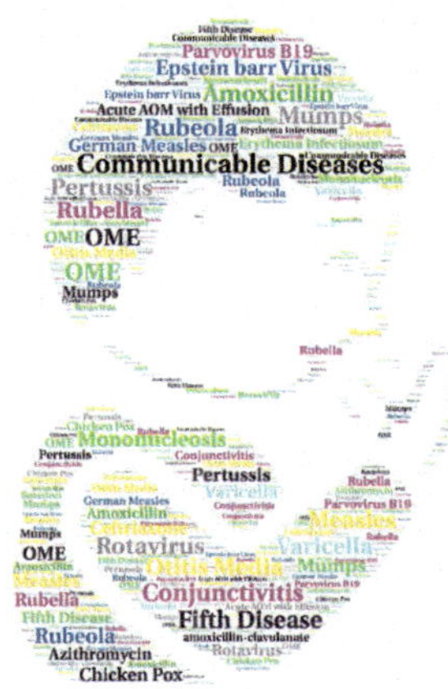


Modified from Shutterstock. Original image © Panda Vector/Shutterstock.com

## LEARNING OUTCOMES

1. Describe the changes in the immune status, as children move from passive immunity into active immunity.
2. Utilize the nursing process to provide safe, comprehensive health care to children with infectious diseases.
3. Recognize significant factors in infection transmission and ways to prevent it.
4. Synthesize data to create a nursing care plan for children with communicable diseases.
6. Recognize the impact of vaccines on reducing the number of cases of communicable diseases.
7. Apply a nursing assessment to a child experiencing anaphylaxis.
8. Teaching/learning principles in providing anticipatory guidance in the prevention and treatment of children with infectious diseases.

# KEY TERMS

Active immunity
Acquired immunity
Airborne precautions
Anterolateral thigh
Antipruritic
Arthralgia
Center for disease control (CDC)
Contact precaution
Droplet precautions
Eustachian tube
Exudate
Humoral immunity
Immunoglobulin A (IgA)
Infectious diseases society of america (IDSA)
Maculopapular
Myringotomy
Natural immunity
Nonpharmacological pain techniques
Orchitis
Otitis media with effusion
Parotitis
Passive immunity
Tympanic membrane
Vastus lateralis

Hippocrates, "the Father of Modern Medicine," described the mumps in his book "*Of the Epidemics*" in 400 BCE (Shulman, S. T. 2004). Human beings have probably been in relationship to these adaptable pathogens for a much longer period. Communicable diseases have evolved along with human civilization, and Western civilization has created vaccines to prevent the transmission of communicable disease since 1790 (Shulman, S. T. 2004).

Communicable diseases originate from microorganisms. Infectious diseases include communicable diseases and non-communicable diseases. Examples of non-communicable diseases, are acquired but not contagious such as Tetanus or E. coli. Communicable diseases are transmittable from person to person through airborne, droplet, or direct contact transmission. Precautions for each mode of transmission (contact, droplet or airborne) are employed by the health-care team. Immunizations, antibiotics, and antitoxins reduce severe complications of communicable diseases. Nurses practice primary prevention to educate and vaccinate children, and secondary prevention to treat infected individuals and control the spread of the disease to others. Immunization recommendations are available at the Center for Disease Control (CDC) website www.cdc.gov/vaccines/schedules (Immunization Schedules 2017).

Infants and children have developing immune systems that make them susceptible to infection. Mothers transfer maternal antibodies through the placenta and breast milk and give the infant passive-immunity, a temporary solution to fight infection. Vaccinated mothers pass on their immunity, and these antibodies are stored in the thymus and influences the infant's T-cells to fight off infections that the mother has fought off. The thymus doubles in size in breastfed babies versus formula fed babies imparting immune modulating effects in both the short term and long-term periods. (Jeppesen, D. L., Hasselbalch, H., Lisse, I. M., Ersbøll, A. K., and Engelmann, M. M. 2004; McDade, T. W., Beck, M. A., Kuzawa, C. W., and Adair, L. S. 2001).

As the infant matures, the infant develops natural and acquired immunity. Natural immunity consists of all of the defenses present at birth. Acquired immunity comes in two types: Humoral immunity and White Blood Cell mediated immunity. Active immunity develops in direct response to fighting off illnesses. Children are susceptible to the respiratory and oral-fecal routes of transmission as personal hygiene techniques are learned. Humoral immunity uses the following Immunoglobulins: IgA, IgD, IgE, IgG, and IgM. IgA, IgG, and IgM attack infections. IgE also targets parasites. IgD's function remains unclear. Antibodies destroy infectious agents and give clues about pathogens. (Warrington, R., Watson, W., Kim, H. L., and Antonetti, F. R. 2011)

# CONDITIONS CAUSED BY BACTERIAL OR VIRAL PATHOGENS

## Conjunctivitis

### Assessment and Interventions

Conjunctivitis or "pink eye" is a bacterial or viral infection that affects the conjunctiva the tissue that covers the white of the eye. Symptoms include itchy, red, irritated, and burning eyes, swelling, an increased amount of tears, a clear, yellow, white or green eye discharge with crusting of the eyelids or lashes, increased sensitivity to light, and a gritty feeling in the eye (see Fig 5-2).

## QSEN Application

According to QSEN, the Informatics competency requires nurses to "[u]se information and technology to communicate, manage knowledge, mitigate error, and support decision making". Nurses can achieve this through the "access to patient care information for all professionals who provide care to patients. Serve as a resource for how to document nursing care at basic and advanced levels, [and] [d]evelop safeguards for protected health information."

The nurse can also "[c]hampion communication technologies that support clinical decision-making, error prevention, care coordination, and protection of patient privacy."

If children have a communicable disease, then nurses report the occurrence to the CDC for national compilations of data. In addition, children change providers frequently, and medical records must follow the child to continue high-quality health care.

From Quality and Safety Education for Nurses http://qsen.org/competencies/pre-licensure-ksas/

Conjunctivitis spreads through direct contact with an infected person. Viral conjunctivitis appears secondarily to a viral infection (see Fig 5-1). It is self-limiting and resolves on its own in 7–14 days. Bacterial conjunctivitis begins unilaterally and then spreads to the other. Interventions include antibiotic ointments and regular cleaning of the eye exudates. Nurses use standard precautions when treating children with conjunctivitis (ATI Testing, 2016).

To prevent the spread of conjunctivitis, the child and family should create proactive habits such as good hand washing, not touching the eyes with fingers, and not sharing makeup, contact lenses, or glasses (CDC 2017).

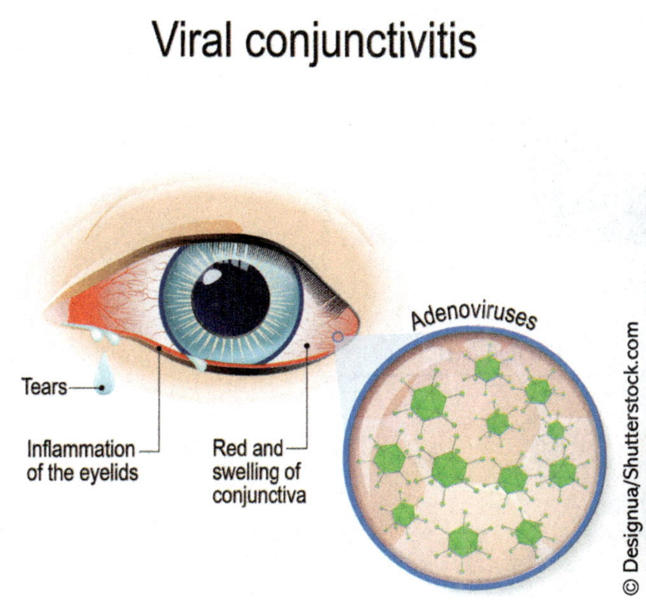


**Fig 5-1** Viral conjunctivitis

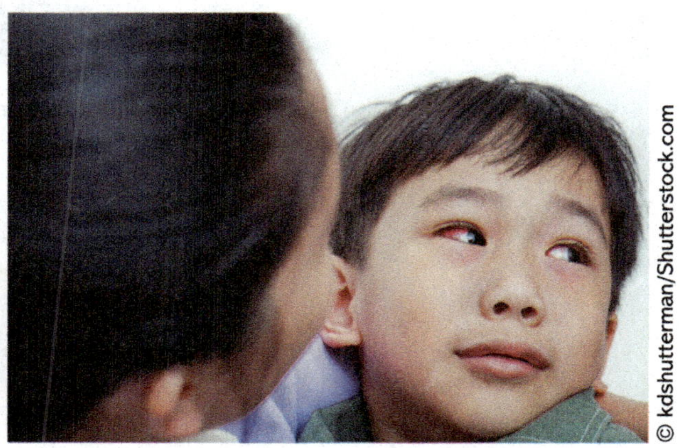


**Fig 5-2** A child with chronic conjunctivitis

## Acute Otitis Media (AOM)

Acute otitis media (AOM) creates a painful infection of the middle ear related to Eustachian tube malfunction (see Fig 5-4). AOM may present with effusion. If so, it is called **Otitis media with effusion** (OME). OME develops when the middle ear collects fluid in the middle ear, but no infection. Repeated infections can cause developmental delays (ATI Testing 2016).

## Assessment and Diagnosis

As the Eustachian tubes in children are shorter and more horizontal than those of adults, and the rise of formula feeding, otitis media commonly presents in the first 24 months of life. It peaks again as children enter school. Otitis media occurs less frequently after 7 years of age (ATI Testing 2016).

Otitis media causes are bacterial or viral. Bacterial origins include *Streptococcus pneumoniae*, *Haemophilus influenzae*, and *Moraxella catarrhalis*, a viral infection includes respiratory syncytial virus (RSV) or influenza, allergies, or enlarged adenoids (ATI Testing 2016).

Breastfed babies develop AOM less frequently than formula-fed babies. This is most likely due to the presence of Immunoglobulin A (IgA) in breast milk that protects against infection (ATI Testing 2016). Breastfeeding also sends milk in a slower flow than a bottle reducing the opportunity for milk to enter the ear. Approximately 80% of non-breastfed babies will develop AOM (Bowatte, G., Tham, R., Allen, K. J., Tan, D. J., Lau, M., Dai, X., and Lodge, C. J. 2015).

AOM risk factors are numerous and include exposure to large numbers of children, exposure to secondhand smoke, cleft lip and/or cleft palate, noncompliance with childhood vaccinations, and Down's syndrome. Assessment findings in AOM include a fever as high as 40° C (104°F), changes in behavior, frequent crying, irritability lethargy, fussiness, or inconsolability. The child may show tugging at the ear (see Fig 5-3), and

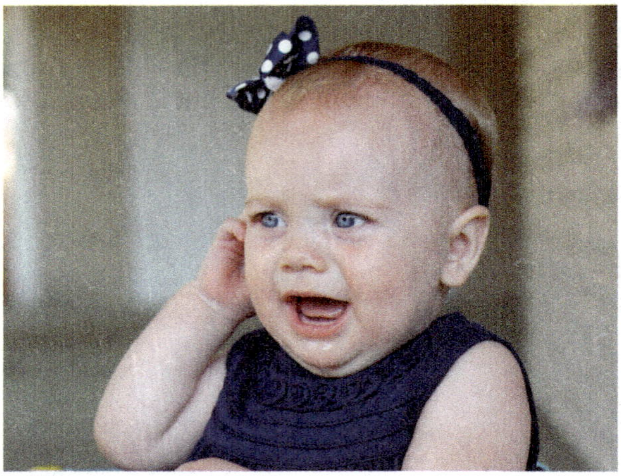

© Dayna More/Shutterstock.com

**Fig 5-3** Sign of an ear infection

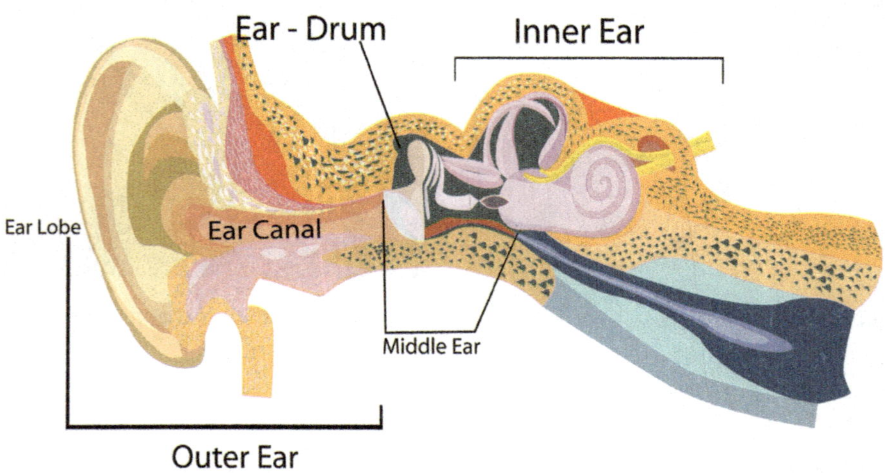


© sanjayart/Shutterstock.com

**Fig 5-4** Anatomy of the ear

have complaints of ear pain, loss of appetite, nausea, vomiting. Upon inspection, the child may have a bulging yellow or red tympanic membrane, purulent drainage in the middle ear, or discharge from the external canal. In addition, the child may present with decreased or no tympanic movement with pneumatic otoscopy, lymphadenopathy of the neck and head, and hearing difficulties and speech delays, if otitis media becomes a chronic condition (ATI Testing 2016).

Assessment findings of OME include a feeling of fullness in the ear, an orange discoloration of the tympanic membrane with decreased movement, rhinitis, cough, diarrhea, and transient hearing loss and balance disturbances (ATI Testing 2016).

A pneumatic otoscope (see Fig 5-5) allows the provider to visualize the tympanic membrane and middle ear structures. The otoscope also assesses tympanic membrane movement. The provider will gently pull the pinna down and back to visualize the tympanic membrane of a child under 3 years of age. For a child older than 3 years, gently pull the pinna up and back. The nurse provides pain and antipyretic medication as needed, comfort measures, and diversional activities (ATI Testing 2016).

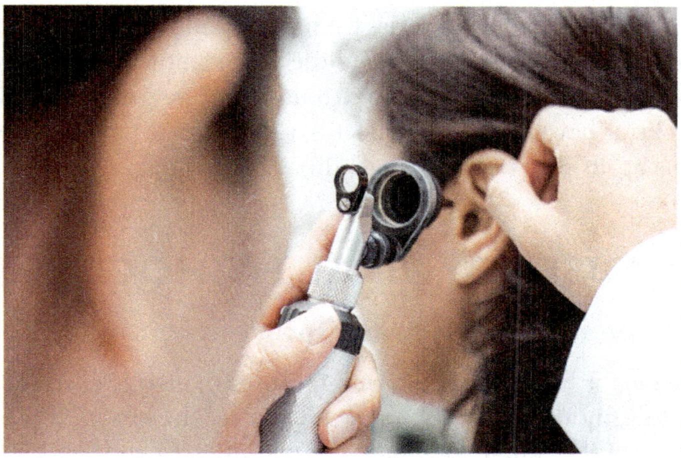



**Fig 5-5** Diagnosis is made by using an otoscope

## Medications and Interventions

The nurse uses age-appropriate techniques to administer medication with consideration to route based on developmental indicators (ATI Testing 2016).

### Pain Medications

Acetaminophen or ibuprofen treat pain and fever (ATI Testing 2016).

### Antibiotics

Antibiotic treatments begin 72 hours after symptoms appear to allow for spontaneous resolution of otitis media. Antibiotics may include amoxicillin, amoxicillin-clavulanate, or azithromycin administered by mouth for 10-14 days.

The provider can administer Ceftriaxone via an IM route, if compliance presents barriers or if the organisms are resistant. The family should complete the total course of treatment (ATI Testing 2016).

### Benzocaine or Lidocaine

Benzocaine or lidocaine ear drops provide topical pain relief; the family will need education regarding administration of the ear drops (ATI Testing 2016).

Xylitol chewing gum also decreases the occurrence of AOM from 30% to 22% of children who do not have respiratory illness. Xylitol has been beneficial in preventing tooth decay and may also provide some protective elements to the child (Azarpazhooh, A., Lawrence. H.P., and Shah, P.S. 2016).

### Surgical Procedures

A myringotomy (a surgical incision in the tympanic membrane) and placement of tympanoplasty tubes may become necessary for a child who has multiple episodes of otitis media. This procedure was modified to use a laser. However, the traditional myringotomy and tympanoplasty tubes are probably more effective (Youssef, T. F. and Ahmed, M. R. 2013).

The provider performs the myringotomy in an outpatient setting under general anesthesia in approximately 15 minutes. The provider makes an incision into the tympanic membrane and places tiny plastic, or metal tubes, into the eardrum to equalize pressure and decrease the effusion. The tubes come out spontaneously in 6-12 months. Parents should limit the child's activities for a few days following the surgery, and notify the provider when tubes come out. The child and family must avoid water in the ears until the tubes fall out.

General health promotion for the family includes feeding the child in an upright position when bottle-feeding or breastfeeding. The nurse should demonstrate to the parents how to clean any drainage in the external ear with a sterile, cotton swabs, and to apply antibiotic ointment. The parents should be aware of risk factors and avoid people who smoke or have respiratory infections. Encourage the parents to continue breastfeeding and to keep immunizations up-to-date (ATI Testing 2016).

## CONDITIONS CAUSED BY VIRAL PATHOGENS

### Mononucleosis Assessment, Diagnosis, and Interventions

The Epstein-Barr virus (EBV), or human herpes virus 4, causes mononucleosis. The virus spreads primarily through saliva because of this, mononucleosis became known as "the kissing disease." It can spread through blood and sexual contact as well. The nurse uses standard precaution to prevent transmission of the EBV virus. The incubation period lasts from 30 to 50 days and makes the origin of the infected person difficult to pinpoint. EBV prevention includes not kissing or sharing personal items, such as drinking cups and toothbrushes with an infected individual (ATI Testing 2016).

In addition, healthy people carry EBV in saliva and can transmit the virus for a lifetime. Individuals who have mononucleosis are contagious for weeks. Symptoms include fatigue, lethargy, fever, headache, an inflamed throat, loss of appetite, swollen lymph nodes in the neck, an enlarged spleen (splenomegaly) that could rupture, swollen liver, and hepatic involvement (see Fig 5-6). A mono spot blood test for EBV antibodies diagnoses past or present infections. Interventions are supportive, acetaminophen and/or ibuprofen and fluids, to treat the fever and pain associated with mononucleosis. A vaccine for EBV does not exist. However, researchers are working on this and may prevent and treat EBV related diseases such as lymphoproliferative diseases or lymphomas. (Infectious Diseases Society of America 2007).

Diagnosis of infectious mononucleosis includes identification of atypical lymphocytes in the blood circulation. Nurses use standard precautions for treating children with EBV (ATI Testing 2016).

### Fifth Disease Assessment and Interventions

Erythema infection (fifth disease) or parvovirus B19 causes a rash that looks, like "slapped cheeks." Although Fifth disease usually manifests as a mild disease, it also occurs in people with a compromised immune system. Fifth disease spread through respiratory secretions, such as saliva, sputum, or nasal mucus droplets, and has an incubation period of 4–21 days. The nurse uses standard precaution to prevent transmission of parvovirus B19. Symptoms include fever, running nose, headache, facial rash, and joint pain. A maculopapular, red rash appears on the face (slapped cheek) from day 1 to day 4. A maculopapular red rash that symmetrically progresses from proximal to distal surfaces occurs through the first week. A secondary rash may appear later on the chest,

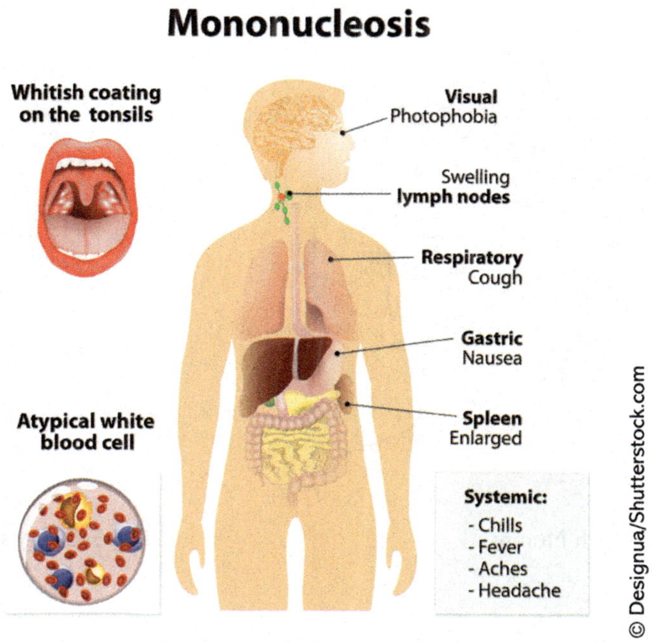


**Fig 5-6** Symptoms of mononucleosis

back, buttocks, or arms and legs. The rash may be itchy, especially on the soles of the feet. Infected persons are contagious once symptoms present but before the rash appears. Treatment includes fluids, antipyretics, and pain relievers. Complications include self-limited arthritis and arthralgia (joint pain, more common in adult women than children (ATI Testing 2016).

## Mumps/paramyxovirus Assessment, Diagnosis, and Interventions

Mumps, or paramyxovirus, causes swelling in the salivary glands. Mumps spread through droplets of saliva or mucus from the mouth, nose, or throat of an infected person. Mumps transmission occurs before the salivary glands swell and five days afterward. Complications are rare in children and more common in adults. They may include inflammation of the testicles (orchitis) in males who have reached puberty, brain inflammation (encephalitis), inflammation of the meningeal covering of the brain (meningitis), inflammation of the ovaries (oophoritis) and/or breast tissue (mastitis), and deafness. Sometimes symptoms are so mild that the infected person shows no symptoms. Symptoms typically appear approximately 14–21 days after infection and include fever, headache, muscle aches, fatigue, anorexia, and swollen and painful salivary glands under the ears on one or both sides (parotitis) (see Fig 5-7 and Fig 5-8), and an earache made worse by chewing (ATI Testing 2016).

Most cases resolve in a few weeks with supportive treatment for fever and pain. Diagnosis includes an oral swab and blood samples. The MMR vaccine will prevent mumps 88% of the time when administered between 12 and 15 months of age, and also at 4 through 6 years of age (CDC 2017; Demicheli, V., Rivetti, A., Debalini, M.G., and Di Pietrantonj, C. 2012).

## Rubella (German Measles)/Rubella Virus Assessment and Interventions

Rubella, or the German measles, causes a mild viral disease that became eradicated in the United States in 2004 (CDC 2017). The disease causes congenital disabilities in the developing fetus. Therefore, pregnant mothers are a vulnerable population. Symptoms of rubella include a low-grade fever, sore throat, headache, malaise, cough, lymphadenopathy, and a red rash that originates on the face and spreads to the rest of the body (see Fig 5-9), that lasts 2–3 days (ATI Testing 2016).

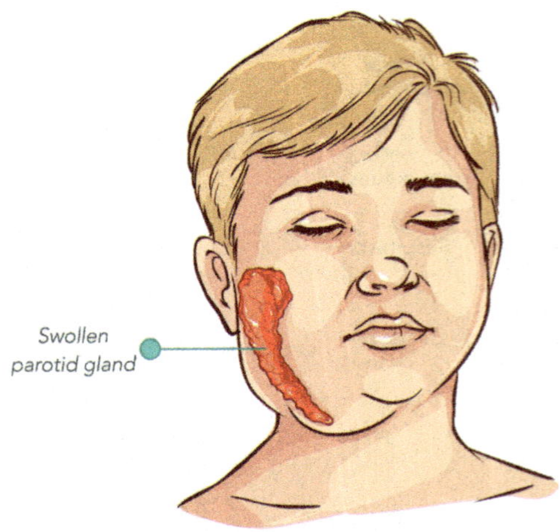


Fig 5-7 A child with Mumps

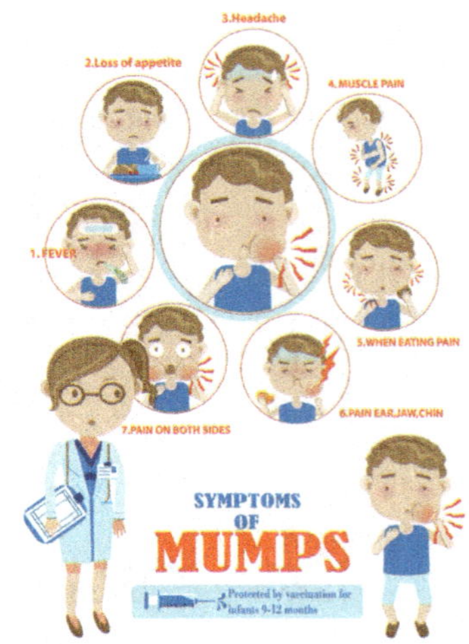
1. FEVER
2.Loss of appetite
3.Headache
4.MUSCLE PAIN
5.WHEN EATING PAIN
6.PAIN EAR,JAW,CHIN
7.PAIN ON BOTH SIDES
SYMPTOMS OF MUMPS
Protected by vaccination for infants 9-12 months
© ann131313/Shutterstock.com

Fig 5-8 Signs and symptoms of mumps

Complications rarely arise with this communicable disease, but may include congenital disabilities (deafness, heart defects, cognitive delays, liver anomalies, and spleen damage) in the fetus of women infected during pregnancy. Incubation for the rubella virus lasts from 14 to 21 days. Children with rubella transmit the virus one week before the rash appears, and remain contagious for up to 5 days. However, 25%–50% of people infected with rubella do not develop a rash or have any symptoms. Rubella spreads through respiratory droplets from direct contact, such as sneezing or coughing. Interventions include supportive care, such as antipyretics and pain relievers (ATI Testing 2016).

The MMR vaccine will prevent rubella 97% of the time when administered between 12 and 15 months of age, and also at 4 through 6 years of age (CDC 2017).

## Rubeola (Measles)/Rubeola Virus Assessment and Interventions

Rubeola virus, or measles, causes a characteristic rash that spreads through direct contact, such as coughing. Rubeola spreads through respiratory droplets that can persist for 2 hours in the air. Rubeola virus is highly contagious. The nurse uses airborne precautions to prevent the transmission of the Rubeola virus. Infected individuals spread the virus 4 days before and 4 days after the rash develops. The incubation period lasts from 10 to 20 days. Three to

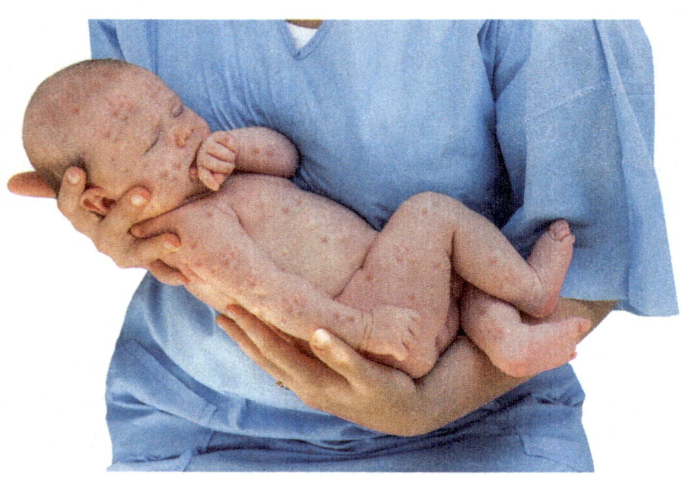


Fig 5-9 A baby with rubella

four days before the rash presents (see Fig 5-11), a child has a mild to moderate fever, conjunctivitis, cough, runny nose, fatigue, and sore throat. Koplik spots (tiny white spots) appear in mouth 2 days before the rash (see Fig 5-10). Once the rash presents a red or reddish-brown rash starts on the face and spreads downward (ATI Testing 2016).

The rash presents with a spike in temperature. The MMR vaccine will prevent measles 97% of the time when administered between 12 and 15 months of age, and also at 4 through 6 years of age (CDC 2017). Interventions are supportive, acetaminophen and/or ibuprofen and fluids, to treat the fever and pain associated with rubeola.

## Varicella (Chickenpox)/Varicella-Zoster Virus Assessment, Diagnosis, and Interventions

Varicella (chickenpox)/varicella-zoster virus causes an easily recognizable, blister-like rash that causes 250–500 itchy lesions (see Fig 5-12). Varicella spreads through touch and breathing the air of an infected person when they eat or talk. The nurse uses airborne precautions to prevent the spread of the virus. Varicella incubation periods span from 2 to 3 weeks. Infected individuals can spread the virus 1 day before lesions appear and until all lesions have formed crusts. Varicella presents 1--2 days before the rash with fever, fatigue, loss of appetite, and headache. The rash begins with macule lesions that start in the center of trunk and spread to the face and proximal extremities. The rash develops from macules to papules, to vesicles, and finally, crust formation. It takes about a week for scabs to form. A varicella-zoster virus diagnosis comes from a positive blood test that may come from a finger stick or venipuncture. Interventions include supportive care, such as fluid administration, antipruritic and pain-relieving drugs, and skin ointments to heal the skin. High-risk clients who have varicella may receive acyclovir (ATI Testing 2016).

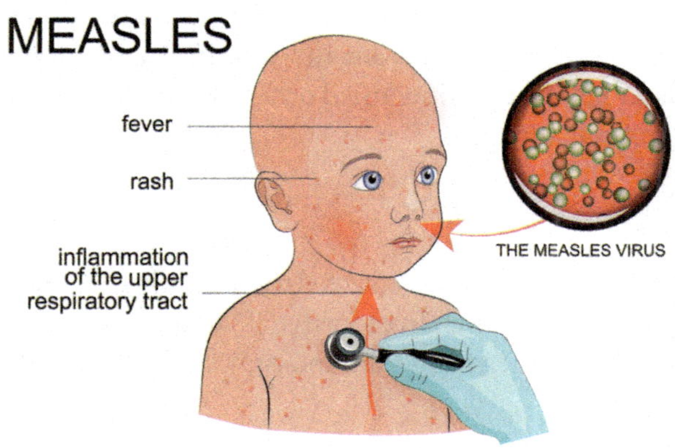



**Fig 5-10** Symptoms of measles

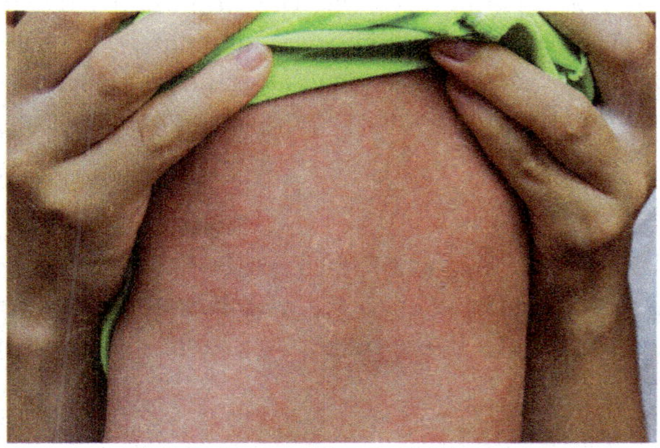


**Fig 5-11** Measles rash in an infant

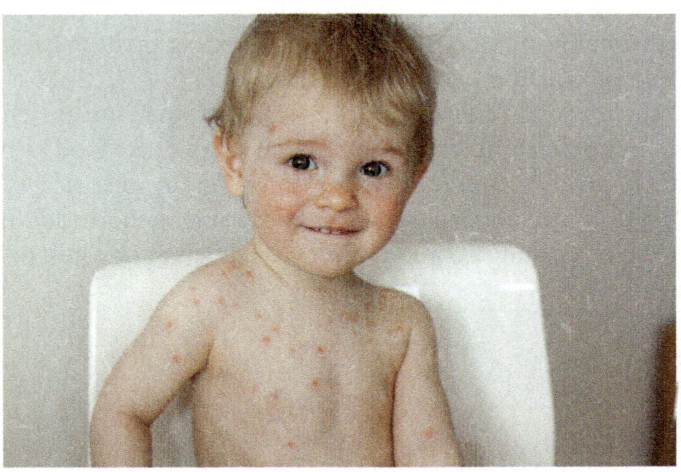


**Fig 5-12** A child with chickenpox

The varicella vaccine will prevent varicella 85% of the time when administered between 12 and 15 months of age, if the child receives a second dose after 10 years from the first the efficacy raises to 98% (CDC 2017).

## Human Immunodeficiency Virus (HIV)

HIV (human immunodeficiency virus) infects a particular subset of T-lymphocytes, the CD-4 T cells, that causes immune dysfunction. HIV produces organ dysfunction and allows a variety of opportunistic illnesses to thrive in its weakened host. Transmission occurs through exposure to blood products or body fluids (blood, semen, pre-seminal fluid, rectal fluids, vaginal fluids, and breast milk) that contain HIV (CDC 2017).

Women can transmit the virus to the fetus or infant perinatally or by breast milk. Risk factors include sexual abuse, unprotected sexual activity, and IV substance use sexually transmitted infections or a knowledge deficit about HIV.

### Assessment

There are three stages of HIV infection and four categories of infection. Stage one for infants consist of a CD-4, T-lymphocyte count of over 1,500. Stage two is 1499- 750. Stage three of HIV infection has CD-4 counts less than 750. As a child's immune system declines, the stages are adjusted. A child over 6 years of age has a range of over 500 CD-4 for stage one, to lower than 200 CD-4 cells in stage three. Each stage is categorized based on wellness measures. The four categories of infection include category N, for non-symptomatic, category A, for mildly symptomatic, category B, for moderately symptomatic, and category C, for severely symptomatic. Children in category N display no symptoms of disease. Mildly symptomatic conditions include lymphadenopathy, hepatomegaly, or recurrent upper respiratory infections. Moderately symptomatic illnesses include oropharyngeal candidiasis, cardiomyopathy, or cytomegalovirus infection. Severely symptomatic disease includes Kaposi's sarcoma, encephalopathy with developmental delays, and wasting syndrome. Assessments must include respiratory status, rate and effort, oxygen saturation, and breath sounds. Complications identified on assessment may include failure to thrive or *Pneumocystis carinii* pneumonia (ATI Testing 2016).

### Diagnosis

Doctors make diagnoses based on age. In infants, under 18 months of age, born to infected mothers who test positive in the polymerase chain reaction (DNA test) and in a virus culture. In children from birth to 18 months or older test positive for HIV in the enzyme-linked immunosorbent assay and Western blot immunoassay (ATI Testing 2016).

### Interventions

Interventions are comprehensive because the virus can affect all body systems. Nurses use standard precautions, use and teach hand hygiene, and teach the family to avoid people with common illnesses, such as flu or cold. Nurses can help prevent respiratory infections by encouraging deep breathing, coughing, and timely immunizations that include vaccinations for flu and pneumonia.

Children need high-quality, high-caloric nutrition rich in protein and enriched with supplements. Total Parental Nutrition (TPN) may become necessary, if the child cannot take food by mouth. The child and family must take meticulous care of oral hygiene, and seek treatment for any disease (ATI Testing 2016).

The nurse should provide non-pharmacological methods of pain relief in addition to pharmacological pain interventions to manage pain by creating a comfortable environment, using heat or ice, and finding distractions for the child (ATI Testing 2016).

### *Medications*

#### Antiretroviral Medications

Antiretroviral medications treat various stages of the HIV cycle, hinder the reproduction of the virus, and slow the progression of the HIV disease process. Most often, combinations of antiretroviral medications are prescribed to minimize the client's development of medication resistance. Antiretroviral medication therapy requires daily treatment for the duration of the child's life.

Nucleoside reverse transcriptase inhibitors include zidovudine, didanosine, stavudine, lamivudine, and abacavir. These medications suppress the synthesis of viral DNA that inhibits reproduction (ATI Testing 2016).

Non-nucleoside reverse transcriptase inhibitors include delavirdine, efavirenz, and nevirapine act to block an enzyme needed to convert RNA to DNA; this causes direct inhibition of viral replication (ATI Testing 2016).

Protease inhibitors, that include indinavir, ritonavir, nelfinavir, amprenavir, saquinavir, and lopinavir, inhibit an enzyme that breaks nonfunctional viral proteins into functional viral proteins. Lab results, such as CBC, WBC, liver function tests need careful monitoring. Antiretroviral medications can increase alanine aminotransferase, aspartate aminotransferase, bilirubin, mean corpuscular volume, high-density lipoproteins, total cholesterol, and triglycerides. Therefore, the nurse or parents must monitor the child to ensure administered antibiotics, such as trimethoprim-sulfamethoxazole are first-line antibiotics given to all infants who are born to infected mothers until the provider rules out HIV infection (ATI Testing 2016) IV gamma globulin prevents recurrent or serious bacterial infections (ATI Testing 2016).

### *Teaching*

The child and parents must learn about the complicated and chronic nature of HIV infection. Parents should verbalize the situations that they must call the provider which include headache, fever, a stiff neck, lethargy, warmth, tenderness, redness at the joints. Older children need teaching to minimize risky lifestyle behaviors like unprotected sex and drug use. The nurse can help the family identify stressors, and appropriate referrals (school/community response to child, finances, access to health care) to support those stressors (ATI Testing 2016).

# CONDITIONS CAUSED BY BACTERIAL PATHOGENS

## Pertussis (Whooping Cough) Assessment and Interventions

*Bordetella pertussis* attaches to respiratory cilia and releases toxins (poisons), which damages the cilia and causes airways to swell. Pertussis spreads through direct droplet contact, such as coughing or sneezing. It may also spread through indirect contact with freshly contaminated articles. The incubation period occurs from 6 to 20 days, usually 7–10 days. The infected person remains contagious for two weeks after a cough manifests. Symptoms may include congestion, a runny nose, sneezing, mild fever, a mild cough that advances to a severe cough in 1 to 2 weeks with violent coughing spells, and a characteristic loud "whooping" sound upon inspiration. Complications from pertussis include ear infections, hernias, weight loss, pneumonia, hemorrhage, seizures, apnea, encephalopathy, and death. Doses are administered at 2, 4, 6, and 15 months (see Fig 5-13) (ATI Testing 2016). The pertussis vaccine has a lesser efficacy than the MMR Supportive interventions to manage pain and fever are indicated and vaccinated people can still contract and transmit the disease (Althouse, B. M. and Scarpino, S. V. 2015).

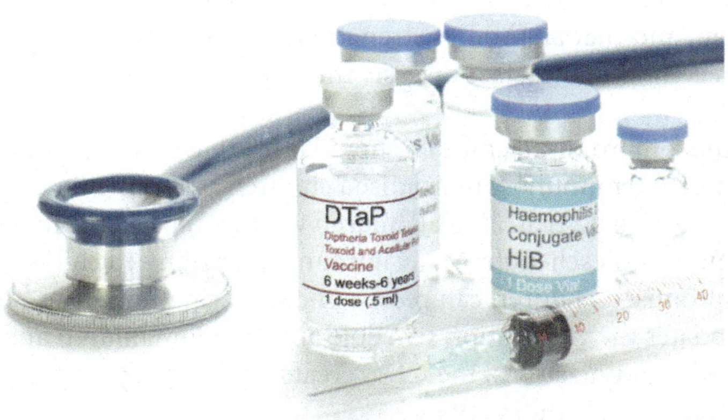


© Sherry Yates Young/Shutterstock.com

**Fig 5-13** Pertussis (whooping cough) or *Bordetella pertussis*

## Influenza

Current information on the influenza shot reveals that in children 2 years of age and older, the nasal spray vaccine made from weakened influenza virus was more effective than the injected vaccines made from killed influenza virus. In children less than 2 years of age, the vaccine was no more effective than a placebo (Jefferson, T., Rivetti, A., Di Pietrantonj, C., Demicheli, V., and Ferroni, E. 2012).

## Interventions for all Communicable Diseases

The nurse and parents follow similar interventions for all communicable diseases. Treatment with antipyretics and pain relievers include acetaminophen or ibuprofen, not aspirin. Aspirin increases the risk for Reye syndrome. Treatment with antipruritic (diphenhydramine, hydrochloride, and hydroxyzine) relieves severe itching. A sore throat benefits from analgesics, lozenges, and saline rinses (ATI Testing 2016).

Skin care includes maintaining clean and dry skin, and the use of calamine lotion for topical relief. Children should be kept cool, and dressed in lightweight, loose clothing. Bathwater temperature should not be hot. Children's nails should be short, and mittens are helpful to prevent scratching in infants. The child needs clean sheets daily (ATI Testing 2016).

The nurse or parents must provide adequate fluids and nutritious foods for healing. The child also benefits from quiet diversional activities and periods of rest.

The nurse should encourage parents to notify the child's school or day care center of the child's infection. Parents can obtain a plan from the school so the child can keep up with school work. The health department receives notification about any new incidences of communicable diseases (ATI Testing 2016).

### Teaching

Infection control has several components that are highly effective when practiced routinely. The nurse reinforces the practice of hand hygiene to prevent the spread of infection and communicable disease. Parents also learn to teach the child to cover the nose and mouth when coughing or sneezing. Parents should change bed sheets daily and wash them with mild detergent. Finally, parents must understand the importance of completing antibiotic or antiviral therapy (ATI Testing 2016).

The pediatric nurse administers and provides teaching for children receiving immunizations. The pediatric nurse needs a balanced clinical understanding of the benefits of immunization, as well as understanding the parents who are concerned about vaccines. The following teaching points are best received when communicated with an open mind and therapeutic communication.

Begin with a biological explanation of the immune system and the mechanism of vaccination. Be sure to explain that vaccines use a substance to elicit a specific antibody response that produces memory cells that can protect the child if exposed to the same pathogen again. The nurse should reinforce that the substance uses an antigen that is weakened or killed to elicit the response. The family must understand the importance of a strong immune system, and that antibodies strengthen the immune system. Families must also understand that if the vaccinated child contracts a disease, the effects may be milder or non-symptomatic (ATI Testing 2016).

The families of immunocompromised children should learn that their children may also receive immunizations. Vaccinations are given to immunocompromised children at specific times according to the Infectious Disease Society of America (Rubin, L. et al. 2013). Children who are born preterm receive the dose of each vaccine according to the immunization schedule. Many immunocompromised children receive vaccinations, and even highly immunocompromised children can receive most vaccinations. The Centers for Disease Control and Prevention website updates the vaccination schedule annually for children and adolescents. For children who have missed scheduled immunizations, the CDC created a "catch-up" schedule, which is also found on the CDC website (Immunization Schedules 2017).

Most importantly, parents need respect and time to understand the complexity in the use of vaccination, personal biases, and the benefits to most children in the United States. Nurses need time to explain these issues, minimize their personal bias, and respect parents who make different choices. The nurse is responsible for delivering the appropriate teaching about vaccines, if the parents refuse.

### Clinical Pearl

There are efforts in research to create immunoglobulins for communicable diseases. There are efforts with measles and chickenpox to create immunoglobulins that can stop disease after exposure (Young, M. K., Cripps, A. W., Nimmo, G. R., and van Driel, M. L. 2015; Macartney, K. and McIntyre, P. 2008).

The exploration of this development could assuage many concerns about the erosion of herd immunity for parents and health-care professionals.

Tetanus exposure treatment currently uses immunoglobulins, or passive immunity, to fight off a tetanus exposure. A dose of IV immune globulin or antibodies fights off the tetanus until the body can make its own antibodies. The same may be done for measles and chickenpox.

Vaccines have prevented disease since the 1790's, and although they are not 100% effective, they are an important way to manage communicable disease on a global level for a global society (Shulman, S. T. 2004).

## Other Adverse Effects, Contraindications, and Precautions

Anaphylaxis can occur in response to any vaccine and becomes contraindicated for that child (see Fig 5-14 and Fig 15). A child experiencing anaphylaxis can have itching, hives, and constriction of the airways. These symptoms can develop into shock where children have a weak, thread pulse and hypotension. A child that has a moderate or severe illness with or without fever may delay that vaccination. However, minor illnesses, such as the common cold are not contraindications to immunizations. A child with a severe febrile illness will not receive vaccinations while ill. Although, most immunocompromised children receive vaccinations, live virus vaccines, such as varicella or MMR, need to comply with the guidelines set out by the Infectious Diseases Society of America (ISDA) (Infectious Diseases Society of America 2007). Contrary to popular belief, severely immunocompromised children benefit from receiving vaccines.

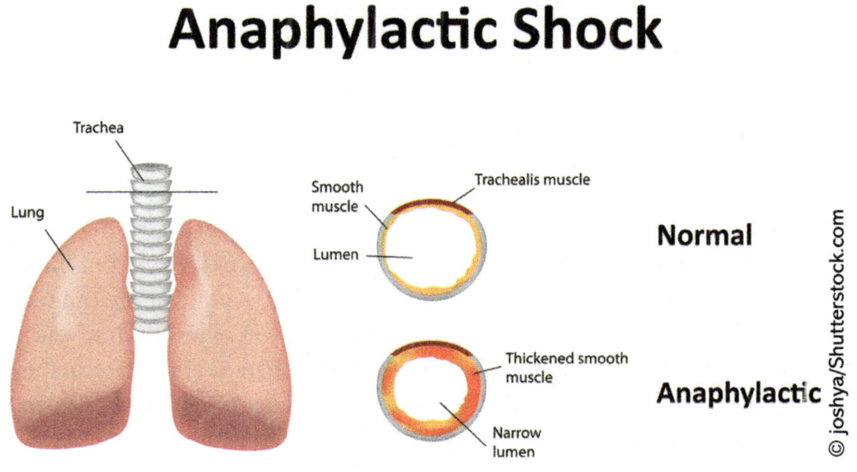


**Fig 5-14** Constriction in anaphylaxis

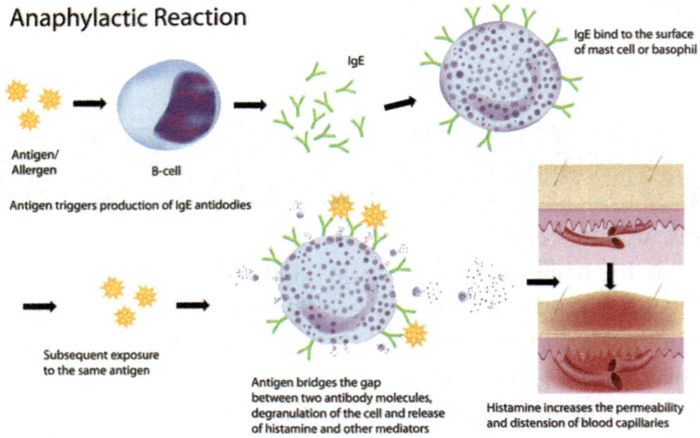




**Fig 5-15** Anaphylactic reaction

## Vaccine Administration

The nurse ensures that the parents or guardian understands the informed consent presented by the doctor or nurse practitioner. The nurse provides his or her name, address, and title. The nurse should review vaccine information sheets (VIS), with parents, legal guardians and older children. The nurse needs to document this important teaching (ATI Testing 2016).

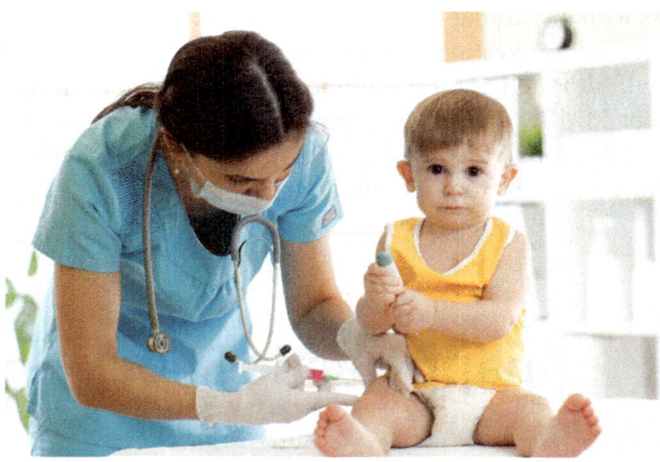



**Fig 5-16** The nurse landmarks the vastus lateralis for an IM vaccine

The nurse administers intramuscular (IM) immunizations in the vastus lateralis but the nurse may use the ventrogluteal muscle if there are contraindications (see 5-16). Children over 3 years of age can receive deltoid injections but the administration of vaccines in the deltoid muscle generally occurs in older children and adolescents. The nurse administers subcutaneous injections in the outer aspect of the upper arm or anterolateral thigh (ATI Testing 2016).

The nurse uses an appropriately sized needle for the route, site, age, and the amount of medication. Adequate needle length reduces the incidence of swelling and tenderness at the injection site. All injections for children use a 23–25-gauge needle (Beirne, P. V., Hennessy, S., Cadogan, S. L., Shiely, F., Fitzgerald, T., and MacLeod, F. 2015). Infants need a 1″ in the anterolateral thigh or vastus lateralis. Toddlers need a 1″–1 1/4″ in the anterolateral thigh. Children can receive a deltoid injection with a 5/8-1″ needle, or a 1–1 1/4″ needle in the anterolateral thigh (ATI Testing 2016).

The nurse should use nonpharmacological pain techniques, such as distraction, cuddling, pacifiers, and a calm demeanor in the providers (Riddell, P. R. R. et al. 2015). Breastfed children should feed, as it provides pain relief (Shah, P.S., Herbozo, C., Aliwalas, L.L., & Shah, V.S. 2012). Children may also receive a topical anesthetic before the injection. Infants may also receive a concentrated oral sucrose solution 2 minutes prior to, during, and 3 minutes after immunization administration (Liddle, M., Bonjour, A., Tyra, C., Kathman, L., and Staab, J. 2013).

After administration of the vaccine, cool compressions ease pain at the injection site. Children should receive praise, a colorful bandage or sticker as a reward.

The nurse must document the administration of the vaccine that includes date, route, and site of injection, type, manufacturer, lot number, and expiration date of the vaccine (ATI Testing 2016).

The nurse encourages parents to remain up-to-date on immunizations for the child. The parents must also understand aspirin should not be used for the child, to treat fever or local reaction following the administration of a live virus vaccine, due to the risk of developing Reye's syndrome. The nurse also instructs the parents and child to observe for complications and notify the provider, if adverse effects occur. If this does occur, the nurse reports any adverse reactions to the Vaccine Adverse Event Reporting System (VAERS) (ATI Testing 2016).

## CHAPTER HIGHLIGHTS

- Newborns have an immature immune system that only contains maternal antibodies.
- Communicable diseases, or infectious diseases, are transmitted via airborne, droplet, or direct contact.
- Natural immunity includes immune defenses that occur from birth.
- Passive immunity includes maternal antibodies passed through the placenta and breast milk.
- Immunizations are not 100% effective and can cause reactions and anaphylaxis.
- Immunizations decrease the occurrence of common communicable diseases.
- Immunocompromised children still receive immunizations.
- The nurse uses a 23–25-gauge needle for all vaccine administration. In infants a 23-gauge needle minimizes local reactions, and is injected into the vastus lateralis muscle. The nurse uses the deltoid muscle after 3 years of age or older.
- Nurses promote wellness through health promotion teaching, handwashing, a diet consistent with the Harvard Healthy Plate, and regular exercise.

## REFERENCES

Althouse, B. M. and Scarpino, S. V. 2015. "Asymptomatic transmission and the resurgence of Bordetella pertussis." *BMC Medicine*, 13(1), 1–12. doi: 10.1186/s12916-015-0382-8.

Azarpazhooh, A., Lawrence, H.P., and Shah, P.S. 2016. "Xylitol for preventing acute otitis media in children up to 12 years of age." *Cochrane Database of Systematic Reviews 2016*, Issue 8. Art. No.: CD007095.

doi: 10.1002/14651858.CD007095.pub3.

Beirne, P.V., Hennessy, S., Cadogan, S.L., Shiely, F., Fitzgerald, T., and MacLeod, F. 2015. "Needle size for vaccination procedures in children and adolescents." *Cochrane Database of Systematic Reviews 2015*, Issue 6. Art. No.: CD010720.

doi: 10.1002/14651858.CD010720.pub2.

Bowatte, G., Tham, R., Allen, K. J., Tan, D. J., Lau, M., Dai, X., and Lodge, C. J. 2015. "Breastfeeding and childhood acute otitis media: a systematic review and meta-analysis." Acta Paediatrica (Oslo, Norway 1992), 104(467), 85–95. doi: 10.1111/apa.13151.

CDC. "Pink Eye: Usually Mild and Easy to Treat". (2017, March 20). Retrieved July 27, 2017, from https://www.cdc.gov/features/conjunctivitis/index.html.

Infectious Diseases Society of America. 2007. Vaccine Shows Promise in Preventing Mono. Science Daily. Retrieved July 27, 2017 from www.sciencedaily.com/releases/2007/12/071210121632.htm.

Demicheli, V., Rivetti, A., Debalini, M.G., and Di Pietrantonj, C. 2012. "Vaccines for measles, mumps, and rubella in children." *Cochrane Database of Systematic Reviews 2012*, Issue 2. Art. No.: CD004407. doi: 10.1002/14651858.CD004407.pub3.

Immunization Schedules. 2017. Retrieved September 10, 2017, from https://www.cdc.gov/vaccines/schedules/hcp/child-adolescent.html.

Jefferson, T., Rivetti, A., Di Pietrantonj, C., Demicheli, V., and Ferroni, E. 2012. "Vaccines for preventing influenza in healthy children." *Cochrane Database of Systematic Reviews 2012*, Issue 8. Art. No.: CD004879.

doi: 10.1002/14651858.CD004879.pub4.

Jeppesen, D. L., Hasselbalch, H., Lisse, I. M., Ersbøll, A. K., and Engelmann, M. M. 2004. "T-lymphocyte subsets, thymic size, and breastfeeding in infancy." *Pediatric Allergy & Immunology*, 15(2), 127–32. doi: 10.1111/j.1399-3038.2004.00032.x.

Liddle, M., Bonjour, A., Tyra, C., Kathman, L., and Staab, J. 2013. Cincinnati Children's Hospital Medical Center, Best Evidence Statement: Reducing Pain for Children and Adolescents Receiving Injections, http://www.cincinnatichildrens.org/svc/alpha/h/health-policy/best.htm, BESt 147, 1–9, 1/16/13.

Macartney, K. and McIntyre, P. 2008. Vaccines for post-exposure prophylaxis against varicella (chickenpox) in children and adults. Retrieved July 27, 2017, from https://www.ncbi.nlm.nih.gov/pubmed/18646079.

McDade, T. W., Beck, M. A., Kuzawa, C. W., and Adair, L. S. 2001. "Prenatal Undernutrition and Postnatal Growth Are Associated with Adolescent Thymic Function." *Journal of Nutrition*, 131(4), 1225.

Rubin, L., Levin, M., Ljungman, P., Davies, E., Avery, R., Tomblyn, M., Bousvaros,A., Dhanireddy, S., Sung,L., Keyserling, H. and Kang, I. 2013. "IDSA Clinical Practice Guideline for Vaccination of the Immunocompromised Host." *Clinical Infectious Diseases*, 58(3), 309–18.

Riddell, P. R. R., Racine, N. M., Gennis, H. G., Turcotte, K., Uman, L. S., Horton, R. E., Ahola Kohut, S., Hillgrove Stuart, J., Stevens, B., Lisi, D. M. 2015. "Non-pharmacological management of infant and young child procedural pain." *Cochrane Database of Systematic Reviews 2015*, Issue 12. Art. No.: CD006275.

doi: 10.1002/14651858.CD006275.pub3.

Shah, P. S., Herbozo, C., Aliwalas, L. L., Shah, V. S. 2012. "Breastfeeding or breast milk for procedural pain in neonates." *Cochrane Database of Systematic Reviews 2012*, Issue 12. Art. No.: CD004950. doi: 10.1002/14651858.CD004950.pub3.

Shulman, S. T. 2004. The History of Pediatric Infectious Diseases. Retrieved July 26, 2017, from http://www.nature.com/pr/journal/v55/n1/full/pr200425a.html?foxtrotcallback=true.

Warrington, R., Watson, W., Kim, H. L., and Antonetti, F. R. 2011. An introduction to immunology and immunopathology. Retrieved September 10, 2017, from https://aacijournal.biomedcentral.com/articles/10.1186/1710-1492-7-S1-S1.

Young, M. K., Cripps, A. W., Nimmo, G. R., and van Driel, M. L. 2015. "Post-exposure passive immunisation for preventing rubella and congenital rubella syndrome." *The Cochrane Database of Systematic Reviews*, (9), CD010586. doi: 10.1002/14651858.CD010586.pub2.

Youssef, T. F., and Ahmed, M. R. 2013. "Laser-assisted myringotomy versus conventional myringotomy with ventilation tube insertion in treatment of otitis media with effusion: Long-term follow-up." *Interventional Medicine & Applied Science*, 5(1), 16–20. http://doi.org/10.1556/IMAS.5.2013.1.3.

CHAPTER 6

# CARING FOR CHILDREN WITH CARDIAC DISORDERS

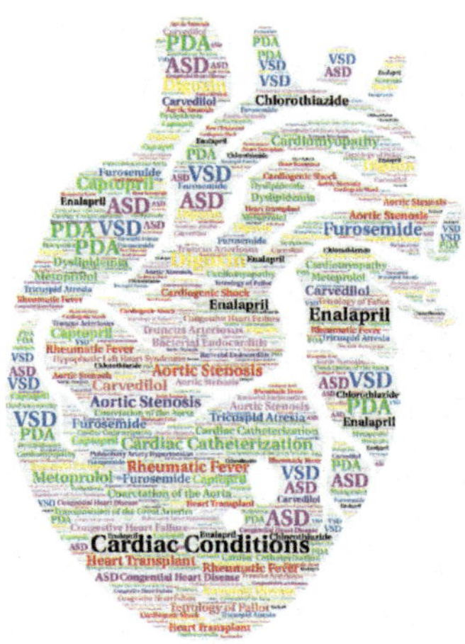


Modified from Shutterstock.
Original image © Alexey Pushkin/Shutterstock.com

## LEARNING OUTCOMES

1. Describe the anatomy of the heart in relations to fetal and adult circulation.
2. Utilize the nursing process to provide safe, comprehensive health care to children with cardiac conditions.
3. Contrast the differences between congenital and acquired heart disease.
4. Synthesize assessment data to create a nursing care plan for children with congenital heart defects.
5. Recognize the signs and symptoms of heart failure and shock in a child.
6. Create a nursing care plan for a child with Kawasaki's disease.
7. Create a nursing care plan for a child with Rheumatic fever.
8. Understand wellness strategies to promote health in the child with congenital heart disease that can create patterns in the adult with congenital heart disease.
9. Teaching/learning principles in providing anticipatory guidance in the prevention and treatment of children with cardiac conditions.

# KEY TERMS

Atrial septal defect (ASD)
Cardiac catheterization
Ductus arteriosus
Ductus venosus
Echocardiography (ECG)
Electrocardiogram (EKG)
Foramen ovale
Indomethacin (NSAID)
Maternal TORCH infections
Patent ductus arteriosus (PDA)
Positive inotrope
Stenosis
"Tet" spells
Ventricular septal defect (VSD)

Many medical breakthroughs have contributed to better ways of managing congenital heart anomalies. Angioplasties, stents, and cardiac catheterization, give pediatric cardiologists tools to attempt to fix most cardiac abnormalities. The critical heart abnormalities in this chapter can result in heart failure in the child. The nurse is responsible for teaching wellness and promoting health and infection control for children with cardiac conditions to prevent heart failure. Due to the chronic nature of congenital heart disease, children need to have short-term goals and long-term goals that extend into adulthood.

Most pathology in the pediatric hearts stems from the incomplete transition from fetal circulation to adult circulation. As the newborn takes its first breath, three fetal shunts close. This event takes the newborn from a high-pressure (right), and low-pressure (left-sided) circulation (Fig 6-1) to a high-pressure (left) and low-pressure (right-sided) circulation (Fig 6-2). If the pediatric heart has any defect, it will inhibit shunt closure, and the child cannot oxygenate and circulate blood efficiently. The **ductus arteriosus** lies between

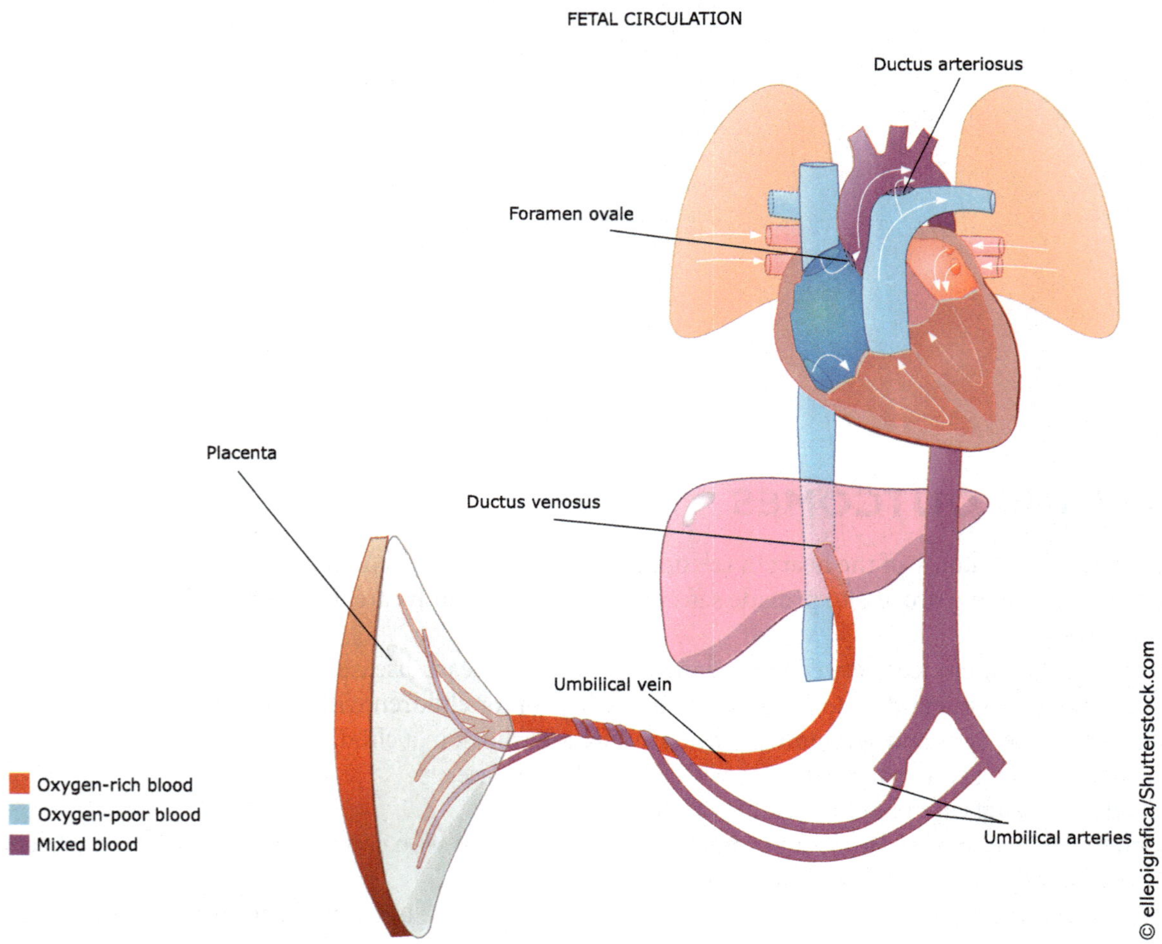


**Fig 6-1** High-pressure (right),

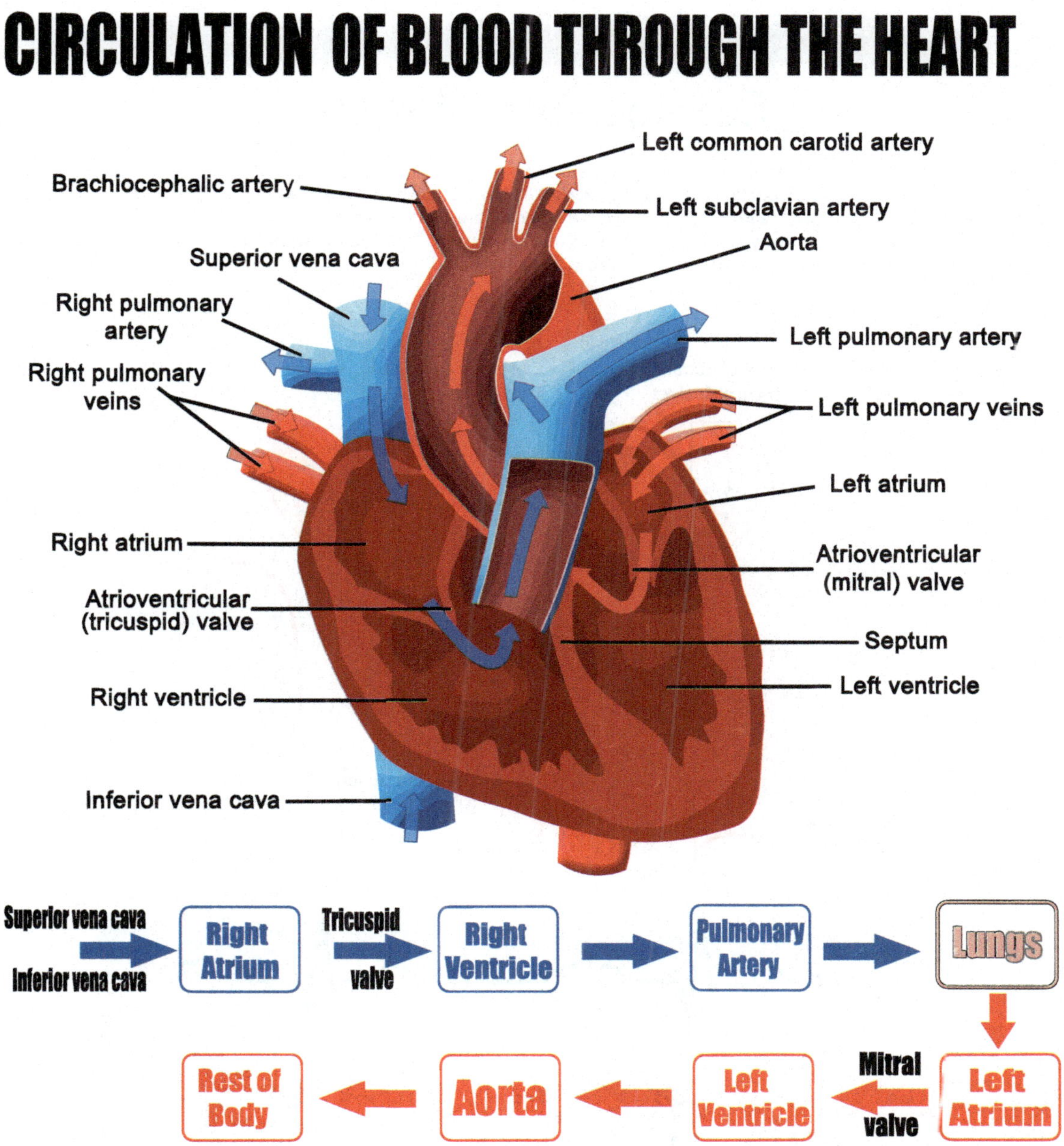




**Fig 6-2** High-pressure (left), low-pressure (left) system pressure left system low-pressure (right) system (adult) (fetus)

the aorta and the pulmonary artery and is the shunt that takes blood past the lungs in fetal circulation. The **ductus venosus** lies between the umbilical vein and the Inferior Vena Cava (IVC) and carries blood around the liver in fetal circulation. The **foramen ovale** sits between the two atria and allows oxygenated blood from the umbilical vein to flow past the right atrium and into the left atrium, from the left ventricle into the aorta (ATI Testing 2016).

Children with cardiac conditions may have congenital or acquired disease. Around 3–4 weeks of gestation the heart begins to beat, and may already have a congenital disease. In addition, anatomic abnormalities can develop into heart disease and heart failure. These defects and most heart defects are detectable through auscultation. Learning the art of auscultation begins with correlating heart sounds to the heart's electrical and pumping activities (see Fig 6-3). Cardiac nurses have opportunities to sharpen their skills working alongside cardiologists (ATI Testing 2016).

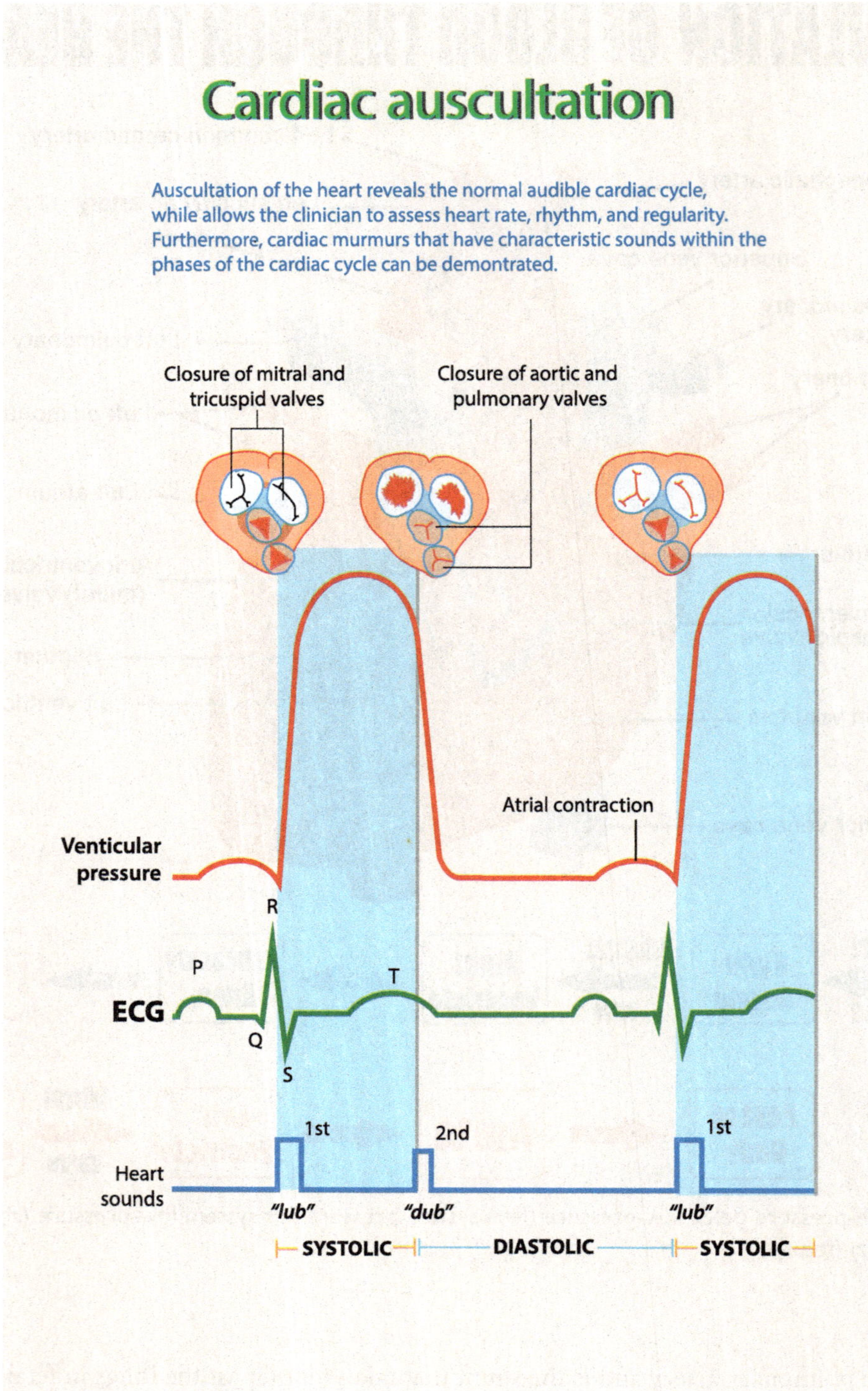




**Fig 6-3** Heart sounds are electrical and mechanical.

Heart failure is the insufficiency of the heart muscle to meet the physical requirements of the body, not that the heart has stopped beating. Heart failure occurs in response to a congenital anomaly or an infection that impairs adult circulation or the valves. Children are currently developing heart failure through an unhealthy lifestyle that results in obesity, increased cholesterol, and inflammation that leads to vascular pathology (ATI Testing 2016).

# CONGENITAL HEART DISEASE

Anatomic anomalies of the heart prevent the transition from fetal circulation to adult circulation and impair the pulmonary system. Defects may be present at any of the fetal shunts, and impair blood flow and perfusion to the lungs (ATI Testing 2016).

Defects that Increase Pulmonary Blood Flow

Cardiac anomalies that increase blood flow to the lungs include: A **Patent Ductus Arteriosus (PDA)**, **Atrial Septal Defects (ASD)**, and **Ventricular Septal Defects (VSD)**. The ASD originates from the failure of the foramen ovale to close, essentially creating one atrium that does not efficiently pump the blood to the ventricles. The patent foramen ovale allows blood to and mix from the left and right sides of the heart. The VSD allows for a significant amount of pressure from the left side of the heart to enter the right side of the heart and cause pulmonary congestion. The PDA redirects blood meant to be oxygenated by the lungs back to the body without being oxygenated. These defects increase blood to the lungs causing congestion, pulmonary hypertension, and pulmonary edema (ATI Testing 2016).

## Defects that Decrease Pulmonary Blood Flow

Defects that decrease blood flow to the lungs obstruct the blood flow from the lungs and have an anatomic anomaly (ASD or VSD). They include Tetralogy of Fallot (TOF) and tricuspid atresia. TOF has pulmonary stenosis as one of the defects that restricts the blood flow to the lungs. Tricuspid atresia obstructs blood from the right atrium to the right ventricle and decreases the amount of blood that reaches the lung (ATI Testing 2016).

In defects that decrease pulmonary blood flow, there is a right to left shift that allows deoxygenated blood to enter the systemic circulation. Defects that obstruct blood flow to the pulmonary or systemic systems include Coarctation of the aorta (COA), pulmonary stenosis, or aortic stenosis. COA impedes blood flow through the descending aorta to the lower body. Aortic stenosis acts as a mini version of a coarctation by constricting the blood flow to the body and causing hypertension from the stenosis. Pulmonary stenosis hinders blood flow to the lungs and causes right ventricular hypertrophy (ATI Testing 2016).

## Defects with Obligatory Mixing

Defects that demand the mixing of blood through the fetal shunts include Transposition of the great arteries (TGA), truncus arteries, and hypoplastic left heart syndrome. TGA is the interchange of the aorta and pulmonary artery. The aorta is attached to the right side of the heart, and the pulmonary artery connects to the left side of the heart. A septal defect or a PDA is kept open as the only means to oxygenate the blood. Truncus arteriosus combines the pulmonary artery and the aorta into one vessel that mixes the circulations. Hypoplastic left heart is a condition, where there is no functional left ventricle (ATI Testing 2016).

Risk factors impact the developing fetus in the first month of gestation and include **maternal TORCH infections** (Toxoplasmosis; syphilis varicella-zoster, parvovirus B-19; rubella; Cytomegalovirus; and Herpes), alcohol or substance abuse, Diabetes mellitus, or genetic factors, such as a family history, or Trisomy 21 (Down's syndrome) (ATI Testing 2016).

## Defects that Increase Pulmonary Blood Flow

### Atrial Septal Defect (ASD)

An ASD occurs from the incomplete formation of the heart that does not seal both atria into separate spaces. Blood flow breaches the septum between the right and left atria and results in increased pulmonary blood flow. This mixing of blood causes blood to flow from the left side of the heart to the right side (left-to-right shunt). Children with an ASD may present asymptomatically, or with a loud, harsh murmur with a fixed, split, second heart sound, or with heart failure (ATI Testing 2016).

### Ventricular Septal Defect (VSD)

A VSD is a hole in the septum between the right and left ventricle that results in increased pulmonary blood flow causing a left-to-right shunt. Children with a VSD present with a loud, harsh murmur auscultated at the left sternal border and/or heart failure. Many VSD's closes spontaneously or can cause sudden cardiac arrest (ATI Testing 2016).

### Patent Ductus Arteriosus (PDA)

A PDA is a condition in which the normal fetal circulation shunt (ductus arteriosus) that lies between the pulmonary artery and the aorta does not close, causing increased pulmonary blood flow, pulmonary congestion, and a left-to-right shunt. Children present with a machine hum murmur, a wide pulse pressure, bounding pulses, and possible heart failure. Children may also present asymptomatically, and may not be diagnosed until older (ATI Testing 2016).

## Obstructive Defects

Obstructive defects are those where blood flow exiting the heart meets an area of narrowing (**stenosis**), which obstructs blood flow. A stenosis causes blood pressure to increase before the defect and decrease behind the stenosis, which decreases cardiac output and leads to heart failure (ATI Testing 2016).

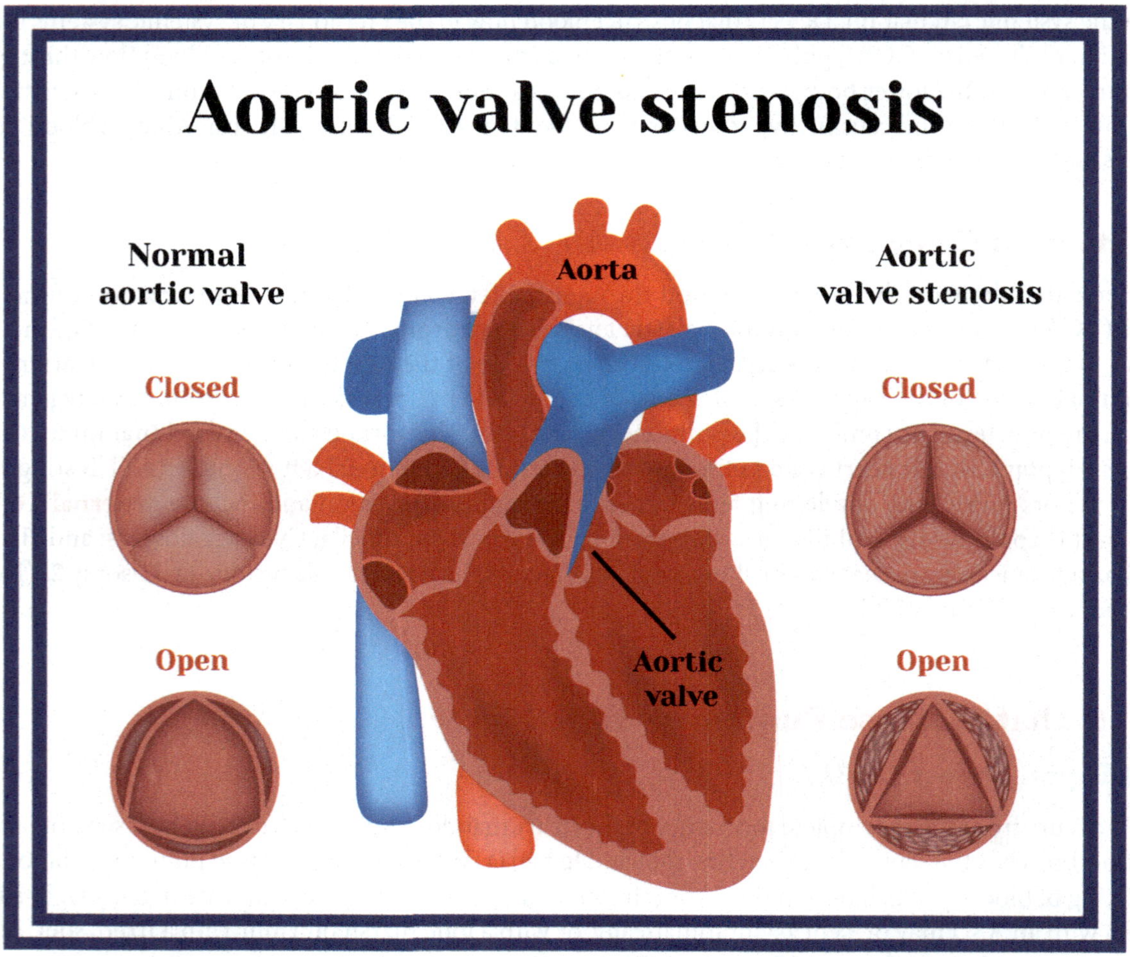




**Fig 6-4 A** stenosis impedes blood flow.

### Pulmonary Stenosis

Pulmonary stenosis is a narrowing of the pulmonary valve or pulmonary artery that impedes blood flow from the ventricles. Children present with a systolic ejection murmur, possible cyanosis (varies with the severity of defect), cardiomegaly, and possible heart failure (ATI Testing 2016).

### Aortic Stenosis

Aortic stenosis is a constriction in the aortic valve (see Fig 6-4). Infants present with faint pulses, hypotension, tachycardia, and poor feeding tolerance. Children show symptoms with exercise and have dizziness, chest pain, and a possible ejection murmur (ATI Testing 2016).

### Coarctation of the Aorta

A COA is a narrowing of the lumen of the aorta, usually, at or near the ductus arteriosus, that obstructs blood flow from the ventricle (see Fig 6-5). Children present with an elevated blood pressure in the arms with bounding pulses, cool skin in the legs, and decreased blood pressure in the legs with weak or absent femoral pulses. COA causes heart failure in infants. Children complain of dizziness, headaches, fainting, or nosebleeds in older children (ATI Testing 2016).

## Defects that Decrease Pulmonary Blood Flow

### Tricuspid Atresia and Tetralogy of Fallot

Children with TOF can present in a "**Tet-Spell**," a hypercyanotic spells characterized by acute cyanosis and hyperpnea. Children with tricuspid atresia have no opening in the tricuspid valve which necessitates the maintenance of a patent ASD to allow blood flow to the left atrium. Infants present with cyanosis, dyspnea, and tachycardia. Children have clubbing of the fingers and are hypoxic (ATI Testing 2016).

Children present with four defects that result in mixed blood flow: pulmonary stenosis, ventricular septal defect, overriding aorta, and right ventricular hypertrophy (see Fig 6-6). Newborns present with cyanosis at birth with worsening cyanosis over the first year of life. They have a systolic murmur and episodes of acute cyanosis and hypoxia or "Tet" spells (ATI Testing 2016).

## Mixed Defects

### Transposition of the Great Arteries (TGA) and Truncus Arteriousus

Infants with TGA present with a murmur, cyanosis, cardiomegaly, and heart failure.

Children with Truncus arteriosus present with a murmur, cyanosis, poor feeding habits, delayed growth, lethargy, and fatigue (ATI Testing 2016).

### Hypoplastic Left Heart Syndrome

Infants with HLH syndrome have a minimally functional left side of the heart (see Fig 6-7). An ASD (patent foramen ovale) allows for oxygenation of the blood. Newborns present with mild cyanosis, cold hands and feet, and lethargy. Once the PDA closes decreased cardiac output, cyanosis and cardiac arrest occur (ATI Testing 2016).

#### *Surgical and Medication Interventions*

### Shunt Closure

The providers can close an ASD during cardiac catheterization using pulmonary artery banding, or a complete repair with a patch. VSD's require a patch closure during the cardiac catheterization (ATI Testing 2016).

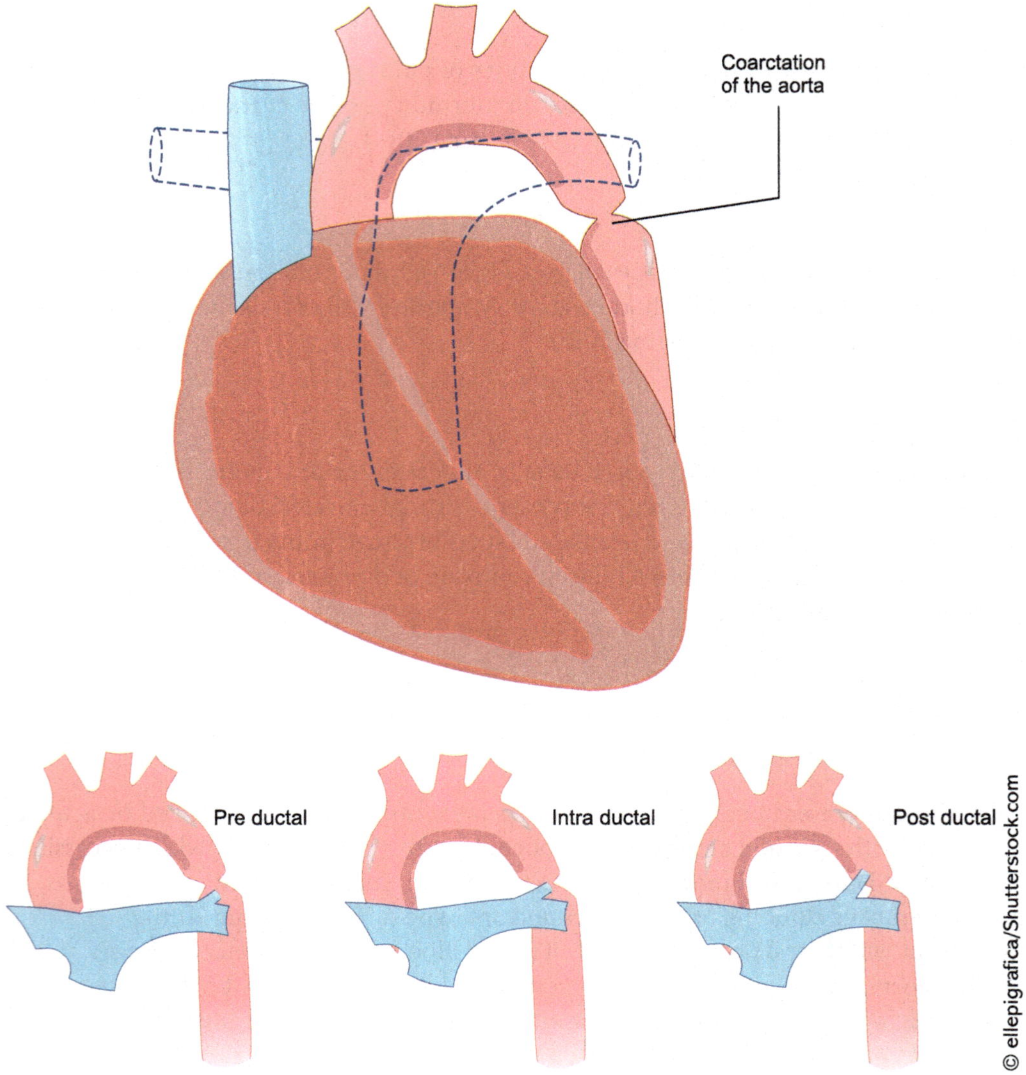


**Fig 6-5** The COA does not allow normal blood flow to the lower body

A PDA is closed pharmacologically or surgically. The provider uses **indomethacin (NSAID)** to close the PDA. If there is recurrence or treatment failure, a procedure that uses coils to occlude the PDA during cardiac catheterization or a thoracoscopic repair is performed (ATI Testing 2016).

## Pulmonary Stenosis

Children with pulmonary stenosis may receive a balloon angioplasty with cardiac catheterization. Infants can undergo a Brock procedure to resect the artery. Or children may undergo a pulmonary valvotomy to enlarge the valve (ATI Testing 2016).

## Aortic Stenosis

Children with aortic stenosis may respond to balloon dilation with cardiac catheterization. Alternatively, they may need a surgical procedure, such as the Norwood procedure or an aortic valvotomy (ATI Testing 2016).

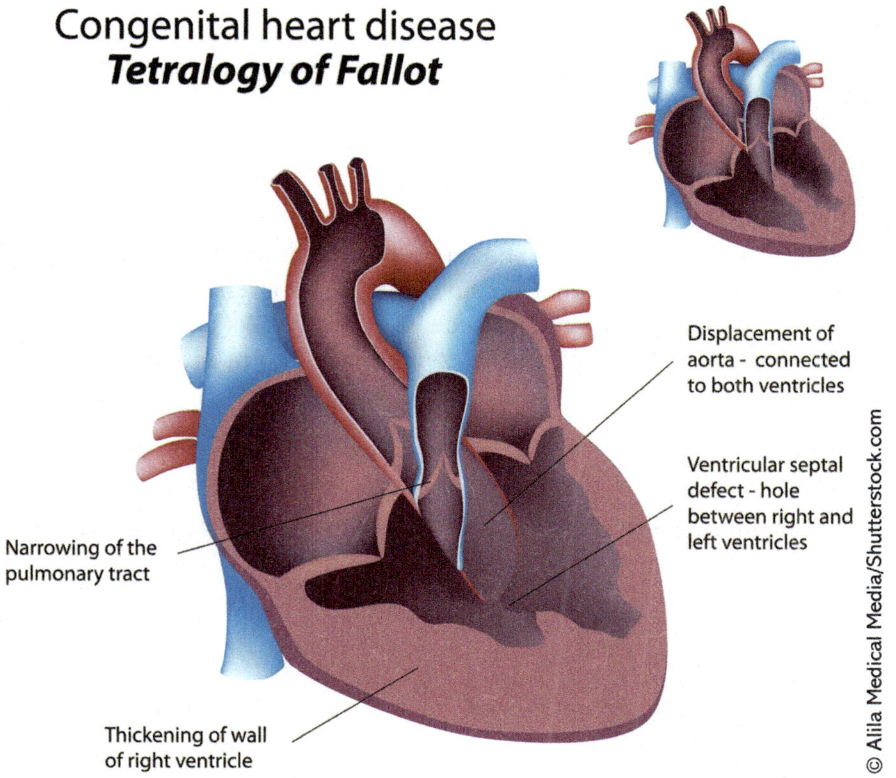


**Fig 6-6** The four defects in the Tetralogy of Fallot

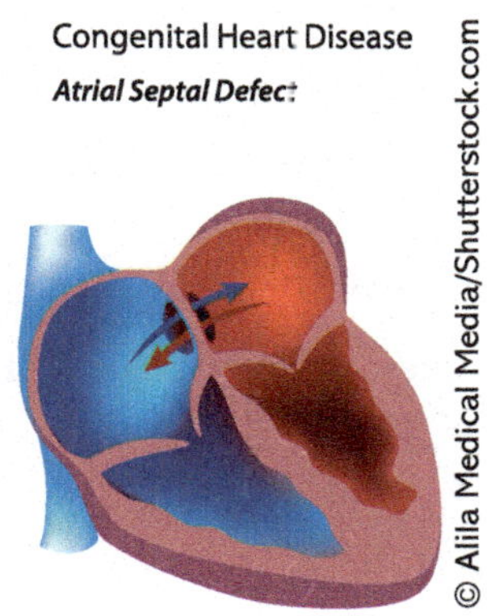


**Fig 6-7** An ASD is kept open to compensate for an underdeveloped left ventricle

## Coarctation of the Aorta

Infants under 6 years of age should have surgical repair. Infants and children receive a balloon angioplasty to dilate the vessel. If the adolescent acquires this coarctation, the provider places a shunt (ATI Testing 2016).

## Tricuspid Atresia

Children with Tricuspid atresia have three surgeries. The first operation creates a shunt from a branch of the aorta to the pulmonary artery (Norwood). Then, the surgeon connects the superior vena cava to the pulmonary artery (Glenn procedure). Finally, the modified Fontan procedure creates a shunt that connects the IVC and the SVC to the pulmonary artery and has a fenestration (hole), so blood can travel from the IVC and into the right atrium (ATI Testing 2016).

## Tetralogy of Fallot (TOF)

A child with TOF has a shunt placed until he or she is robust enough to undergo the primary repair. A complete repair takes approximately a year (ATI Testing 2016).

## Transposition of the Great Arteries (TGA)

A neonate with TGA has surgery to swap the arteries within the first 2 weeks of life (ATI Testing 2016).

## Truncus Arteriosus

A child with Truncus arteriosus requires surgical repair within the first month of life (ATI Testing 2016).

### Hypoplastic Left Heart Syndrome

A child with Hypoplastic left heart syndrome has three surgeries, like the child with Tricuspid atresia. The Norwood, the Glenn shunt, and the Fontan procedure (ATI Testing 2016).

## Pulmonary Artery Hypertension

Pulmonary hypertension (PAH) is excessive blood pressure in the arteries of the lungs that results in high pressure from the left side leaking into the low-pressure pulmonary side. PAH is a progressive and eventually fatal disease, as hypertension causes the accumulation of pulmonary edema in the alveoli (see Fig 6-8). There is no cure for PAH. Children with PAH present with dyspnea with exercise, chest pain, and syncope (ATI Testing 2016).

### Diagnosis

A chest x-ray, **electrocardiogram**, **echocardiography**, and cardiac catheterization confirm the diagnosis (ATI Testing 2016).

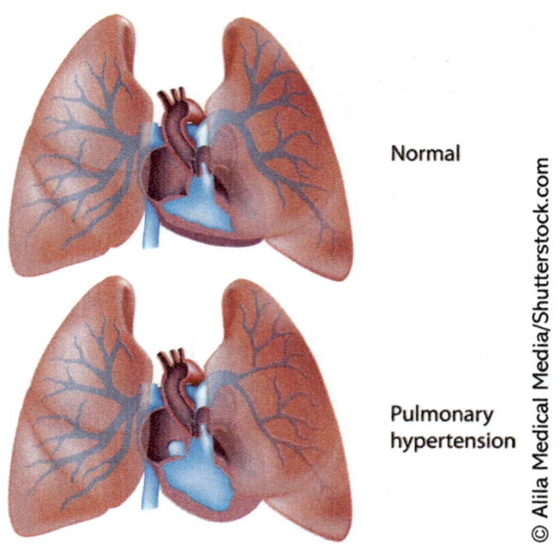


**Fig 6-8** PAH creates a back-up in the right ventricle that causes pulmonary edema

### Interventions and Teaching

Parents and the child should learn about supplemental oxygen, administering prostacyclin (vasodilator) without interruptions, and the importance of maintaining a strict medication schedule. Parents should also keep children out of high altitude areas. The nurse supports the child and family regarding diagnosis and decisions about treatment options and prepares the family for possible lung transplantation (ATI Testing 2016).

## Infective (Bacterial) Endocarditis

Infective endocarditis is an infection of the inner lining of the heart (endocardium) and the valves mostly caused by Streptococcus viridans or Staphylococcus aureus. Children who require prophylaxis treatment includes children who have artificial heart valves; a previous diagnosis of infective endocarditis, and congenital heart disease. Risk factors include a congenital or acquired heart disease and indwelling pulmonary artery catheters. Complications include heart failure, myocardial infarction, or embolism (ATI Testing 2016).

### Assessment

Children present with fever, malaise, a new murmur, myalgias, arthralgias, headache, diaphoresis, and weight loss. Newborns have feeding problems, respiratory distress, tachycardia, heart failure, and possible septicemia. The nurse draws labs and monitors the CBC, ESR, Urinalysis, and blood cultures results (ATI Testing 2016).

### Diagnosis

An electrocardiogram (ECG), echocardiogram, chest x-ray, CT and MRI scans confirm the diagnosis (ATI Testing 2016).

### Clinical Pearl

Medical breakthroughs in pediatric cardiac surgery have increased survival for children with cardiac conditions. However, the life of a child with a chronic cardiac condition can have physical, motor, cognitive and neurological alterations related to their chronic disease. In addition, he/she can have academic difficulties, behavioral problems, speech delay, and lack of attention and hyperactivity issues.

The best outcomes come from ongoing medical monitoring and the proper use of medications. Decreased hospitalizations promote self-esteem and self-image of children and adolescents. These important skills are the building blocks to completing normal development tasks.

The maintenance of health in children with CHD still requires care from parents and medical staff with nutrition, immunization, winter disease prevention and prophylaxis of bacterial endocarditis.

In addition, the child with a cardiac condition benefits from daily wellness strategies. A rehabilitation program of daily exercise, psychological interventions create a healthy lifestyle pattern.

Nurses can promote and praise the continued efforts a child and family make to maintain the health of the child. (Bertoletti, J., Marx, G. C., Hattge, S. P., and Pellanda, L. C. 2014).

### Interventions and Teaching

High dose IV antibiotics are necessary for an extended length of time (2–8 weeks) usually via a peripherally inserted central catheter (PICC). The nurse should focus on prevention and wellness, by reinforcing the need for the child to take prophylactic antibiotics before dental and surgical procedures (ATI Testing 2016).

Regular dental appointments reduce the risk of infection from caries. The family should also verbalize the signs and symptoms of infection and endocarditis (low-grade fever, malaise, decreased appetite with weight loss) and know to call the provider as soon as symptoms appear (ATI Testing 2016).

## Cardiomyopathy

A child with cardiomyopathy has lost the contractility of the myocardium which decreases cardiac output (see Fig 6-9). Risk factors include genetic factors, infection, metabolic conditions, collagen diseases, drug toxicity, and dysrhythmias. If untreated, cardiomyopathy progresses to cardiac shock (ATI Testing 2016).

### Assessment

Children with cardiomyopathy present with tachycardia, dysrhythmias, dyspnea, fatigue and poor growth, and hepatosplenomegaly (ATI Testing 2016).

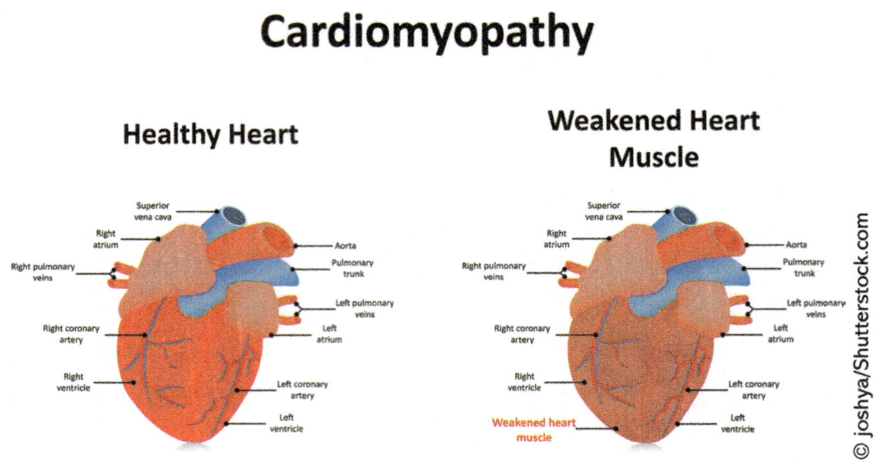


**Fig 6-9** A weakened heart muscle cannot contract properly

## Diagnosis

The provider diagnoses a child with cardiomyopathy through a chest x-ray, ECG, echocardiogram, and cardiac catheterization (ATI Testing 2016).

# Shock

Cardiogenic shock results from impaired cardiac function that leads to a decrease in cardiac output (ATI Testing 2016) (see Fig 6-10).

A child experiences anaphylactic shock as a hypersensitivity to a foreign substance that leads to systemic vasodilation and subsequent edema. Anaphylaxis, or anaphylactic shock can occur in response to an allergy (latex or peanuts), drugs, insect stings, or blood transfusions. Risk factors include cardiac surgery, acute dysrhythmias, congestive heart failure, trauma, or cardiomyopathy. Anaphylaxis develops from an allergy, asthma, or a family history of anaphylaxis (ATI Testing 2016).

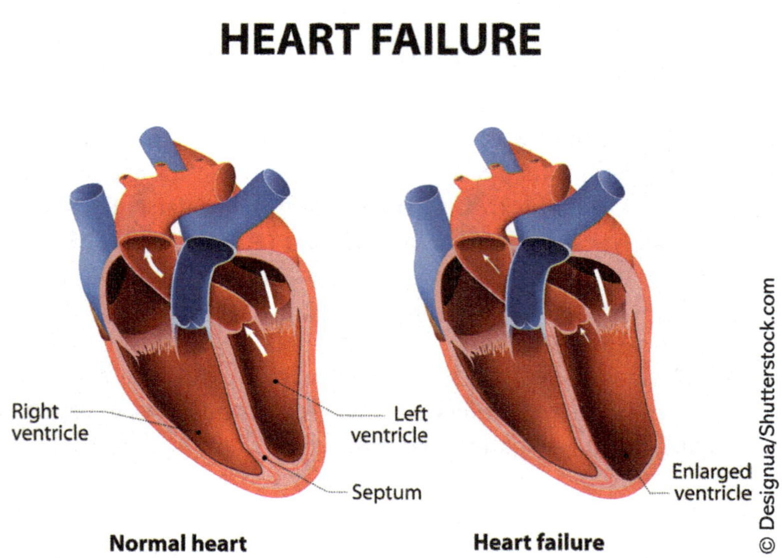


**Fig 6-10** An overstretched heart muscle from inappropriate pressures results in cardiogenic shock

## Assessment

The infant in shock presents with dyspnea and crackles, grunting, tachycardia, hypotension, and weak peripheral pulses (ATI Testing 2016).

As the heart is failing, the baby displays sweating, tachycardia, a gallop rhythm, a murmur, fatigue, pallor, cool extremities with weak pulses, a narrowed pulse pressure and cardiomegaly. Pulmonary symptoms include tachypnea, dyspnea, retractions, nasal flaring, grunting, wheezing, crackles, cyanosis, cough, and orthopnea. Signs of systemic venous congestion include ascites, neck vein distention, periorbital edema, weight gain, peripheral edema, and hepatomegaly. Signs of hypoxemia also develop as tachypnea, dyspnea, cyanosis, poor weight gain, polycythemia, and clubbed fingers (ATI Testing 2016).

## Diagnosis

Lab tests to determine oxygen carrying capacity and acid base balance include hemoglobin, hematocrit, serum electrolytes, and an ABG (ATI Testing 2016).

The nurse applies an ECG monitor to identify dysrhythmias. A chest x-ray determines heart size and blood flow through the heart (ATI Testing 2016).

## Interventions

The goal of treatment in cardiogenic shock is to maintain oxygenation of the red blood cells and compensate for the third spacing of fluid from the vascular compartment. Oxygen is a pulmonary dilator and could worsen pulmonary edema in heart conditions with right sided pathology. Therefore, only small amounts (bolus) of fluids (5-10ml/kg) is given to prevent pulmonary edema (Kar, S.S. 2015). Loop diuretics, dobutamine (or milrinone) and norepinephrine regulate third spacing, help the heart muscle contract, and tighten the vasculature to promote perfusion (Brissaud, O., Botte, A., Cambonie, G., Dauger, S., de Saint Blanquat, L., Durand, P., Kuteifan, K. 2016; Kar, S. S. 2015).

### *Medications*

Dobutamine is an adrenergic drug (neurotransmitter) that works through the stimulation of beta-1 receptors in the heart. It is a positive inotrope. Dobutamine has the side effect of tachycardia and can cause dysrhymias and fatal arrhythmia. It is given at 5–20μg/kg/min (Kar, S. S., 2015).

Milrinone is used for children with right side heart dysfunction in continuous perfusion of 0.5–0.75μg/kg/min. It is a phosphodiesterase-3 inhibitor, that increases the hearts contractility (**positive inotrope**), and vasodilates the vasculature decreasing afterload (Kar, S.S. 2015).

Norepinephrine constricts blood vessels, and is an alpha-adrenergic and also dilates the coronary arteries and is a beta-adrenergic (Kar, S. S., 2015).

## QSEN Application

### Quality Improvement

The advances made in cardiac surgery, require nurses to pay attention to quality improvement. QSEN defines quality improvement as the ability to "[u]se data to monitor the outcomes of care processes and use improvement methods to design and test changes to continuously improve the quality and safety of health care systems". The behaviors nurses can engage in "[d]esigning and using databases as sources of information for improving patient care, select and use relevant benchmarks". Using a system to integrate nursing research at the bedside is critical to maintain best practices for patients.

From Quality and Safety Education for Nurses http://qsen.org/competencies/pre-licensure-ksas/

## *Extracorporeal membrane oxygenation (ECMO)*

An extracorporeal membrane oxygenation (ECMO) is a machine that by passes the lungs through central venous access, oxygenates and warms the blood before returning the hemodynamically stable blood back to the child (see Fig 6-11). Fig 6-12 shows tubing coming from the left side of the heart, and the other tube delivers oxygenated and warmed blood to the right side of the heart. It is used as a temporary reprieve for the child in surgery, or as a bridge to transplantation (Kar, S. S. 2015).

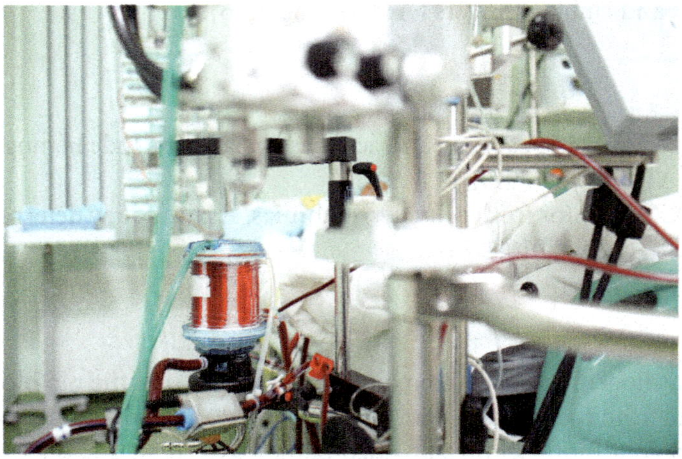



**Fig 6-11** ECMO Machine

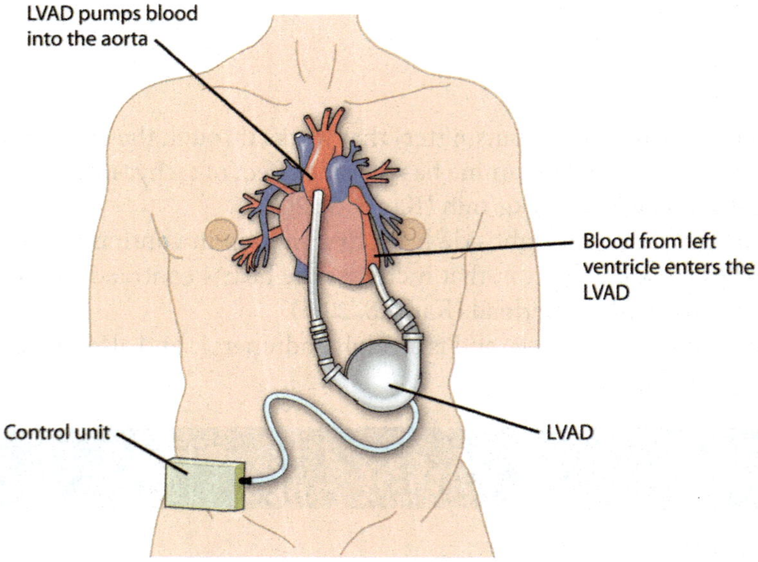




**Fig 6-12** A VAD for the left ventricle (LVAD)

## *Ventricular-Assist Device (VAD)*

A Ventricular-Assist Device (VAD) is a pump that can act as one or both ventricles (see Fig 6-12). There are benefits to a VAD, over ECMO that, it doesn't require an oxygenator and requires a lower dose of anticoagulation medication reducing the risk of cardiovascular events. However, a VAD requires four sites of cannulation into directly into the heart, where ECMO has to sites into the venous circulation (Kar, S.S. 2015).

### *Cardiac catheterization*

A cardiac catheterization can diagnose, but also evaluates dysrhythmias and allows the opportunity for some repairs (ATI Testing 2016).

The child has a radiopaque catheter inserted into the femoral artery and threaded into the heart with the use of fluoroscopy (see Fig 6-13). A contrast medium (can be iodine-based) illuminates the vasculature, so images of the blood vessels and heart as the contrast medium circulates through the cardiovascular system. Complications include nausea, vomiting, a low-grade fever, loss of the pulse in the catheterized extremity, transient dysrhythmias, and acute hemorrhage from the entry site (ATI Testing 2016).

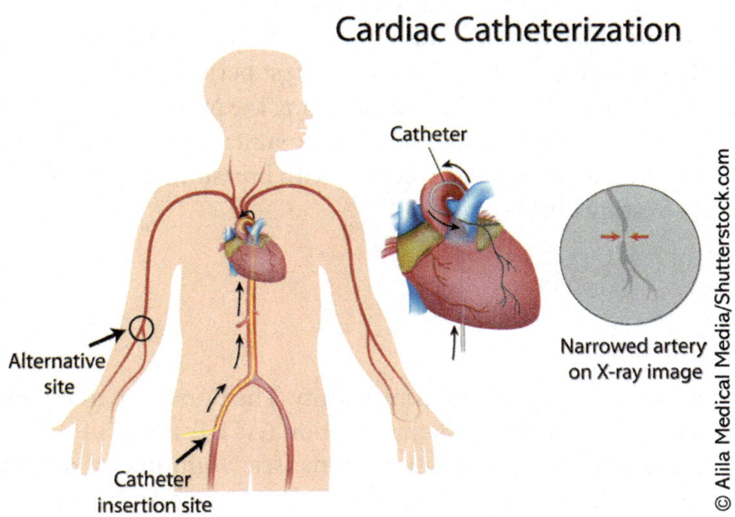


**Fig 6-13** The tunneling of the catheter into the heart

#### *Preprocedural Interventions*

The nurse assesses the child, takes vitals, and looks for signs of infection (severe diaper rash) which can cancel the procedure. The nurse checks the child for allergies to iodine and shellfish. The child is also kept in "nothing by mouth" or "nil per os" (NPO) status for 4 to 6 hours before the procedure by the nurse (inpatient) or by the parents (outpatient). The nurse marks the dorsalis pedis and posterior tibial pulses on both extremities for quick assessments. The nurse provides pre-sedation as ordered (ATI Testing, 2016).

#### *Post procedure Interventions*

The child needs continuous cardiac monitoring and pulse ox assessments for signs of bradycardia, dysrhythmias, hypotension, and hypoxemia. The nurse takes the child pulse and respirations for a 1 full minute. The nurse monitors the pulses for equality and symmetry. The nurse closely monitors the temperature and color of the affected extremity. A child with a cool leg and skin that blanches, are signs of an arterial obstruction. A call to the provider is necessary. The nurse applies direct, continuous pressure at 2.5 cm (1") above the entry site of the vessel, and applies a pressure dressing. The nurse monitors the insertion site (femoral or antecubital area) for bleeding or hematomas and maintains the dressing (ATI Testing 2016).

The child must remain in a flat position, with the legs extended for 4–8 hours to prevent embolism and hemorrhage. The nurse encourages the child to drink and void to excrete the contrast medium and to monitor hydration status. The child can develop hypoglycemia from the procedure, and may need an infusion with dextrose. The nurse may administer replacement fluids and/or medication to control emesis (ATI Testing 2016).

## Cardiac Interventions

The nurse aims to conserve the child's energy by clustering care and providing frequent rest periods. The nurse offers small, frequent meals, and minimizes bathing to keep the child calm and requiring less work from the heart. The nurse monitors inputs and outputs (I&O) fluid status and daily weight for nutritional status interventions.

Complications manifest as tachycardia, unstable blood pressure, serum electrolyte imbalances, and oliguria. Infants should receive cool, humidified oxygen via an oxygen hood (or tent), mask, or nasal cannula. The nurse monitors the oxygen saturation and suctions the airways, if necessary (ATI Testing 2016).

## Teaching

Parents should monitor the child for signs of infection and limit activity for the first 24 hours. They should also learn the techniques to minimize cardiac output. Interventions such as bedrest, choosing a soft preemie nipple or a high flow nipple for feedings every 3 hours, and rest periods during feedings.

Parents can promote breathing in their child by positioning the infant in a car seat at a 45° angle and allowing the child to sleep with several pillows while asleep and maintaining a semi-Fowler's or Fowler's position while awake. If a child is too weak to feed, gavage feeding with breast milk (possibly fortified) or high-density formula is appropriate (ATI Testing 2016).

## Medications

### *Digoxin*

Digoxin is an inotrope that increases myocardial contractility. The nurse or parent holds digoxin, if an infant's pulse is less than 90/min, or a child's pulse is less than 70/min (ATI Testing 2016).

Signs of toxicity include bradycardia, dysrhythmias, nausea, vomiting, or anorexia. If the child vomits, then do not repeat the dose. The therapeutic serum digoxin levels range from 0.8 to 2 mcg/L. The child takes digoxin every 12 hours. Therefore, a reasonable medication schedule is necessary (8 am and 8 pm; not 3 am and 3 pm). The nurse or parent guides the oral elixir toward the side and back of mouth when administering, and gives water to flush the medication and prevent oral decay. Missed doses are not made up; never give an extra dose or a higher dose in subsequent doses (ATI Testing 2016).

### *Captopril or Enalapril*

Captopril or enalapril are Angiotensin-converting enzyme (ACE) inhibitors that vasodilate the pulmonary and systemic vessels and decrease afterload. The nurse completes a blood pressure assessment before and after administering the medication and looks for signs of hyperkalemia (ATI Testing 2016).

### *Metoprolol or Carvedilol*

Metoprolol or carvedilol are beta-blockers that decrease heart rate and blood pressure and promote vasodilation. The nurse takes a blood pressure and pulse before administration. Adverse effects include dizziness, hypotension, and headache (ATI Testing 2016).

### *Furosemide or Chlorothiazide*

Furosemide or chlorothiazide are potassium-wasting diuretics rid the body of excess fluid and sodium. The nurse can mix the medication in a small amount of juice to disguise the bitter taste and minimize intestinal irritation (ATI Testing 2016).

Children should eat a potassium rich diet (great northern beans, sweet potatoes, tomatoes, watermelon, edamame), and stay hydrated while on diuretic therapy.

Signs of potassium imbalance include muscle weakness, irritability, excessive drowsiness, and increased or decreased heart rate. Daily weights inform the nurse if edema develops. Adverse effects include hypokalemia, nausea, vomiting, and dizziness. Worsening effects of heart failure include increased sweating, and decreased urinary output (ATI Testing 2016).

## Rheumatic Fever

Rheumatic fever originates as a Group A beta-hemolytic streptococcus (GABHS) infection of the throat and manifests as inflammation of the myocardium, endocardium, and epicardium and vegetative growths predominantly on the mitral valve (see Fig 6-14). Rheumatic fever affects the heart, joints, and the Central Nervous System (CNS). The risk factors for Rheumatic fever is an untreated GABHS infection, and not finishing the antibiotic prescribed for the infection (ATI Testing 2016).

### Assessment

Rheumatic fever presents within 2–6 weeks following an untreated or partially treated upper respiratory infection (strep throat) with GABHS (ATI Testing 2016).

Children present with fever, tachycardia, cardiomegaly, prolonged PR interval, a new or changed heart murmur, muffled heart sounds, a pericardial friction rub, or a report of chest pain, (carditis). The child develops nontender, subcutaneous nodules over bony prominences, and moving polyarthritis (painful swelling) in the large joints (wrists, shoulders, elbows, knees, ankles) that can migrate from joint to joint (ATI Testing 2016).

Children have a pink, non-pruritic macular rash (erythema marginatum) on the trunk and inner surfaces of extremities that appears and disappears (ATI Testing 2016).

Central nervous system involvement (chorea) develops after a few months of no treatment and includes involuntary, purposeless muscle movements, muscle weakness, involuntary facial movements; impaired fine motor development, labile moods, and random, uncoordinated movements of the extremities. Children are irritable, have poor concentration, and exhibit behavioral problems. The mitral valve can become stenotic as a complication (ATI Testing 2016).

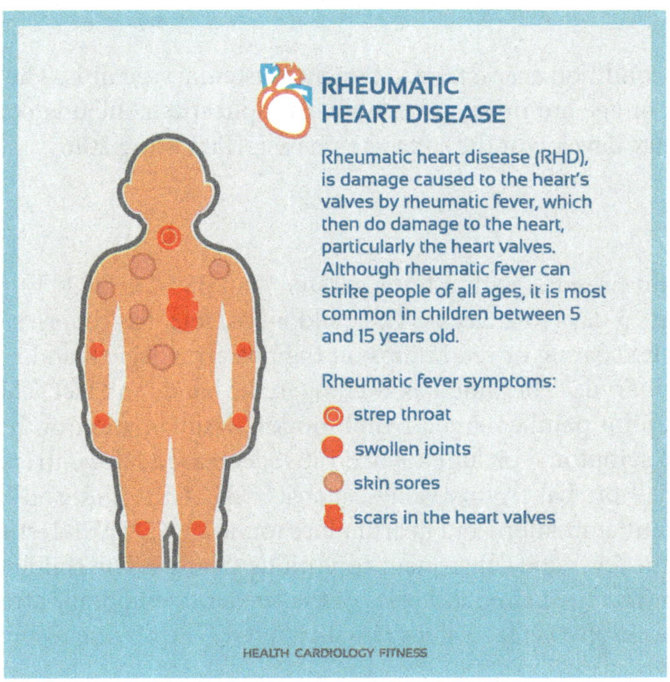




**Fig 6-14** Symptoms of Rheumatic fever

### Diagnosis

#### *Jones criteria*

Rheumatic fever used the Jones criteria to diagnose rheumatic fever. The child with Rheumatic fever presents with two major criteria or the presence of one major and two minor criteria following a GABHS infection. The major criteria include carditis, subcutaneous nodules, polyarthritis, rash (erythema marginatum), and chorea. The minor criteria include fever and arthralgia (joint pain). Children also have a positive throat culture for GABHS and a serum antistreptolysin-O titer that is elevated or rising, elevated C-reactive protein (CRP), and Erythrocyte sedimentation rate (ESR) for inflammation. An ECG and an echocardiograph determine cardiac function (ATI Testing 2016).

### Interventions

The nurse administers an antibiotic as prescribed, delivers supportive care, offers a high nutrient diet, encourages bedrest, and offers developmentally distraction activities (ATI Testing 2016).

### Medications

After the acute phase of the disease is over a regimen for antibiotic prophylaxis begins. Prophylaxis options include a daily oral dose of 1 g sulfadiazine, a monthly intramuscular injection of 1.2 million units of penicillin G, or two daily oral doses of 200,000 units of penicillin. The length of treatment ranges from 5 years to indefinitely, if there is permanent damage to the valves (ATI Testing 2016).

### Teaching

The nurse encourages compliance with the medication regimen as it is essential to the favorable outcome of the disease. The family should understand the signs of chorea, and understand its self-limiting nature. They should also know the signs of infection in case, reinfection occur (ATI Testing 2016).

## Kawasaki Disease

Kawasaki disease (KD) is a condition characterized by acute systemic vasculitis. The cause of KD is unknown, and children under 5years of age are most susceptible. Complications include coronary artery dilation or aneurysm formation that may develop in the subacute phase (ATI Testing 2016).

### Assessment

In the acute phase, the child presents with a fever greater than 38.9° C (102° F) that does not respond to (see Fig 6-15). The fever lasts 5 days to 2 weeks. The child is irritable, has red eyes, bright red, chapped lips, strawberry tongue with white coating or red bumps on the posterior aspect, and red, inflamed oral mucous membranes, including the pharynx. The child has swelling in the hands and feet. They develop red palms and soles, a nonblistering rash, joint pain, enlarged lymph nodes, desquamation of the perineum, and cervical lymphadenopathy. Cardiac symptoms include myocarditis, decreased left ventricular function, pericardial effusion, and mitral regurgitation. Laboratory values, such as CBC, CRP, ESR, and BNP evaluate white blood cell count, anemia, signs of inflammation, and heart failure found in KD (ATI Testing 2016).

In the subacute phase, the fever and subsequent conditions resolves. The child remains irritable, has peeling skin around the nails and on the palms and soles of the feet, and temporary arthritis. In the convalescent phase all physical symptoms resolve yet lab values remain altered. The disease resolves in 6–8 weeks from the onset (ATI Testing 2016).

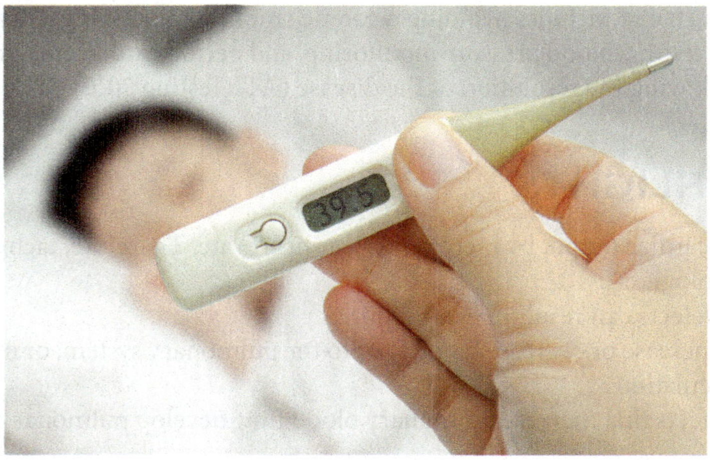


© all_about_people/Shutterstock.com

**Fig 6-15** A very high fever is a hallmark sign of Kawasaki's disease

## Diagnosis

A chest x-ray, echocardiogram and/or ECG indicate myocarditis, pericarditis, arthritis, meningitis, or inflammation (ATI Testing, 2016).

## Interventions

The nurse monitors vital signs and cardiac function, I&Os, and obtain a daily weight. The nurse begins an IV and gives IV gamma globulin (IVIG) to inhibit the child's immune response and fluids to prevent dehydration. The child should take clear liquids and soft foods by mouth. The nurse administers high dose aspirin which has a synergistic effect with IVIG (ATI Testing 2016).

Nursing care, such as cool cloths to the skin, moisturizing lotion for the skin, and the maintenance of oral hygiene, benefits the patient. The nurse should cluster nursing activities to ensure a calm environment to minimize cardiac stress (ATI Testing 2016).

## Medications

Gamma globulin

The nurse administers Gamma globulin 2 g/kg over 8–12 hours via IV infusion. Outcomes are best, if given within the first 7 days of illness (ATI Testing 2016).

### *Aspirin*

The child receives high dose aspirin 80–100 mg/kg/day divided every 6 hours, until the child is afebrile. Then, the dosage is reduced to 3–5 mg/kg/day to continue until platelet count returns to the expected range (approximately 6–8 weeks). Coronary sequelae may develop that requires indefinite aspirin therapy (ATI Testing, 2016).

## Teaching

The family should learn about the disease progression and resolution, including that child irritability can last 2 months, arthritic symptoms can last several weeks, and skin manifestations are painless, but the skin could be tender (ATI Testing 2016).

Follow up appointments are essential to optimal outcomes (ATI Testing 2016).

The family should help the child with passive ROM exercises in the bathtub (ATI Testing 2016).

Wellness care after discharge includes avoiding cigarette smoke, maintaining a healthy diet and a healthy weight, serum cholesterol testing, blood pressure monitoring, and period cardiac imaging. Live immunizations are held for 11 months following the resolution of the disease (ATI Testing 2016).

## CHAPTER HIGHLIGHTS

- Children increase cardiac output by increasing their heart rate. Therefore, tachycardia is often the first sign in many pathologies.
- Congenital heart defects can result in heart failure.
- Heart defects can increase or decrease blood flow to the pulmonary system, or may decrease blood flow to the systemic circulation.
- Newborns with defects that increase pulmonary blood flow develop pulmonary hypertension and pulmonary edema.
- Newborns with defects that decrease systemic blood flow have low cardiac output and poor perfusion to the organs.
- Signs of heart failure are tachycardia, tachypnea, pallor, crackles and cyanosis.
- Defects that continue to deteriorate create cardiomyopathy in children and subsequent heart failure.
- ECMO and VADs can maintain a child's cardiac output and oxygenation while awaiting transplant.

## REFERENCES

ATI Testing. 2016. Nursing Care of Children. Retrieved from http://www.atitesting.com/ati_next_gen/DisplayResources.aspx?Name=rm_rn_ncc_2016_ebook_20170417.pdf.

Bertoletti, J., Marx, G. C., Hattge, S. P., and Pellanda, L. C. 2014. "Quality of Life and Congenital Heart Disease in Childhood and Adolescence." *Arquivos Brasileiros de Cardiologia*, 102(2), 192–8. http://doi.org/10.5935/abc.20130244.

Brissaud, O., Botte, A., Cambonie, G., Dauger, S., de Saint Blanquat, L., Durand, P.,Kuteifan, K. et al. 2016. "Experts' recommendations for the management of cardiogenic shock in children." *Annals of Intensive Care*, 6, 14. http://doi.org/10.1186/s13613-016-0111-2.

Kar, S. S. 2015. "Pediatric cardiogenic shock: Current perspectives." *Arch Med Health Sci*, 3, 252–65.

## CHAPTER 7

# CARING FOR CHILDREN WITH GASTROINTESTINAL CONDITIONS

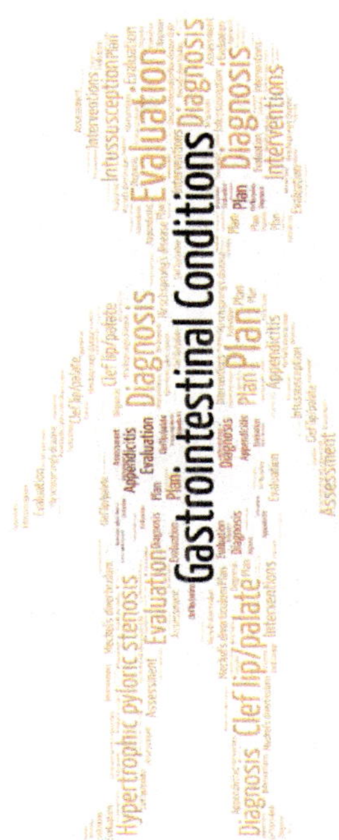


Modified from Shutterstock. Original image © eveleen/Shutterstock.com

## LEARNING OUTCOMES

1. Describe the changes in immune status as children move from passive immunity into active immunity.
2. Utilize the nursing process to provide safe, comprehensive healthcare to children with gastrointestinal conditions.
4. Recognize signs and symptoms of gastrointestinal disorders.
5. Synthesize data to create a nursing care plan for children with gastrointestinal disorders.
6. Contrast treatment for gastrointestinal disorders of bacterial versus viral origin.
7. Understanding the difference between gastrointestinal disorders that need surgical procedures versus the disorders that respond to medication, and do not require surgery.
8. Recognize the close relationship between the GI system and the airway, and propose nursing interventions to maintain the child's airway.
9. Teaching/learning principles in providing anticipatory guidance in the prevention and treatment of children with gastrointestinal conditions.

# KEY TERMS

Bile
Folic acid deficiency
Harvard Healthy Plate
H2-receptor antagonist
Hypotonic dehydration
Hypertonic dehydration
Isotonic dehydration
McBurney's point
Mild dehydration
Moderate dehydration
Lactation consultant
Neurological sequelae
Nissen fundoplication
Nonnutritive sucking
Rebound tenderness
Oral replacement solution (ORS)
Patient controlled anesthesia (PCA)
Proton pump inhibitor
Scintigraphy
Severe dehydration
Sunken fontanels
Teratogens
Urinary 5-hydroxyindoleacetic acid (U-5-HIAA) levels

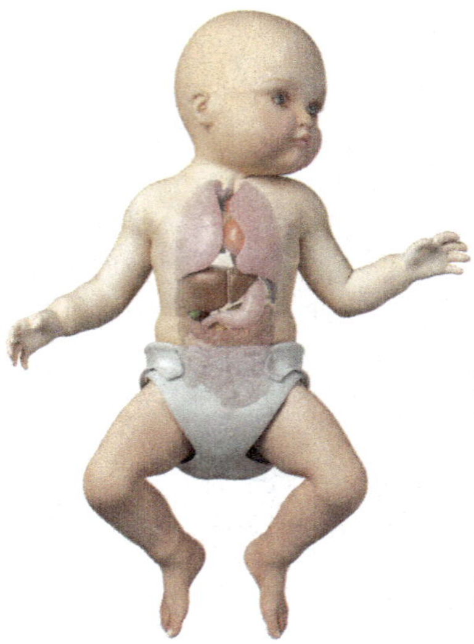



The gastrointestinal (GI) system is essential to maintain, as it absorbs and eliminates food, and provides immune support for infectious diseases. However, new research indicates that the gut produces neurotransmitters that affect the emotional well-being of the child as well as supports a microbiome of bacteria that number $3.8 \times e^{13}$ (Sender, R., Fuchs, S., and Milo, R. 2016). This sophisticated organ system also includes approximately 200–600 million neurons (Furness, J. B., Callaghan, B. P., Rivera, L. R., and Cho, H. J. 2014). These new insights create new relationships between microbiology, immunology, neurology, and nutrition (Joscelyn, J. and Kasper, L. H. 2014).

## Clinical Pearl

Newborns have a small stomach capacity of approximately 20 ml. Newborns who bottle feed in the hospital are routinely given over 60 ml of formula per feeding. Overfeeding newborns stresses them, causes spitting up, reflux and hypoglycemia especially for low birth weight babies. Feeding and sleeping should alternate in 1-hour intervals, based on cues from the newborn (Bergman, N. J. 2013).

There are differences in the infant and child's digestive tracts, when compared to an adult's digestive system Newborns have more peristalsis that suggests frequent, small feedings (1–2 hours) are beneficial. Newborns also lack amylase and trypsin that breaks down starch and protein respectively. Therefore, the infant is not ready to eat food until 6 months or when the enzyme concentration increases. Liver function has also not developed, as bilirubin and bile breakdown take a few weeks to occur. These organs completely developed by two years of age (ATI Testing 2016).

# CLEFT LIP AND PALATE

## Assessment and Interventions

Cleft lip originates from the incomplete fusion of the oral cavity (see Fig 7-1). Cleft palate derives from the incomplete closure of the palettes (see Fig 7-2). These structural anomalies occur during the first trimester of fetal life. If a pregnant woman comes in contact with **teratogens**, such as cigarette smoke, alcohol, anticonvulsants, retinoids, or steroids this defect may occur. Cleft lip and clef palette can present together, or as separate abnormalities. **Folic acid deficiency** or family histories are also risk factors. The anomalies can present unilaterally (on one side of the face), or bilaterally (on both sides of the face) (ATI Testing 2016).

Assessment of a cleft lip reveals a visible separation from the upper lip toward the nose. A cleft palate appears as a visible or palpable opening of the palate connecting the mouth and the nasal cavity (ATI Testing 2016).

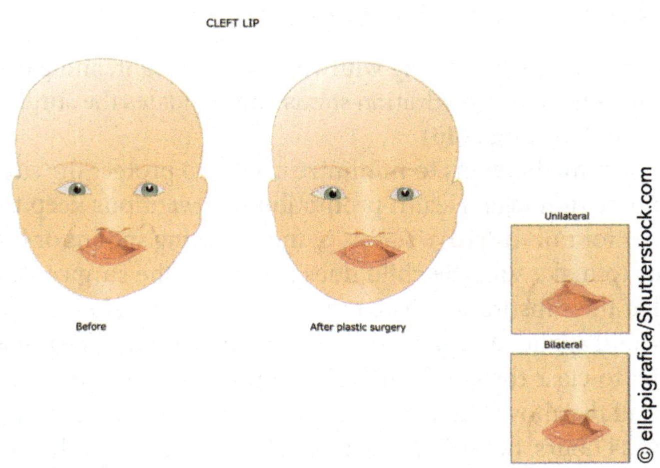


**Fig 7-1** Cleft lip: an opening in lip

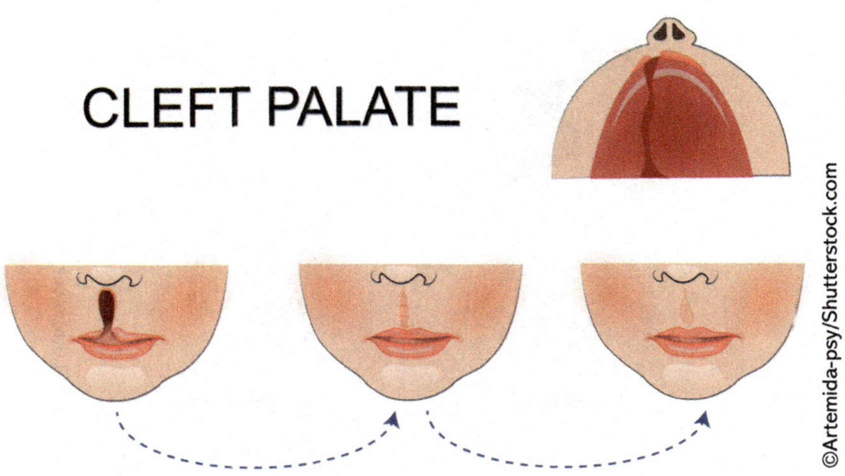


**Fig 7-2** Cleft palate: an opening in the mouth

### *Surgical Procedures*

Children have surgery for cleft lip repair at 2–3 months of age. Children who need cleft palate repair must wait until they are 6 to 12 months of age. Severe defects may require several revisions (ATI Testing 2016).

The neonatal pre-procedure assessment includes a baseline weight, inspection of the lip and palate, followed by palpation of the palate. The nurse assesses the strength of the infant's suck to determine the best feeding technique. The nurse should assess the baby's ability to feed. The nurse should then evaluate the child and family for coping skills and outside support, and note the level of bonding and attachment (ATI Testing 2016).

A child with an isolated cleft lip should attempt to breast feed. Mothers need extra support and confidence. The nurse should also coordinate a **lactation consultant**. If the child cannot latch on to the breast, a wide-based bottle may help. The nurse or parent can also occlude the gap with a finger while feeding the child in an upright position (ATI Testing 2016).

The nurse or parent uses a specialized bottle with a one-way valve and a specially cut nipple for children with a cleft palate or a cleft lip and palate while feeding the infant in an upright position. The nurse should burp the infant frequently. The nurse may start syringe feedings if bottle feeding is unsuccessful. Parents are encouraged to feed children, so they learn in a supportive environment, and are successful once discharged (ATI Testing 2016).

With both conditions parents should have referrals to community resources and support groups. A consultation with social services can identify the issues concerning finances or insurance (ATI Testing 2016).

## Postoperative Assessment and Interventions

The nurse initiates postoperative care beginning with vital signs, weight, and pain scores using an age-appropriate tool. The nurse monitors the child's hydration status and evaluates the surgical site for crusting, bleeding, and infection (see Fig 7-3) (ATI Testing 2016).

Interventions include pain medications to minimize crying to protect the surgical site and an upright, or side-lying position to facilitate drainage. Health promotion interventions keep the surgical sutures intact by avoiding nipples or a pacifier for **nonnutritive sucking**, and not using spoons or forks inside of the mouth. The nurse uses elbow restraints to make sure the child does not injure the surgical site and uses range of motion exercises per the protocol at their institution. The nurse cleans the incision site with normal saline, water, or diluted hydrogen peroxide and applies antibiotic ointment as prescribed. The nurse gently aspirates secretions of mouth and nasopharynx to clear the child's airway and prevent respiratory complications. A child with a cleft palate repair includes all the above and placing the infant in a prone position post-procedure, maintain a clear liquid diet for the first 24 hours, not using a suction catheter in the mouth and using a face mask to deliver

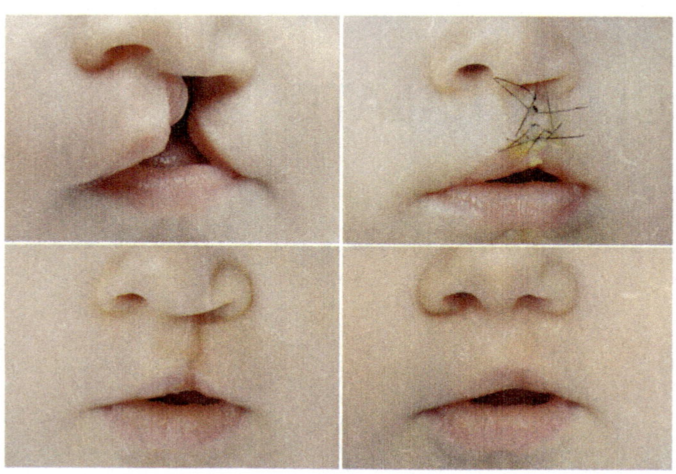



**Fig 7-3** Child with a cleft lip and cleft palate repair

oxygen. A child with a cleft palate repair may have pressure-equalizing tubes inserted to promote fluid drainage from the ears and to prevent otitis media or middle ear effusion. Parents should also keep up on routine dental care, as tooth eruption may not typically occur and need orthodontia (ATI Testing 2016).

## QSEN Application

GI disorders are multidisciplinary in nature. According to QSEN, Teamwork and Collaboration means to "function effectively within nursing and inter-professional teams, fostering open communication, mutual respect, and shared decision-making to achieve quality patient care" To be an effective team member, nurses can "[d]emonstrate awareness of own strengths and limitations as a team member, continuously plan for improvement in use of self in effective team development and functioning, and act with integrity, consistency and respect for differing views." From Quality and Safety Education for Nurses http://qsen.org/competencies/graduate-ksas/#teamwork_collaboration

Nurses are a part of a multidisciplinary team that includes surgeons, gastroenterologists, and nutritionists. Acquiring the skills to think broadly promotes teamwork across the disciplines.

## Teaching

The nurse explains the use of restraints, and the need for them until the lip or palate heals. Parents learn feeding techniques to maintain the skin integrity of the surgical site. Parents must understand the importance of monitoring the child's temperature for possible infection at the site or in the ear. If the child has a cleft palate, hearing and speech problems need early identification and early intervention (ATI Testing 2016).

The child requires a multidisciplinary health care team that includes a plastic surgeon, orthodontist, otolaryngologist, speech-language pathologist, pediatrician, nursing, audiologist, orthodontist, social worker and a psychologist (ATI Testing 2016).

# GASTROESOPHAGEAL REFLUX DISEASE (GERD)

Gastroesophageal Reflux (GER) and Gastroesophageal Reflux Disease (GERD) originate from the backing up of gastric juices into the esophagus (GER), and the erosion of the lining of the esophagus (see Fig 7-4). Risk factors of GER include prematurity, bronchopulmonary dysplasia, neurological impairments, asthma, cystic fibrosis, cerebral palsy, or scoliosis. Risk factors of GERD include neurologic impairments, hiatal hernia, and morbid obesity (ATI Testing 2016).

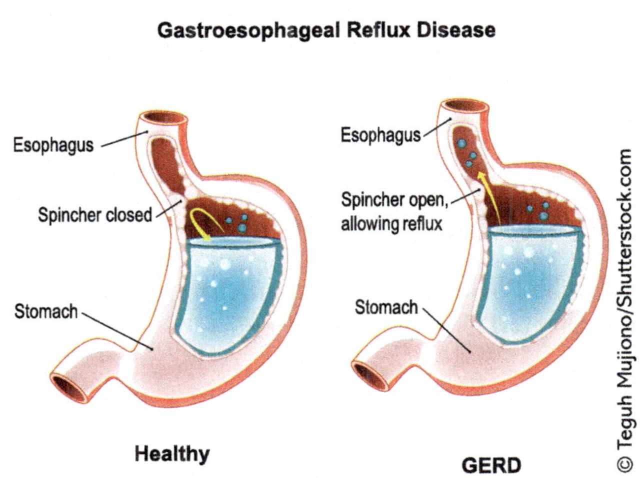


**Fig 7-4** The mechanism for reflux

## Assessment

Infants may present with excessive spitting up or forceful vomiting, irritability, excessive crying, blood in vomitus, arching of the back while or after eating or stiffening of the body, respiratory distress, and failure to thrive. Children may complain of heartburn, abdominal pain, difficulty swallowing, chronic cough, and noncardiac chest pain (ATI Testing 2016).

## Diagnosis

An upper GI endoscopy detects GI structural abnormalities such as esophagitis and strictures. The child needs a 24-hr intraesophageal pH study to measures the amount of gastric acid reflux, and a **scintigraphy** using a radioactive tracer to obtain an image of the esophagus) to determine the composition of the gastric secretions (ATI Testing 2016).

## Interventions

Interventions for GER include small, frequent meals and head elevation after feeding. Feedings may need thickening with 1 teaspoon rice cereal. However, thickened feeds are only moderately effective at managing GER (Horvath, A., Dziechciarz, P., and Szajewska, H. 2008). In fact, there is no evidence to support or refute the effectiveness of thickened feeds; it is not an evidence-based intervention as of yet (Huang, R.C., Forbes, D., Davies, and M.W. 2002). Children should not consume reflux inducing foods, such as caffeine, citrus, peppermint, spicy or fried foods that relax the lower esophageal sphincter. Weight control will keep pressure off of the esophagus in older children. The nurse positions the child supine with the head elevated after meals (ATI Testing 2016).

The classic interventions for GERD, include the above interventions for GER, plus the administration of a **proton pump inhibitor** (esomeprazole, omeprazole, pantoprazole, and rabeprazole), or an **H2-receptor antagonist**, cimetidine, famotidine, or ranitidine) lack support in the current research findings. Although, these medications are currently used, acid suppression does not decrease reflux. Nonpharmacological interventions are more effective for GER than medications, and most GER resolves without intervention as the LES sphincter develops (Rosen, R. 2014). Breastfed infants have shorter durations of reflux than formula-fed babies (Heacock, H. J. 1992).

## Surgical Procedures

Surgery may become necessary for severe cases. Children undergo the **Nissen fundoplication, a** laparoscopic surgical procedure that wraps the fundus of the stomach around the distal esophagus to decrease reflux. However, complications such as recurrent pneumonia, weight loss, and failure to thrive may arise (ATI Testing 2016).

# HYPERTROPHIC PYLORIC STENOSIS

Hypertrophic pyloric stenosis is the thickening of the pyloric sphincter, which creates an obstruction that presents in the first few weeks of life (ATI Testing 2016).

## Assessment

The child presents with a nonbilious, potentially blood-tinged vomit immediately or several hours following a feeding. As the obstruction worsens, the child projectile vomits (ATI Testing 2016).

The constant vomiting leaves the child in constant hunger, and irritable. With the infant lying supine, an olive-shaped mass appears in the right upper quadrant of the abdomen and may have a peristaltic wave that moves from left to right when lying flat (ATI Testing 2016).

This lack of nourishment results in dehydration as evidenced by pale, cool, dry skin,, dry mucous membranes, decreased skin turgor, decreased urinary output, concentrated urine, thirst, tachycardia, and sunken eyes. This child also fails to gain weight (ATI Testing 2016).

## Diagnosis

An ultrasound that reveals an elongated, mass surrounding an elongated pyloric canal confirms the diagnosis (ATI Testing 2016).

## Interventions

### Surgical Procedures

The child undergoes a laparoscopic pylorotomy to create an incision in the pylorus that allows food to pass into the small intestine (ATI Testing 2016).

### Preoperative Interventions

The nurse takes a set of vitals, including weight, starts IV fluids and electrolyte imbalances based on lab findings. She monitors Input and output status. The nurse drops an NG tube into the baby for decompression not feeding. The child takes nothing by mouth. The nurse administers IV fluids for correction of dehydration and electrolytes imbalances (ATI Testing 2016).

### Postoperative Interventions

The nurse takes a new set of vitals, including weight and compares them to the child's baseline. The nurse monitors for bleeding or signs of infection. The nurse also administers IV fluid and pain medications to keep the child hydrated and comfortable (ATI Testing 2016).

The child starts clear liquids 4–6 hours after surgery. The provider advances to breast milk or formula as tolerated 24 hours after surgery. The nurse documents the child's ability to tolerate feedings (ATI Testing 2016).

# HIRSCHSPRUNG'S DISEASE

Hirschsprung's disease (congenital aganglionic megacolon) describes a structural anomaly of the GI tract, caused by lack innervation in the colon that results in decreased motility and mechanical obstruction (see Fig 7-5) (ATI Testing 2016).

## Assessment

Since the newborn does not pass meconium for 24–48 hours, the nurse cannot discharge the infant. The infant may also vomit bile, refuse to eat, have abdominal distension. The newborn will undergo diagnostic testing.

The signs and symptoms in an infant include failure to thrive, constipation, vomiting, or incidents of diarrhea and vomiting (ATI Testing 2016).

A child with Hirschsprung's disease will appear undernourished, and with an anemic appearance. The child has abdominal distention, a palpable fecal mass, visible peristalsis, constipation, and foul-smelling, ribbon-like stool (ATI Testing 2016).

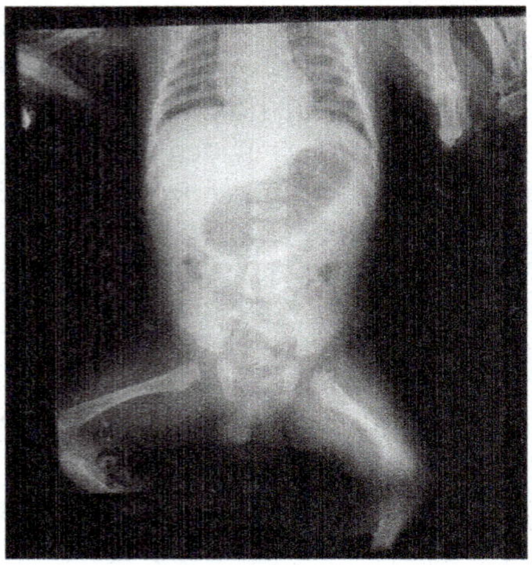


**Fig 7-5** An infant with Hirschsprung's disease showing megacolon

## Diagnosis

A rectal biopsy confirms the absence of ganglion cells in a segment of the colon (ATI Testing 2016).

## Interventions

The nurse maximizes the nutritional status of the child in addition to helping the family and child adapt and prepare for the upcoming surgery. The child needs a high-protein, high-calorie, low-fiber diet. In severe cases, the child may need total parenteral nutrition (ATI Testing 2016).

### Surgical Procedures

The doctor excises the aganglionic section of the bowel and might place a temporary colostomy (ATI Testing 2016).

### Preoperative Interventions

The nurse explains the surgery to the family and child, and guides the child through a bowel preparation procedure with a saline enema bowel prep with saline enemas and oral antibiotics as and oral antibiotics, as ordered. The nurse takes vitals, and a baseline GI assessment, including abdominal girth, and administers maintenance IV fluids and electrolytes (ATI Testing 2016).

### Postoperative Interventions

The nurse does a physical assessment with vital signs and evaluates them with the child's baseline. The child receives supplemental oxygen as prescribed. The nurse administers pain medications, provides Foley catheter care and ostomy care, if necessary. The nurse monitors for signs and symptoms of complications, such as enterocolitis, peritonitis, and shock. Treatment includes resolving inflammation, preventing bowel perforation, maintaining hydration, and initiating antibiotic therapy. Complications of the ostomy can manifest as anal stricture or incontinence that require more interventions, such as dilatation or Bowel-retraining therapy (ATI Testing 2016).

## Teaching

The family needs to learn to care for the surgical site and possible ostomy. They should understand the signs and symptoms of dehydration (ATI Testing 2016).

# INTUSSUSCEPTION

Intussusception occurs when the proximal portion of the bowel telescopes into a more distal portion, resulting in edema, lymphatic and venous obstruction, and ischemia (see Fig 7-6). It usually presents at the junction of the small and large intestine. As the obstruction lingers, edema progresses, and increased mucous enters the intestines. Infants and children belonging to ages 3 months to 6 years are at the highest risk (ATI Testing 2016).

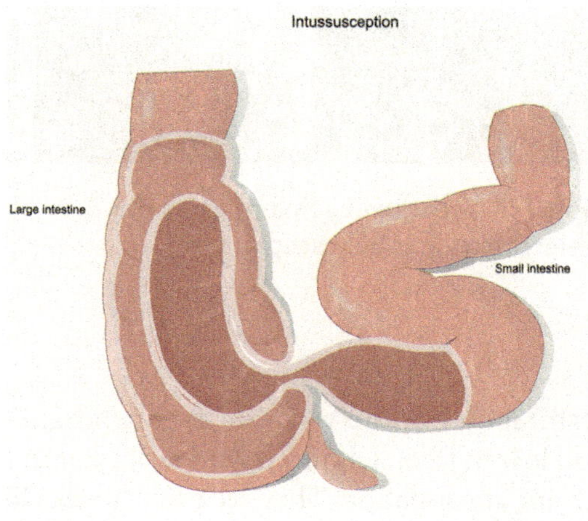


© ellepigrafica/Shutterstock.com

**Fig 7-6** Telescoping of intestines

## Assessment

The child presents with fever, vomiting, sudden episodic abdominal pain, crying while in knees to chest position, and a sausage-shaped abdominal mass. The stools combine with blood and mucus to produce stools the consistency of red currant jelly. The child has a tender, distended abdomen (ATI Testing 2016).

## Diagnosis

An abdominal ultrasound confirms the telescoped intestines.

## Interventions

The health-care team works together to stabilize the child before the procedure. The nurse runs IV fluids to correct and prevent dehydration. A nasogastric (NG) tube to decompresses the abdomen (ATI Testing 2016).

An air enema with or without contrast (barium) expands the telescoped intestine and allows the body to re-establish perfusion (see Fig 7-7). If the intussusception becomes chronic, the child will need surgery (ATI Testing 2016).

## Teaching

Parents need information about the diseases as well as the possibility of surgery, and to support the child and family with developmentally appropriate interventions.

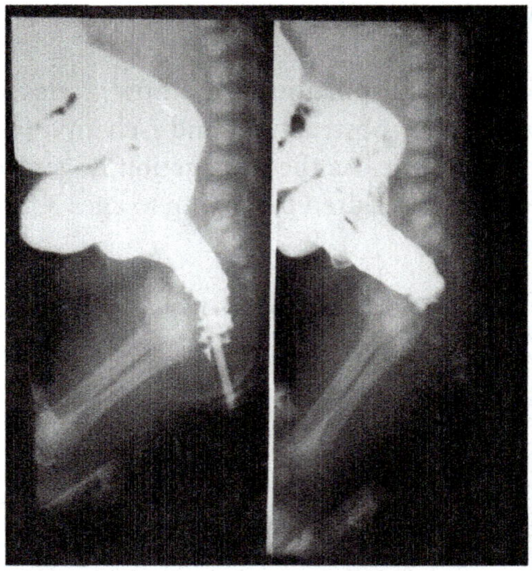



**Fig 7-7** A barium enema releases the telescoping in Intussusception

# APPENDICITIS

Appendicitis results from the inflammation of the vermiform appendix. (see Fig 7-8). The appendix may become blocked when the diet is too low in fiber. Children who lack fiber in their diets, in particular through fruits and vegetables, experience chronic constipation. They are prone to **fecaliths** (stony fecal matter). Fecaliths can lodge in the lumen of the appendix causing obstruction, edema, and infection. Children who suffer chronic viral disease can develop hyperplasia of the lymphoid tissue that occludes the lumen of the appendix. This presents mostly in school-aged children (Swischuk, L., Chung, D., Hawkins, H., Jadhav, S., Radhakrishnan, R., Swischuk, L. E., and Jadhav, S. P. 2015).

## Assessment

A child presents with many general assessment findings, such as fever, diarrhea or constipation, possible vomiting, anorexia, decreased or absent bowel sounds, lethargy, tachycardia, rapid, shallow breathing. Several assessment points help diagnose appendicitis. Abdominal pain, from the inflamed appendix, in the Right

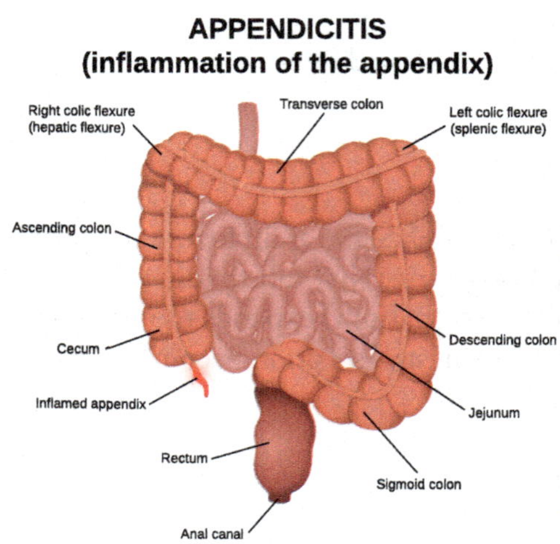




**Fig 7-8** An inflamed appendix

Lower Quadrant (RLQ) that is one-third of the length from the anterior iliac spine to the umbilicus, is known as, **McBurney's point**. Tenderness at McBurney's point alerts the nurse to a potential appendix rupture. A traditional test for appendicitis includes **rebound tenderness**, or Blumberg's sign, where pressure on the left side of the abdomen, produces pain on the right side. Another sign has been used that is less traumatic to the child, the **pinch-an-inch test**. This test pinches and slightly pulls the skin at McBurney's points and creates pain (Adams, B. D., Rickett, D., Albaneze, P. A., Jones, M. D., and York, G. 2005). Appendicitis may also present with a rigid abdomen and no pain.

## Diagnosis

A Computed tomography (CT) scan shows an enlarged diameter of the appendix, as well as thickening of the appendiceal wall. These findings are consistent with appendicitis.

Appendicitis may present with an increase in **urinary 5-hydroxyindoleacetic acid (U-5-HIAA) levels**. The nurse can measure this lab value through the collection of a 24–hour urine samples. Classic laboratory tests include a CBC to evaluate WBC, neutrophil percentage and C-reactive protein (CRP), and a urinalysis to differentiating appendicitis versus a urinary system issue (ATI Testing 2016).

## Interventions

### Pre-Procedure Interventions

The nurse prepares the family and child for immediate surgery. The nurse should closely monitor the child for rupture of the appendix as evidenced by a decrease or alleviation in pain. To prevent rupture, the nurse avoids the use of the nonpharmacological intervention, and heat. The nurse also avoids enemas or laxatives that may stimulate peristalsis (ATI Testing 2016).

### Surgical Procedures

The child undergoes a laparoscopic surgical procedure to remove the nonruptured appendix (ATI Testing 2016).

### Preoperative Interventions

The nurse takes vitals, monitors GI function and administers IV fluid replacement as prescribed and IV antibiotics (ATI Testing 2016).

### Postoperative Interventions

The nurse monitors vital signs and GI function and the surgical site. The child receives fluid and electrolyte replacement, antibiotics, and pain medication preferably with Patient Controlled Anesthesia (PCA). The nurse continues the NG tube to low continuous suction, with the child kept NPO. The child receives wound care with irrigation (saline or antibacterial solution) for the surgical sites in addition to drain care. The nurse looks for complications like fever and peritonitis (ATI Testing 2016).

Peritonitis symptoms include fever, a sudden increase in pain, irritability, a rigid abdomen, abdominal distention, tachycardia, rapid, shallow breathing, pallor, or chills (ATI Testing 2016).

## Teaching

Preoperatively, the family should learn incision care and signs of infection. The child and parents must understand the need to maintain NPO status and how to use a PCA machine (ATI Testing 2016).

Postoperatively, the child and parent should verbalize understanding about postoperative care, such as early ambulation, the advancement of the child's diet, and wound care. The parent and child should feel competent to administer pain medication through the PCA (ATI Testing 2016).

## Clinical Pearl

It was common practice to withhold opioids to children with appendicitis in fear of masking their symptoms. However, the literature does not support that assumption. Treating children when they were in pain kept them more comfortable and did not mask rebound tenderness (Aghamohammadi, D., Gholipouri, C., Hosseinzadeh, H., Khajehee, M. A., Ghabili, K., and Golzari, S. E. 2012).

Finally, parents must understand how to prevent another bout of appendicitis. They need encouragement and support to identify sources of fiber, they can introduce into the family diet to minimize fecaliths formation, and infection control techniques to minimize viral infections. Assure the family, that a healthy diet high in fiber and low in processed foods are as essential to their family routines as holiday celebrations and family traditions (ATI Testing 2016).

# INFECTIOUS GASTROENTERITIS

Several pathogens cause infectious gastroenteritis rotavirus, E-coli, salmonella, C. difficile, C. botulinum, staphylococcus, G. lamblia, shigellosis, caliciviruses, Yersinia enterocolitis, or Enterobius vermicularis. Gastroenteritis is an inflammation of the stomach lining (see Fig 7-9). The child's diagnosis depends on samples of stool and blood samples evaluated in the lab (ATI Testing 2016).

## Assessment

The nurse obtains a baseline height, weight, and vital signs. A dehydration assessment (dry mucous membranes, poor skin turgor, delayed capillary refill, lack of tears) indicates the severity of the problem (ATI Testing 2016).

A rectal temperature is contraindicated. Strict I&Os that include urine and stool are kept to determine hydration status. Dehydration presents as mild, moderate, or severe (ATI Testing 2016).

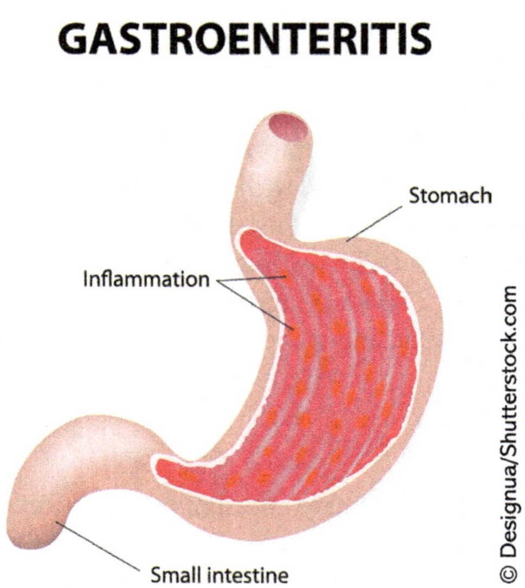


**Fig 7-9** Gastroenteritis is inflammation of the stomach lining

## Interventions

The nurse administers IV fluids and an **oral replacement solution (ORS)** of 75 to 90 sodium mEq/L at 40 to 50 mL/kg over 4 hr. The nurse follows this with maintenance therapy with ORS of 40 to 60 sodium mEq/L and limit to 150 mL/kg/day. The nurse also replaces each diarrhea stool with 10 mL/kg of ORS for ongoing diarrhea. Children with mild dehydration receive 50 mL/kg rehydration fluid every 4 to 6 hours.

Children with moderate dehydration need 100 mL/kg rehydration fluid every 4 to 6 hours (ATI Testing 2016).

The provider orders antibiotics for Shigella, C. difficile, and G. lamblia, but not for C. botulinum, E. coli, and Salmonella. Infants may receive breastmilk or formula, if supplementary hydration becomes necessary. Infants may receive water, breast milk, or lactose-free formula, if additional fluids become necessary. Isotonic parental fluids are bolused at 20ml/kg for isotonic and hypotonic dehydration. Rapid fluid replacement can cause cerebral edema in hypertonic dehydration. If the child was hypokalemic IV potassium may be started after the child urinated to confirm kidney function. If the child cannot avoid, the potassium may reach hyperkalemic levels and cause dysrhythmias (ATI Testing 2016).

## Medications

The antibiotics metronidazole, tinidazole, and beta-lactams treat C. difficile, G. lamblia and Shigella respectively. Probiotics, such as Lactobacillus rhamnosus or Saccharomyces boulardii at 5 to 40 billion colony forming units/day prevent watery diarrhea associated with antibiotic use (Goldenberg, J.Z., Lytvyn, L., Steurich, J., Parkin, P., Mahant, S., and Johnston, B.C. 2015).

The treatment of parasitic worms (Enterobius vermicularis) includes mebendazole, albendazole, and pyrantel pamoate (ATI Testing 2016).

## Teaching

The nurse can simplify the teaching by creating "a do and don't list." The "do's" include informing the child's school or day care of the infection/infestation, and understanding about using commercially prepared ORS for diarrhea. Parents should also change the bed linens and the child's underwear daily for several days. Parents must cleanse toys and child care areas thoroughly to prevent further spread or reinfestation.

The "don'ts" includes giving space between juices, gelatin, sodas, and gelatin. These options have high carbohydrate content, low electrolyte content, and a hi osmolality. Children should refrain from caffeine, due to its mild diuretic effect; chicken or beef broth, which is high in sodium and low in carbohydrates; the BRAT diet (bananas, rice, applesauce, and toast) is inadequate related to a negligible nutritional value, high carbohydrate content, and low electrolyte content. Parents should make sure the family does not share dishes and utensils, and they must thoroughly wash them in hot, soapy water or in the dishwasher. Parents should discourage nail biting, and the family should understand prevention measures, including hand washing and the rotavirus vaccine (ATI Testing 2016).

The main complication to gastroenteritis is dehydration. Dehydration can present as isotonic, hypotonic, and hypertonic based on the deficit the child develops (ATI Testing 2016).

**Isotonic dehydration** simply means that the child lost water and sodium in nearly equal amounts. There is a significant loss of extracellular fluid that creates a volume deficit in the vascular compartment and sodium levels are in the normal range. Hypovolemic shock will eventually develop, if not treated.

**Hypotonic dehydration** means the child has lost more electrolytes than water. This creates a gradient that forces water into the cells, which creates less circulating volume. Electrolyte imbalance compounds the hypovolemia and puts the child at risk for **neurological sequelae** (change in the level of consciousness, irritability, hyperreflexia, and seizures). Serum sodium levels drop below 130 mEq/L. A child with hypotonic dehydration has a high likelihood of being in hypovolemic shock. **Hypertonic dehydration** refers to a water loss that exceeds an electrolyte loss and creates a fluid shift from inside of the cells to outside of the cells. The child is less likely to develop hypovolemic shock. Hypertonic dehydration may also produce neurologic changes as the serum sodium concentration elevates to levels greater than 150 mEq/L (ATI Testing 2016).

The process of dehydration has three stages and treatment is guided by the amount of fluid loss. **Mild dehydration** causes a weight loss of 3%–5% in infants and 3%–4% in children. The signs and symptoms include behavioral changes, dry mucous membranes, a depressed anterior fontanel, increased pulse, with a blood pressure within normal limits, and a capillary refill greater than 2 seconds. **Moderate dehydration** causes a weight loss of 6%–9% in infants and 6%–8% in children, with a capillary refill between 2 and 4 seconds, and possible thirst and irritability. The child's pulse increases but the blood pressure remains normal. The child may have episodes of orthostatic blood pressure. Other symptoms include dry mucous membranes, decreased tears, and declining skin turgor, with slight tachypnea. Infants present with a normal to sunken anterior fontanel. **Severe dehydration** is defined by a greater than 10% loss in infants, and 10% loss in children, with a capillary refill greater than 4 seconds. The child has tachycardia, hyperpnea, and orthostatic blood pressure can quickly progress to shock. Children are thirsty, have very dry mucous membranes, no tears, sunken eyeballs, **sunken fontanels**, and tenting skin. Children produce little (oliguria) to no urine (anuria). All parents should encourage oral hydration. The child's diet advances from clear fluid to a normal diet as they get better (ATI Testing 2016).

# MECKEL'S DIVERTICULUM

Meckel's diverticulum is a complication that results in the incomplete closure of the omphalomesenteric duct in the fetus. This results in an outpouching by the ileocecal valve (see Fig 7-10). Complications include GI hemorrhage and bowel obstruction, if left untreated (ATI Testing 2016).

## Assessment

Children present with usually painless rectal bleeding, abdominal pain, and bloody stools with mucus (ATI Testing 2016).

## Diagnosis

The healthcare provider makes a diagnosis through radiographic evidence from the Meckel's scan, a radionucleotide scan that confirms Meckel's diverticulum. A CBC confirms the loss of blood (ATI Testing 2016).

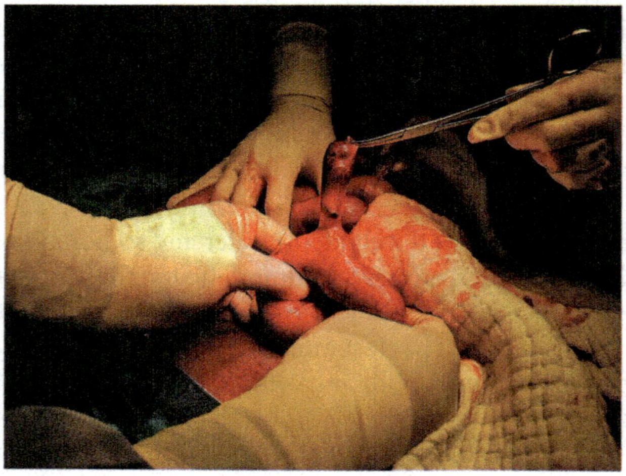



**Fig 7-10** Meckel's diverticulum is an outpouch that needs surgical removal

## Interventions

### Surgical Removal of the Diverticulum

The nurse prepares the child and family for surgery using developmentally appropriate techniques (ATI Testing 2016).

### Preoperative Interventions

The nurse provides oxygen, administers IV fluids and blood transfusions to correct hypovolemia as ordered. The child rests, and the nurse monitors the amount of blood loss in the stools (ATI Testing 2016).

### Postoperative Interventions and Teaching

The nurse monitors the airway, the respiratory status, initiates oxygen therapy, if necessary, and begins antibiotic and fluids. The nurse also monitors the surgical site for hemorrhage and the return of bowel and bladder function. The nurse maintains the child on an NG tube to low continuous suction, and keeps the child NPO. The nurse teaches the child and family about the procedure and the complications of surgery, such as hemorrhage and infection (ATI Testing 2016).

# FAILURE TO THRIVE

Failure to thrive (FTT) results from the inability of a child to absorb calories necessary for growth and development. An infant who is under the 5th percentile for weight with a consistent pattern of weight loss fits the clinical definition of FTT. Causes may include inadequate caloric intake, inadequate absorption, increased metabolism, or defective processing of food. Risk factors include intrauterine growth restriction, disturbed parent-child interactions, dysfunctional parenting behaviors, poverty, family stress, and ineffective breastfeeding (ATI Testing, 2016).

FTT may occur secondarily to cerebral palsy, congenital heart disease, hepatic disease, cystic fibrosis, Down syndrome, gastroesophageal reflux, and premature birth. Complications include extreme malnourishment that requires an NG or OG tube to feed the child (ATI Testing 2016).

## Assessment

Children who are less than 5th percentile on growth chart, with a malnourished appearance, who appear withdrawn needs further assessment. The nurse looks for a decreased activity level, and no fear of strangers. Children may also present with minimal smiling, withdrawal behavior, developmental delays, a wide-eyed gaze, a stiff or flaccid body, and a feeding disorder. The nurse assesses for dehydration, such as decreased urine output, dry mucous membranes, and decreased feeding (ATI Testing 2016).

## Interventions

The nurse reviews the nutrition history of the child with the parents and observes for parent-child interaction. The nurse measures height and weight without clothing or a diaper. Observe for low weight, malnourished appearance, and manifestations of dehydration (ATI Testing 2016).

The nurse establishes a feeding schedule and meets I&O and caloric needs. The nurse teaches the parents feeding cues of early and late hunger.

The nurse gives support, if the mother is breastfeeding, including proper positioning, latching on, and timing. The nurse may also give formula. All children receive a multivitamin. The nurse teaches the parents about mixing formula and potential electrolyte imbalances. The nurse models developmentally appropriate interactions; the parents can reflect back as a sign they are bonded to the infant through eye contact and face-to-face posture during feedings. Parents can also talk to the infant while feeding, and to burp the infant frequently. The nurse should keep the environment calm without distractions. This requires persistence as infants may refuse at first. Try 10–15 minutes of feeding time, and take a break. The nurse should never force the infant to eat (ATI Testing 2016).

If necessary, an NG tube is placed to facilitate feeding. Children at risk for aspiration need a radiographic image to confirm placement. Otherwise, aspirate pH testing with a value of 5 or below indicated the correct placement. The nurse measures the tube length from age-related height-based methods, rather than nose-ear-xiphoid or nose-ear-mid-xiphoid-umbilicus measurements (Cincinnati Children's Hospital Medical Center 2011).

## CHAPTER HIGHLIGHTS

- The gastrointestinal system has digestive, immunological, neurological, and microbiological functions.
- Ideally, newborns receive breast milk. Formula-fed infants need no more than 1 oz. feedings per hour with time for sleep in between.
- Cleft lip and cleft palate are congenital anomalies that require surgery and a multidisciplinary team for the best outcome.
- GER and GERD treatment is most effective through non-pharmacological interventions.
- Hypertrophic pyloric stenosis creates projectile vomiting in infants.
- Hirschsprung's disease produces distention and failure to pass stool.
- Intussusception is a condition where the intestine telescopes back on itself and causes obstruction.
- Appendicitis occludes the lumen of the appendix. Appendicitis is caused by a low fiber diet and/or serial viral infections.
- Gastroenteritis is a common cause for gastrointestinal upset and may result in fluid and electrolyte imbalances.

## REFERENCES


Adams, B. D., Rickett, D., Albaneze, P. A., Jones, M. D., and York, G. 2005. Pinch-an-inch test for appendicitis. Retrieved August 03, 2017, from https://www.ncbi.nlm.nih.gov/pubmed/16440921.

Aghamohammadi, D., Gholipouri, C., Hosseinzadeh, H., Khajehee, M. A., Ghabili, K., and Golzari, S. E. 2012. "An Evaluation of the Effect of Morphine on Abdominal Pain and Peritoneal Irritation Signs in Patients with Acute Surgical Abdomen." *Journal of Cardiovascular and Thoracic Research*, 4(2), 45–8. http://doi.org/10.5681/jcvtr.2012.011.

ATI Testing. 2016. Nursing Care of Children. Retrieved from http://www.atitesting.com/ati_next_gen/DisplayResources.aspx?Name=rm_rn_ncc_2016_ebook_20170417.pdf.

Bergman, N. J. 2013. Neonatal stomach volume and physiology suggest feeding at 1-h intervals. Retrieved August 02, 2017, from https://www.ncbi.nlm.nih.gov/pubmed/23662739.

Cincinnati Children's Hospital Medical Center Best Evidence Statement (BESt). 2011. Retrieved from https://www.cincinnatichildrens.org/-/media/cincinnati%20childrens/home/service/j/anderson-center/evidence-based-care/recommendations/type/confirmation%20of%20nasogastric%20tube%20ngt%20placement.

Furness, J. B., Callaghan, B. P., Rivera, L. R., and Cho, H. J. 2014. The enteric nervous system and gastrointestinal innervation: integrated local and central control. Retrieved August 02, 2017, from https://www.ncbi.nlm.nih.gov/pubmed/24997029.

Goldenberg, J. Z., Lytvyn, L., Steurich, J., Parkin, P., Mahant, S., and Johnston, B. C. 2015. "Probiotics for the prevention of pediatric antibiotic-associated diarrhea." *Cochrane Database of Systematic Reviews*, Issue 12. Art. No.: CD004827. doi: 10.1002/14651858.CD004827.pub4.

Heacock, H. J. (1992). "Influence of breast vs. formula milk in physiologic gastroesophageal reflux in health newborn infants." *J Pediatr Gastroenterol Nutr.* 14(1):41–6.

Horvath, A., Dziechciarz, P., and Szajewska, H. 2008. The Effect of Thickened-Feed Interventions on Gastroesophageal Reflux in Infants: Systematic Review and Meta-analysis of Randomized, Controlled Trials. Retrieved July 31, 2017, from http://pediatrics.aappublications.org/content/122/6/e1268.

Huang, R.C., Forbes, D., and Davies, M. W. 2002. Feed thickener for newborn infants with gastro-oesophageal reflux. Cochrane Database of Systematic Reviews 2002, Issue 3. Art. No.: CD003211. DOI: 10.1002/14651858.CD003211.

Joscelyn, J., and Kasper, L. H. 2014. "Digesting the emerging role for the gut microbiome in central nervous system demyelination." *Multiple Sclerosis (Houndmills, Basingstoke, England), 20*(12), 1553–9. doi: 10.1177/1352458514541579.

Rosen, R. 2014. "Gastroesophageal Reflux in Infants More Than Just a phenomenon." *Jama Pediatrics*, 168(1), 83–9.

Sender, R., Fuchs, S., and Milo, R. 2016. "Revised Estimates for the Number of Human and Bacteria Cells in the Body." *PLoS Biology*, *14*(8), e1002533. http://doi.org/10.1371/journal.pbio.1002533.

Swischuk, L., Chung, D., Hawkins, H., Jadhav, S., Radhakrishnan, R., Swischuk, L. E., Jadhav, S. P. et al. 2015. "Non-fecalith-induced appendicitis: etiology, imaging, and pathology." *Emergency Radiology*, 22(6), 643–649. doi: 10.1007/s10140-015-1338-1.

## CHAPTER 8

# CARING FOR CHILDREN WITH URINARY CONDITIONS

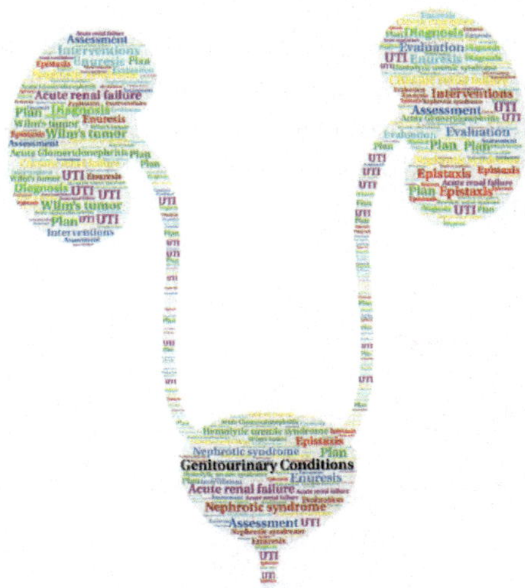




## LEARNING OUTCOMES

1. Describe the functions of the kidney and urinary system.
2. Recognize signs and symptoms of urinary or renal conditions.
3. Synthesize assessment data to create a nursing care plan for children with urinary or renal conditions.
4. Contrast pre-renal, intrinsic, and post-renal causes of acute renal failure.
5. Create a nursing care plan for a child with Chronic Renal Failure that promotes growth and development and optimizes nutrition.
6. Recognize the close relationship between the renal system and the cardiovascular system and develop wellness strategies that care for the whole child.
7. Utilize the nursing process to provide safe, comprehensive healthcare to children with urinary conditions.
8. Teaching/learning principles in providing anticipatory guidance in the prevention and treatment of children with urinary conditions.

# KEY TERMS

Anticholinergics
Antidiuretic hormone
Autoimmunity
Azotemia
Beta-blockers
Clean-catch urinalysis
Diphenhydramine
ESRD
GFR
Hemolytic anemia
Hyperkalemia
Nephrons
Proteinuria
Pyelonephritis
Recombinant growth hormone
Suprapubic aspiration
Tricyclic antidepressants
Urinalysis
Vasodilators

The urinary system removes waste products from the body, regulates fluid and electrolytes and acid-base balance, in addition to regulating calcium levels and producing erythropoietin. The urinary system includes the kidneys, ureters, bladder, and urethra. Children possess all of the **nephrons** (tubules that filter urine) they will have, but they are smaller with a smaller surface area and absorb less water until the ureters reach adult size in adolescence. Children have a lower **glomerular filtration rate (GFR)** that is approximately 20 ml/hr when normal adult GFR is 90–120 ml/hr. Children reach adult rates by 18 months of age. Children also do not concentrate urine as well as an adult and cannot eliminate electrolytes as effectively. Children can concentrate urine by two years of age. The kidneys maintain acid–base balance by secreting or storing H+ that creates bicarb, and through the absorption of bicarb from the urine. The kidneys absorb or excrete calcium in response to parathyroid hormone and vitamin levels. The kidneys transform vitamin D into calcitriol that cues intestinal absorption of calcium. The kidneys also create erythropoietin the hormone that stimulates red blood cell formation (ATI Testing 2016).

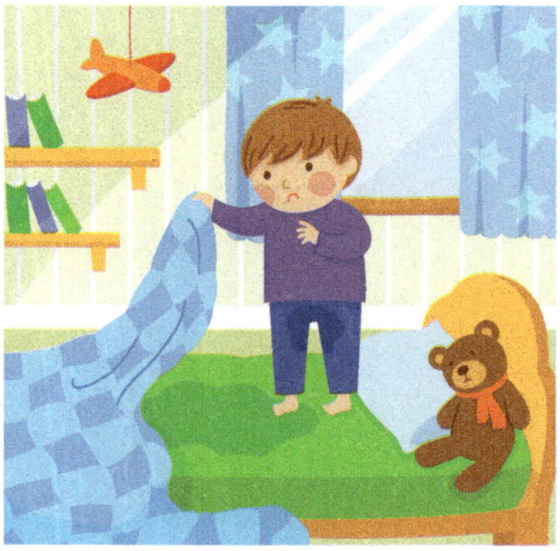

© ayelet-keshet/Shutterstock.com

# ENURESIS

## Assessment

Enuresis is a condition where a child cannot control urination, even though the child is old enough to have bladder control (ATI Testing 2016).

## Diagnosis

Involuntary urination must occur at least twice a week for at least 3 months. In addition, the child must be at least 5 years of age for a diagnosis. Organic causes related to genitourinary dysfunction are ruled out before the diagnosis of enuresis is made. (ATI Testing 2016).

A primary enuresis diagnosis describes a child who has never been free of bed-wetting. Secondary enuresis diagnosis describes a child who started bed-wetting after the development of urinary control. Enuresis risk factors include a family history of enuresis, disorders associated with bladder dysfunction, boys, and psychosocial disturbances (ATI Testing 2016).

To obtain an enuresis diagnosis, involuntary urination must occur at least twice a week for at least 3 months. In addition, the child must be at least 5 years of age. Organic causes related to genitourinary dysfunction are ruled out before the diagnosis is made. There are two types of enuresis primary and secondary (ATI Testing 2016).

A primary enuresis diagnosis describes a child who has never been free of bed-wetting. Secondary enuresis diagnosis describes a child who started bed-wetting after the development of urinary control. Enuresis risk factors include a family history of enuresis, disorders associated with bladder dysfunction, boys, and psychosocial disturbances. Complications of the diagnosis include low self-esteem, altered body image, social isolation, and fear. Support for the child and family includes listening to concerns and correcting misperceptions. Early interventions can prevent long-term emotional issues (ATI Testing 2016).

## Interventions and Teaching

The home environment should have an accessible bathroom, possibly through the use of a night light and a clear path from the bedroom. The child should void before bedtime as part of the bedtime routine, and take adequate fluids during the day (with none before bed) to prevent dehydration. The parent may have to wake the child once at night. The child should keep a calendar of wet and dry days (and total intake and output) with praise for dry days, but no punishment for wet days. On wet days the child should change the bedding. Children with psychosocial issues need positive reinforcement. Parents should refrain from punishing, scolding, or teasing the child following an incident. The child should wear regular sleep wear and not diapers. A healthy diet high in fiber prevents constipation which can exacerbate enuresis (ATI Testing 2016).

## Medications

Medications are the last interventions and may include oral or nasal administration of **antidiuretic hormone**, Desmopressin acetate what reduces the production of urine. Nasal desmopressin is kept refrigerated. Parents administer medications before bed (ATI Testing 2016).

**Tricyclic antidepressants,** such as imipramine hydrochloride also inhibit urination. However, there are adverse effects, such as an increase in suicidality. Children take the medication for 6–8 weeks followed by a gradual withdrawal. Parents should administer this medication with food, 1 hour before bedtime. Children should refrain from sun exposure, and parents should not use over the counter medications with this drug (ATI Testing 2016).

**Anticholinergics,** such as oxybutynin chloride, relax the bladder (ATI Testing 2016).

# UTI

Children with urinary tract infections (UTI) have bacteriuria (or bacteria in the urine), asymptomatic bacteriuria (or bacteriuria with no manifestations of UTI), or symptomatic bacteriuria (bacteriuria with manifestations) of UTI. UTI can become recurrent, if not completely treated or if lifestyle behaviors do not change. UTI can be present as recurrent, persistent, or febrile (ATI Testing 2016).

Recurrent UTIs are multiple occurrences of bacteriuria or symptomatic bacteriuria. Persistent UTIs are unresolved bacteriuria with antibiotic therapy. Febrile UTIs are symptomatic bacteriuria and present with fever. Children may have cystitis or inflammation of the bladder or urethritis or inflammation of the urethra. If a UTI goes untreated, **pyelonephritis** or inflammation of the upper urinary tract and the kidneys can develop (see Fig 8-1). The urinary tract may be the origin for sepsis or urosepsis. Risk factors include urinary stasis, urinary tract anomalies, reflux within the urinary tract system, constipation, onset of toilet training, uncircumcised males with inadequate hygiene. In women, synthetic, tight underwear, and wet bathing suits, or sexual activity are additional risk factors (ATI Testing 2016).

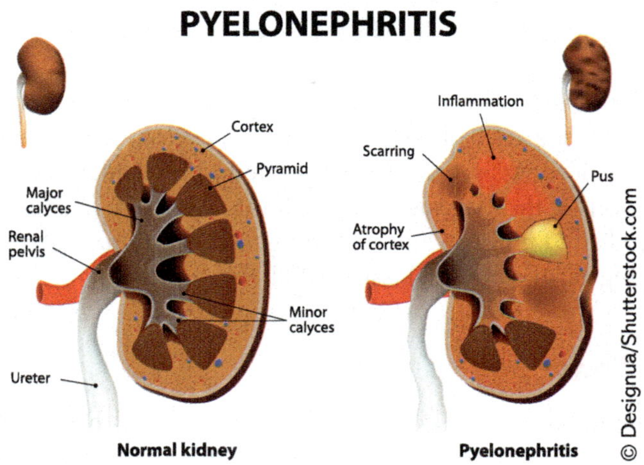


**Fig 8-1** Pyelonephritis occurs when a UTI spreads to the kidney

## Assessment

Infants may present with irritability or crying upon urination. They may also show signs, such as poor feeding, vomiting, or failure to gain weight, increase in thirst, frequent urination and straining with urination, foul-smelling urine, fever and diaper rash, dehydration, pallor, or seizure. Children may present with abdominal or back pain or pain with urination. They may also show a poor appetite, vomiting, slowed growth, thirst, enuresis, frequent urination, facial edema, seizures, pallor, fatigue, blood in the urine, edema in the extremities, hypertension, and tetany. Complications include progressive kidney injury and urosepsis (ATI Testing 2016).

## Diagnosis

### Laboratory Tests

A **clean-catch urinalysis** and urine culture with sensitivity can confirm the pathogen. Sterile catheterization and **suprapubic aspiration** are the most accurate methods for sampling urine for urinalysis and culture in children less than 2 years of age. Catheterization is less painful (Badiee, Z., Sadeghnia, A., and Zarean, N. 2014).

## Interventions and Teaching

If a suprapubic aspiration occurs, the nurse needs confirmation of informed consent. The nurse should keep urine somewhat concentrated, and should not administer large amounts of oral fluids to prevent a false-negative in the urine specimen (ATI Testing 2016).

A urine culture differentiates between *Escherichia coli*, *Proteus*, *Pseudomonas*, *Klebsiella*, *Haemophilus*, or *Staphylococcus aureus*.

A **urinalysis** determines pH (weak acid or neutral alkaline), protein, glucose, ketone, or nitrite levels (ATI Testing 2016).

If the site of the primary infection site or to locate anatomic defects, a percutaneous kidney tap procedure can reveal the site (ATI Testing 2016).

An ultrasonography or a voiding cystourethrogram (an x-ray during urination), an IV pyelogram (diagnoses blood) or a dimercaptosuccinic acid scan (radionucleotide scan) allows for the visualization of the kidney (ATI Testing 2016).

Educate the child and family about any procedures needed for the child. The nurse will assess the child for allergy to iodine or shellfish if a contrast medium is used. The nurse sedates infants and young children, if necessary, and may assist older children to remain quiet during the examinations (ATI Testing 2016).

The child is kept on NPO status after midnight in preparation for a cystoscopy and IVP. IVP requires bowel preparation. The nurse monitors the child post-procedure, according to facility protocol (ATI Testing 2016).

Interventions for all renal patients include frequent voiding and complete emptying of the bladder, oral fluid hydration, and input and output amounts monitored through catheterization (ATI Testing 2016).

## Medications

Antibiotics are selected upon findings of the urine culture and sensitivity testing and might include penicillins, sulfonamide, cephalosporins, and nitrofurantoin. The nurse or parent administers the entire course of antibiotics (ATI Testing 2016).

The family needs education about signs and symptoms of UTIs, such as dysuria, frequency, and urgency. Personal hygiene techniques are genitalia-specific. Females wipe the perineal area from front to back, and males must retract and clean the foreskin of male infants. The child and parents must work together to keep underwear dry. Cotton underwear is most breathable and is best for the child. The parents should encourage oral hydration, and refrain from bubble baths. A healthy diet high in fiber prevents constipation and straining. Adolescents who are sexually active must learn to void immediately after intercourse (ATI Testing 2016).

# ACUTE POST-STREPTOCOCCAL GLOMERULONEPHRITIS

Acute post-streptococcal glomerulonephritis (APSGN) elicits an antibody-antigen affect that results from certain strains of the Group A β-hemolytic streptococcal (GABHS) infection. The infection induces **autoimmunity** causing the immune system to attack the glomerulus and decrease glomerular filtration rate (GFR) (see Fig 8-2 and 8-3). APSGN presents in children between the ages of 5 and 8 years of age.

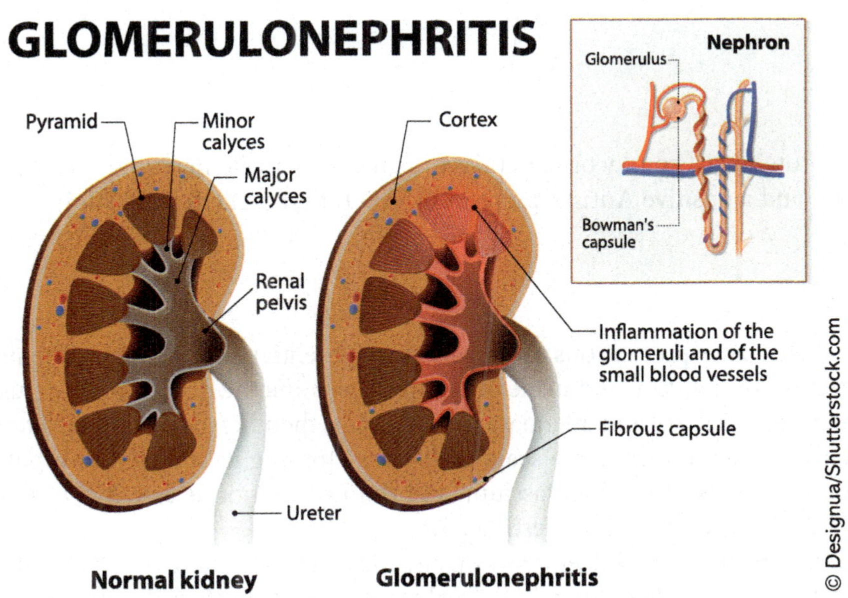


**Fig 8-2** Acute glomerulonephritis is an inflammatory disease

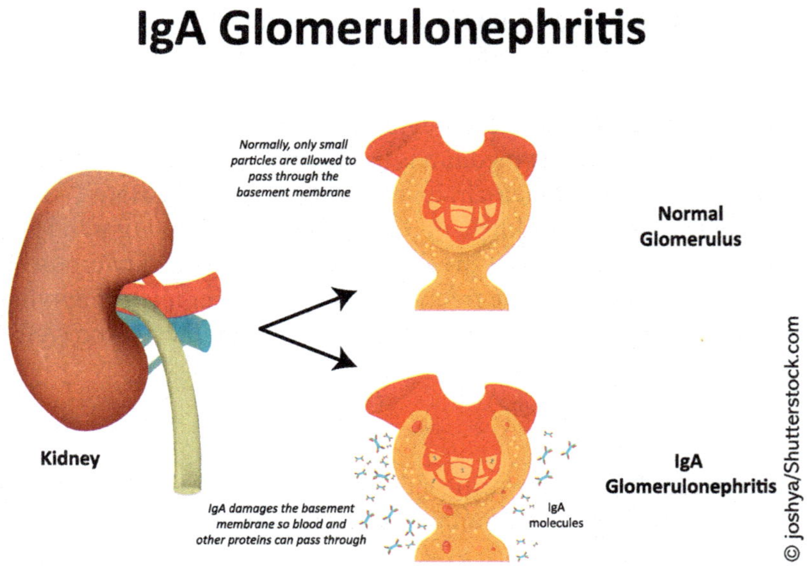


**Fig 8-3** Autoimmune damage to the glomerulus

Children exhibit hallmark symptoms, such as oliguria, edema, hypertension and circulatory congestion, hematuria, and proteinuria after an Upper Respiratory Infection (URI) or a streptococcal infection (ATI Testing 2016).

## Assessment

Children have a range of blood pressures from mild to severe hypertension, cloudy, frothy (**proteinuria**), tea-colored urine, and decreased urine output, irritability, malaise, lethargy, anorexia, headache, abdominal pain, dysuria, and periorbital edema (ATI Testing 2016).

The child's facial edema increases in the morning but then spreads to extremities and abdomen with the progression of the day. The child's vital signs, including daily weights and physical assessment, are focused on cardiovascular status, infection, electrolyte imbalance, fluid overload, and neurological changes (ATI Testing 2016).

## Diagnosis

A urinalysis shows proteinuria, smoky or tea-colored urine, hematuria increased specific gravity, an elevated BUN and creatinine, and a positive Antistreptolysin O (ASO) titer (ATI Testing 2016).

## Interventions

The nurse implements seizure precautions to prepare for a potential seizure event. The nurse monitors children's vital signs, change in the skin, and urine output to determine the dehydration status of the child. If the child has a normal blood pressure and adequate urine output, then he/she is managed at home. The parents should monitor daily weights on the same scale with same clothing in addition to input and output status. Proper nutrition that includes sodium, potassium, and fluid restriction is essential to the health promotion and wellness of a child with APSGN (ATI Testing 2016).

Children should consume small, frequent, meals. Meals should be low protein, if **azotemia** presents (increased BUN and creatinine), low salt, whole food meals. Children should not consume processed foods. The nurse maintains fluid restriction during periods of edema and hypertension. The child is frequently turned and inspected for skin breakdown. The child's edematous body parts are elevated and the nurse may need to pad bony prominences to prevent skin breakdown. The child may require a specialty mattress. The nurse provides frequent rest periods and periods of activity as tolerated by the child. It is beneficial to cluster nursing care to achieve this balance. The nurse promotes the child's health through hand washing and infection control and using age-appropriate diversional activities. Allow the child to verbalize feelings about body image. The nurse should provide emotional support to the child and family (ATI Testing 2016).

## Medications

The nurse may administer antibiotic therapy as prescribed for children with a persistent streptococcal infection. Diuretics and anti-hypertensives decrease swelling and manage hypertension. Educate the child and family about the dizziness associated with the use of anti-hypertensives and diuretics (ATI Testing 2016).

## Teaching

The nurse should emphasize the importance of follow up care: the monitoring of daily weight and blood pressure readings, and the identification of hypertension symptoms (blurry vision, headaches, and low urine output). Children should avoid others with illnesses and practice infection control strategies (ATI Testing 2016).

# MINIMAL CHANGE NEPHROTIC SYNDROME

Children from 2-3 years of age are most likely to develop nephrotic syndrome. Nephrotic syndrome produces many of the same symptoms of APSGN, but the mechanism of the disease is quite different. The child's glomerular membrane changes, so that proteins (mainly albumin) are lost to the urine, resulting in decreased serum osmotic pressure that results in edema. It can present as primary, secondary, or congenital (ATI Testing 2016).

Primary nephrotic syndrome occurs as a metabolic, biochemical, or physiochemical disturbance in the basement membrane of the glomeruli that allows for increased permeability to large, molecules like protein to escape.

Secondary nephrotic syndrome occurs because of a chronic disease like diabetes or lupus that causes damage to the kidney (ATI Testing 2016).

Children can inherit nephrotic syndrome through mutated genes. Although this disease is rare, the disease can manifest at birth in families of Finnish origin (ATI Testing 2016).

## Assessment

The child presents with weight gain over a period of days or weeks, facial and periorbital edema, edema to lower extremities and genitalia, ascites and increased abdominal girth, anorexia, diarrhea, irritability, lethargy, decreased frothy urine, and blood pressure within expected reference range or slightly below (see Fig 8-4). Complications include circulation insufficiency, thromboembolism, sepsis and infection (ATI Testing 2016).

## Diagnosis

A urinalysis with 24-hour urine collection shows proteinuria or a protein greater than 2+ on the dipstick, hyaline casts, some RBC's, and oval fat bodies.

A serum chemistry test reveals hypoalbuminemia or reduced serum protein and albumin; hyperlipidemia or elevated serum lipid levels; hemoconcentration or elevated hemoglobin (Hgb), hematocrit (Hct), and platelets; and/or hyponatremia or reduced sodium levels. The child's GFR is normal or high.

The child may need a kidney biopsy, if nephrotic syndrome is unresponsive to steroid therapy. A biopsy shows any damage to the basement membrane of the kidney (ATI Testing 2016).

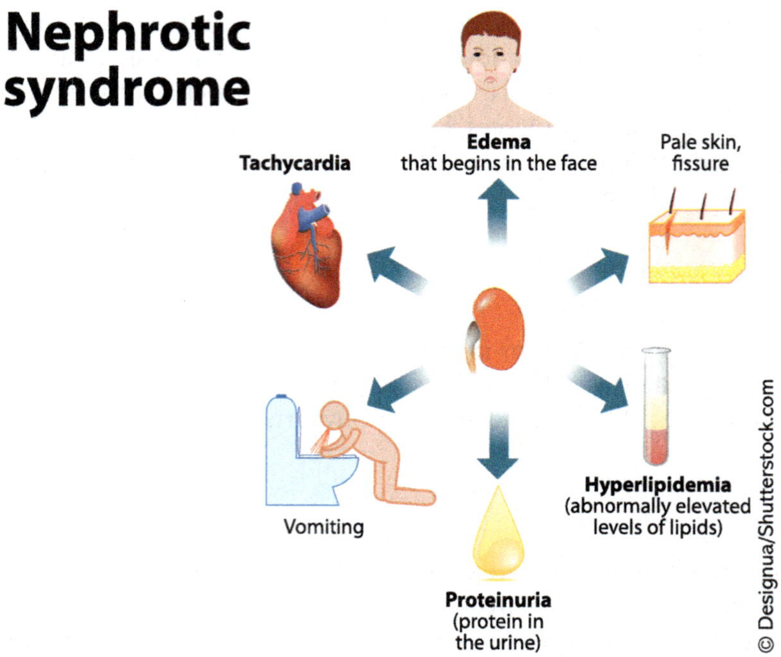


**Fig 8-4** Nephrotic syndrome originates from injury to the glomerular membrane

## Interventions

The nurse clusters care to promote rest, monitors I&Os, and watches lab values for proteinuria. The child's daily weight is evaluated on the same scale with the same clothes daily, for signs of increased edema. The nurse evaluates edema regarding pitting, color of skin and texture. The nurse takes a daily abdominal girth at the widest area at or above the umbilicus to monitor for ascites, and encourages the client to turn, cough, and deep breathe to prevent pulmonary involvement. Clustering nursing care helps to provide for rest periods. Infection control strategies that include hand washing help keep the child infection-free (ATI Testing 2016).

The nurse should encourage whole food intake with fluid and salt restriction, if the child has edema. Potassium restriction is also necessary.

The nurse maintains the child's skin through padding bony prominences, or the use of a specialty mattress to reduce breakdown of skin. The nurse should ensure that the child repositions frequently and that the skin is kept dry.

Elevate edematous body parts. Children with fragile skin should not have a urinary collection bag as the adhesive is too harsh (ATI Testing 2016).

## Medications

The nurse administers antibiotic therapy, if infection presents.

Oral corticosteroids, like prednisone, are first-line treatments (Nishi, S. et al. 201Children with nephrotic syndrome who receive 5–7 days of prednisone at the onset of a viral infection have a lower incidence of relapse (Hahn, D., Hodson, E. M., Willis. N. S., and Craig, J. C. 2015).

Ordered dosages are 60 mg/m$^2$/day for 4 to 6 weeks followed by 40 mg/m$^2$ every other day for 2–5 months with tapering dosages (ATI 2016). The child takes prednisone with food. The nurse evaluates the child for adverse effects, such as hirsutism, slowed linear growth, hypertension, GI bleeding, infection, and hyperglycemia. Prednisone decreases immune function, so the child should avoid large crowds. Corticosteroids have side effects, like increased appetite, weight gain, lowered immunity, and mood swings (ATI Testing 2016).

The child also receives a diuretic, like furosemide, to manage fluid overload. The child should add foods that are high in potassium to balance the loss of potassium from the diuretic (ATI Testing 2016).

The nurse monitors serum electrolyte levels and alerts the provider with any critical values. If the child has significant edema, a solution of 25% albumin increases plasma volume and decreases edema. Urine output should increase as edema decreases (ATI Testing 2016).

### Cyclophosphamide

IV Cyclophosphamide treats patients resistant to prednisone or who cannot tolerate prednisone and have repeated relapses of MCNS (Pravitsitthikul, N.,Willis, N. S.,Hodson, E. M.,Craig, J.C. 2013).

## Teaching

The nurse teaches each the family how to monitor blood pressure, daily weight, and protein in the urine. Instruct the family to notify the provider, if symptoms worsen, the child has relapsed (ATI Testing 2016).

The nurse educates the family and child about administration and side effects of medication. The nurse supports the family and child regarding appropriate dietary management, and promotes rest. The nurse informs the family of strategies to decrease the risk of infection, good hand washing hygiene, up-to-date immunizations, and avoidance of infected people. Allow the child to verbalize feelings about body integrity or image. The nurse provides support to families and makes appropriate referrals as needed. Relapses can cause physical, emotional, and financial stress for the client and family (ATI Testing 2016).

# HEMOLYTIC UREMIC SYNDROME (HUS)

HUS is an acute renal disease that precipitates the breakdown of red blood cells by a pathogen that clogs the kidneys resulting in acute renal failure, **hemolytic anemia,** and thrombocytopenia after an incidence of diarrhea (E-coli, Shigella, or campylobacter or a virus) (see Fig 8-5). HUS is a leading cause of acute renal failure in children 6 months of age to 3 years of age. It occurs primarily in Caucasian people in South Africa, Argentina, and the west coasts of North and South America (ATI Testing 2016).

Diarrhea-positive (D+) HUS accounts for 90% of the cases where the Shiga toxin produces Escherichia coli, E. coli 0157: H7 (ATI Testing 2016).

Diarrhea-negative (D-) or atypical HUS is related to intestinal infections, disturbances in the complement system, malignancies, or genetic disorders (ATI Testing 2016).

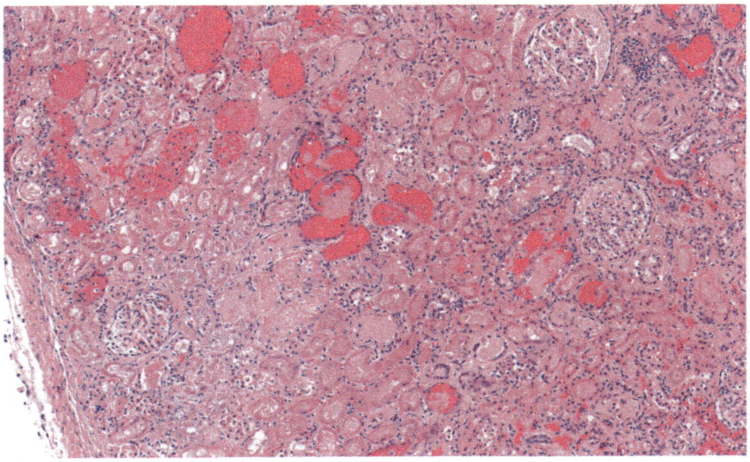


**Fig 8-5** Red blood cells clog the circulation of the kidney in a child with HUS

## Assessment

The child's history includes a prodromal period of diarrhea and vomiting, typically with varicella, measles, or a UTI. The child may have a loss of appetite, irritability, lethargy, pallor, bruising, purpura, or rectal bleeding. Children become anuric and hypertensive in its most severe form.

A CBC reveals decreased hemoglobin and hematocrit, and an elevated reticulocyte count. The urine presents with hematuria, proteinuria, an elevated BUN and serum creatinine, thrombocytopenia, and fibrin split products. Split products also appear in the serum (ATI Testing 2016).

## Interventions

The nurse implements seizure precautions related to hemoconcentration, metabolic disturbances, and/or hypertension. For intravascular dehydration, fluid administration with an isotonic fluid is essential (ATI Testing 2016).

The nurse monitors daily weights. Children receive blood transfusions with fresh, washed packed cells for severe anemia. The nurse administers anti-hypertensives and corrects acidosis and electrolyte imbalances. Total input and output values guide fluid administration values. In severe cases, hemodialysis, peritoneal dialysis (see Fig 8-6 and 8-7), and continuous hemofiltration becomes necessary ATI Testing 2016).

If a child with HUS becomes anuric for 24 hours or has oliguria with uremia, hypertension seizures may present. Once vomiting and diarrhea subside, enteral feedings begin. Children who have severe, persistent colitis and marked tissue catabolism may need parenteral nutrition (ATI Testing 2016).

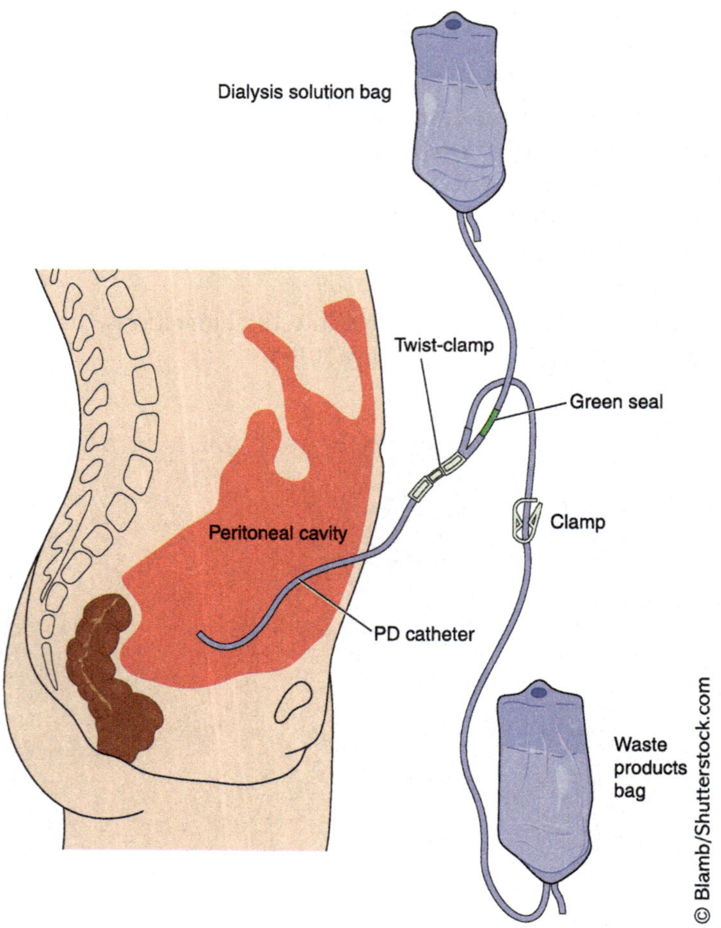


**Fig 8-6** The mechanism for peritoneal dialysis

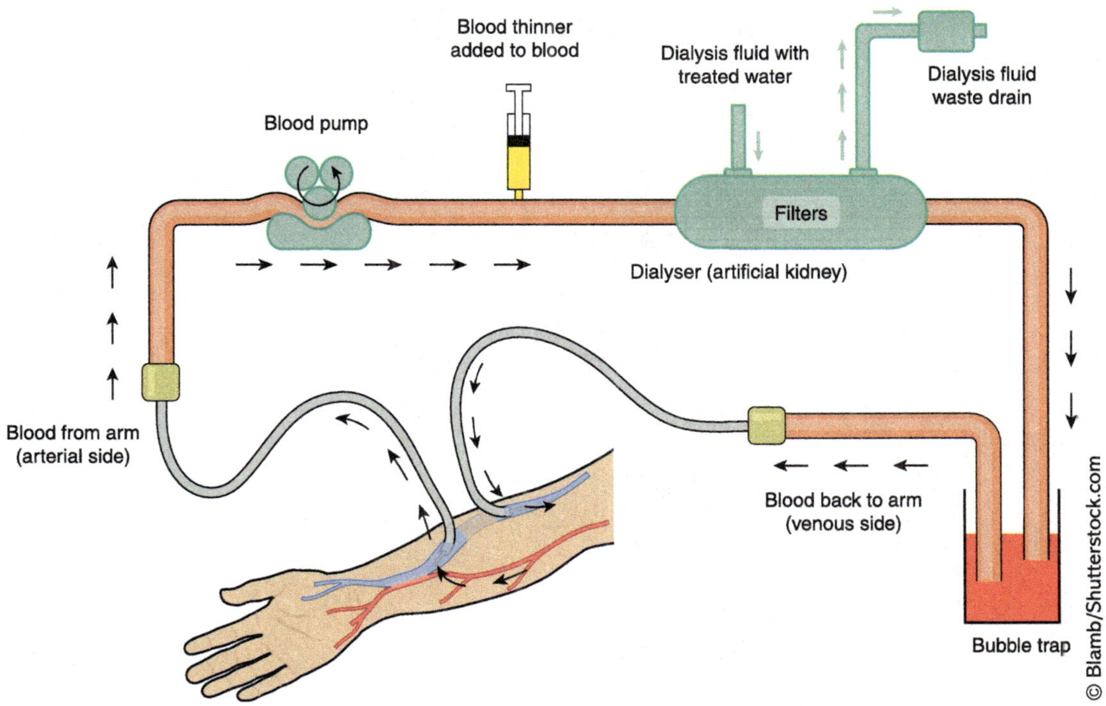


**Fig 8-7** The mechanism for hemodialysis

## Medication

There is no evidence that heparin, corticosteroids, or fibrinolytic agents promote positive outcomes. Researchers are looking at plasma infusion as a treatment (ATI Testing 2016).

## Teaching

Parents are advised to refrain from anti-motility medications for diarrhea. Lifestyle changes to promote wellness and minimize bacterial exposure include no undercooked meat, especially ground beef. The internal temperature of meat products should be at least 74° C (165° F). Parents are advised to also avoid unpasteurized apple juice, unwashed raw vegetables, and alfalfa sprouts. Parents should also avoid public pools (ATI Testing 2016).

Intrinsic causes: nephrotoxic drugs and inflammation and vasculitis

# ACUTE RENAL FAILURE

Renal failure can present as acute or chronic. Acute renal failure (ARF) is precipitated by the inability of the kidneys to excrete waste material, concentrate urine, and conserve electrolytes. ARF can originate from prerenal, intrinsic renal, and postrenal causes. Prerenal or cardiovascular changes are the most common cause of ARF (ATI Testing 2106) (see Fig 8-8). Issues with hypertension, liver failure, dehydration, or shock create prerenal causes. Intrinsic renal causes are structural changes inside of the kidney. Postrenal causes obstruct the drainage of urine beyond the kidney (ATI Testing 2016).

## Assessment

Children present with oliguria followed by an abrupt diuresis with a return to normal urine volumes, edema drowsiness, circulatory collapse, and cardiac arrhythmia: from **hyperkalemia**, seizures (related to hyponatremia or hypocalcemia). Prolonged oliguria precipitates neurological sequelae (ATI Testing 2016).

# Acute Kidney Injury

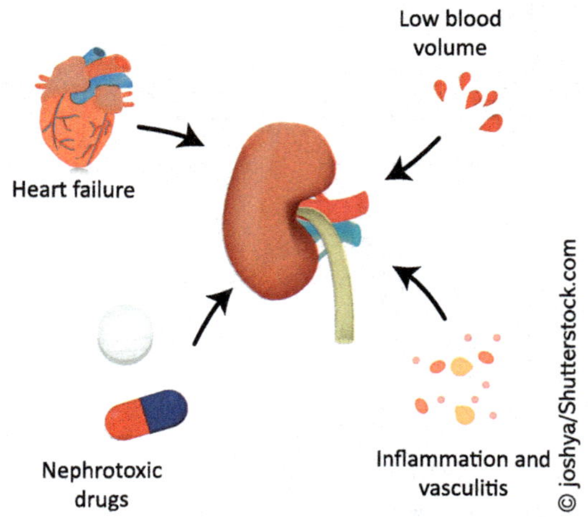


**Fig 8-8** Prerenal causes: heart failure or low blood volume

## Diagnosis

Laboratory tests for hyperkalemia, hyponatremia, metabolic acidosis, hypocalcemia, anemia, azotemia, elevated plasma creatinine, elevated BUN, ECG for cardiac arrhythmias. Treatment plans for prerenal acute renal failure focus on treating the underlying problem (ATI Testing 2016).

## Interventions

The child gains admission to a pediatric intensive care unit (PICU). The nurse tracks vital signs for hypertension complication and to maintain a neutral temperature. The nurse corrects fluid and electrolyte imbalances through strict I&O monitoring (indwelling catheter). The nurse monitors the Central Venous Pressure (CVP) probe to watch for overhydration. A declining neurological assessment calls for seizure precautions (ATI Testing 2016).

The nutritional goal for a child with ARF; maximizes calories while minimizing tissue catabolism, metabolic acidosis, hyperkalemia, and uremia. The child should eat concentrated foods without fluids. If nourishment is via IV route, the nurse should look for complications of fluid overload.

The nurse teaches the family about the medication administration for their child and keeps the family informed as to the status of the child (ATI Testing 2016).

## Medications

The diuretics mannitol and furosemide pull fluid into the kidney to increase urine output in children who with oliguria and no lower tract obstruction.

Calcium gluconate 0.5 mL/kg IV, every 2–3 minutes with continuous ECG monitoring, protect the heart from high levels of serum potassium levels.

Sodium bicarbonate 2–3 mEq/kg IV every 30–60 minutes, elevates serum pH and transient fluid shift to drive potassium into the cell and reduce serum potassium levels (ATI Testing 2016).

Glucose 50% and insulin 1 unit/kg IV moves glucose and potassium into the cells. Insulin transports glucose into cells and decreases serum potassium levels (ATI Testing 2016).

Sodium polystyrene sulfonate 1g/kg orally or rectally binds potassium for excretion. A child may need dialysis or continuous hemofiltration.

Anti-hypertensives that treat encephalopathy include labetalol IV or sodium nitroprusside IV with close monitoring (ATI Testing 2016).

For moderate hypertension, anti-hypertensives may include hydralazine IV, clonidine IV, verapamil IV. The child may need antiepileptic drugs, if a seizure presents (ATI Testing 2016).

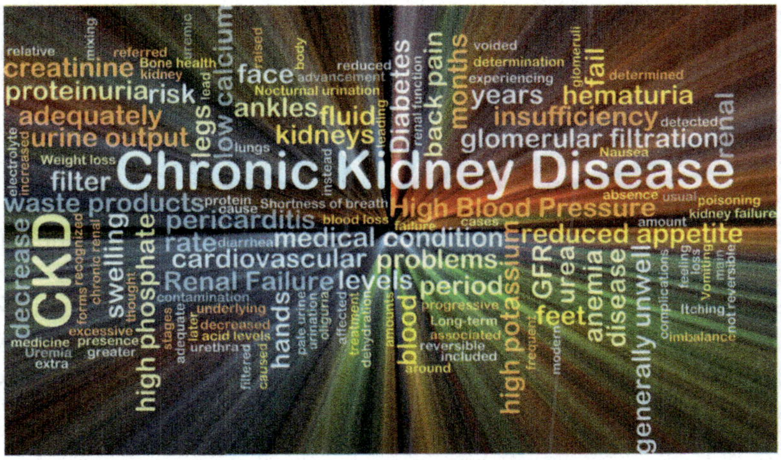




## CHRONIC RENAL FAILURE

Chronic Renal Failure (CRF) or insufficiency occurs when dysfunctional nephrons can no longer filter body fluids and maintain homeostasis. CRF results from many causes. Infants may have congenital renal malformations under five years of age. Children 5-15 years of age often present with glomerular and hereditary renal disease (ATI Testing 2016).

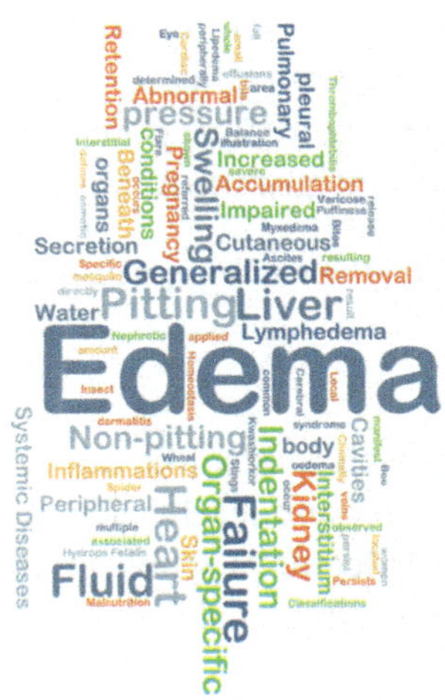




### Assessment

Children present with lethargy, a decreased interest in activities, an increase in fatigue on exertion, and pallor. There are occasional episodes of elevated blood pressure, delayed growth, anorexia, nausea, and vomiting, decreased or increased urinary output and a compensatory increase in fluid intake. A child may have anemia, headache, muscle cramps, nausea, weight loss, puffiness to face, malaise, bone or joint pain. The skin becomes, itchy, and bruised. Adolescent girls may develop amenorrhea. Signs of fluid overload include hypertension, congestive heart failure, and pulmonary edema, confusion, dulling of sensorium and coma are findings of neurologic involvement. Tremors, muscle twitching, and seizures are also findings of neurologic involvement. Complications include **end-stage renal disease (ESRD)**, progressive deterioration, or an irreversible progress of renal insufficiency (ATI Testing 2016).

## Diagnosis

Elevated BUN and creatinine levels point to CRF. Blood tests include serum calcium, CBC, serum creatinine, and electrolytes. In addition, urine tests, imaging, or a kidney biopsy provide information for a diagnosis (ATI Testing 2016).

## Interventions

The nurse evaluates vital signs to monitor hypertension, daily weights, and input and output of fluids to track changes in edema (ATI Testing 2016).

The nutritional goal for a child with CRF is to provide adequate calories and protein for growth. A low protein diet doesn't slow the progression to ESRD and may under nourish a growing child over time (Chaturvedi, S. and Jones, C. 2007). However, dietary phosphorus is restricted, and potassium is limited, if oliguria or anuria presents (ATI Testing 2016).

### QSEN Application

According to QSEN, "Quality Improvement-Identify gaps between local and best practices. Appreciate that continuous quality improvement is an essential part of the daily work of all health professionals. Value own and others' contributions to outcomes of care in local care settings. Appreciate the value of what individuals and teams can do to improve care".

Nurses should "[u]se a variety of sources of information to review outcomes of care and identify potential areas for improvement. Propose appropriate aims for quality improvement efforts. Assert leadership in shaping the dialogue about and providing leadership for the introduction of best practices". Chronic disease is a multidimensional problem that requires an appropriate diet and light, regular exercise for the best outcome. Quality improvement means integrating nursing interventions that serve the whole child.

From Quality and Safety Education for Nurses http://qsen.org/competencies/pre-licensure-ksas/

Children should not consume phosphorus rich foods, like fast foods and processed foods. High levels of phosphorus are difficult for the kidneys to filter and leach calcium from the bones. A diet made up of many fruits and vegetables (folic acid and iron), fish, legumes, whole grains, and fibers and minimal amounts of red meat, sodium, and refined sugar comprise a healthy renal diet (Rysz, J., Franczyk, B., Ciałkowska-Rysz, A. and Gluba-Brzózka, A. 2017).

Fluids are restricted when the child has edema. The nurse practices infection-control strategies, like hand washing and monitors for signs of infection. The child needs a balance of rest and exercise. Exercise creates cardiovascular toning and a sense of well-being (ATI Testing 2016).

## Medication

The nurse administers thiazide and loop diuretics, such as furosemide for hypertension. If the child develops severe hypertension, **beta-blockers** and **vasodilators** can decrease blood pressure (ATI Testing 2016).

### Clinical Pearl

A calcium-phosphorus binding agent helps reduce serum levels of phosphate and benefits children with growing bones when also supplemented with vitamin D (Langman, C. B. and Cannata-Andía, J. B., 2010). However, this medication must count towards total daily calcium intake to avoid hypercalcemia.

A calcium-phosphorus binding agent helps reduce serum levels of phosphate.

If the child develops acidosis, sodium bicarbonate and potassium citrate can re-balance the levels (ATI Testing 2016).

Children with anemia receive folic acid and recombinant human erythropoietin (ATI Testing 2016).

If children have delayed growth, **recombinant growth hormone** may help.

Children with CRF are susceptible to infections and may require antibiotics.

Children with severe liver failure may experience seizures, due to the buildup of toxins that impair the brain's electrical conduction and receive anti-epileptics (ATI Testing, 2016).

Uremia causes pruritus in children and **diphenhydramine** can relieve this symptom (ATI Testing 2016).

## Teaching

Educate the family about the long-term therapeutic regimen, and coordinate a dietary consult. Wellness strategies like exercise and dental care promote health in children with CRF (ATI Testing 2016).

# CHAPTER HIGHLIGHTS

- The urinary system functions to eliminate waste products, maintains fluid and electrolyte balance, produces erythropoietin, regulates calcium and acid-base balances.
- Enuresis is a physiologic and psychosocial problem that requires a holistic framework to allow the child to learn how to gain control over the urinary function.
- Children are vulnerable to UTI infections as they learn personal hygiene routines, and gain bladder control.
- Acute post-streptococcal glomerulonephritis is the result of an immune response to Group A β-hemolytic streptococcal infection and is reversible.
- Nephrotic syndrome results from damage to the glomerulus and is a chronic condition characterized by weight gain, facial and periorbital edema, edema to lower extremities and genitalia, ascites and increased abdominal girth, anorexia, diarrhea, irritability, lethargy, and decreased frothy urine.
- Hemolytic uremic syndrome (HUS) results from a particular E, coli strain 0157:H7 that causes hemolysis, thrombocytopenia, and acute renal failure. If left untreated, chronic renal failure manifests.
- Acute renal failure is reversible when the underlying cause is treated.
- Chronic renal failure progresses to end-stage renal disease.

# REFERENCES

ATI Testing. 2016. Nursing Care of Children. Retrieved from http://www.atitesting.com/ati_next_gen/DisplayResources.aspx?Name=rm_rn_ncc_2016_ebook_20170417.pdf.

Ardissino, G., Daccò, V., Testa, S., Civitillo, C., Tel, F., Possenti, I., Chidini, G. et al. 2015. "Hemoconcentration: a major risk factor for neurological involvement in hemolytic uremic syndrome." *Pediatric Nephrology*, 30(2), 345–52. doi: 10.1007/s00467-014-2918-0

Badiee, Z., Sadeghnia, A., and Zarean, N. 2014. "Suprapubic Bladder Aspiration or Urethral Catheterization: Which is More Painful in Uncircumcised Male Newborns?" *International Journal of Preventive Medicine*, 5(9), 1125–30.

Bitsouri, M. 2012. Essentials in Pediatric Urology. Kerala, India: Research Signpost.

Chaturvedi, S., Jones, C. 2007. "Protein restriction for children with chronic kidney disease." *Cochrane Database of Systematic Reviews 2007*, Issue-4. Art. No.: CD006863. doi: 10.1002/14651858.CD006863.

Couser, W. G. and Johnson, R. J. 2014. "Review: The etiology of glomerulonephritis: roles of infection and autoimmunity." *Kidney International*, 86, 905–14. doi: 10.1038/ki.2014.49.

Hahn, D., Hodson, E. M., Willis. N. S. and Craig, J. C. 2015. "Corticosteroid therapy for nephrotic syndrome in children." *Cochrane Database of Systematic Reviews*, Issue 3. Art. No.: CD001533.doi: 10.1002/14651858. CD001533.pub5.

Langman, C. B. and Cannata-Andía, J. B. 2010. "Calcium in Chronic Kidney Disease: Myths and Realities." *Clinical Journal of the American Society of Nephrology.* 5(1) S1–S2, doi: 10.2215/CJN.06140809.

Nishi, S., Ubara, Y., Utsunomiya, Y., Okada, K., Obata, Y., Kai, H., Matsuo, S. et al. 2016. "Evidence-based clinical practice guidelines for nephrotic syndrome 2014." Clinical & *Experimental Nephrology*, 20(3), 342. doi: 10.1007/s10157-015-1216-x

Pravitsitthikul N., Willis N. S., Hodson E. M., Craig J. C. 2013. "Non-corticosteroid immunosuppressive medications for steroid-sensitive nephrotic syndrome in children." *Cochrane Database of Systematic Reviews 2013*, Issue10. Art. No.: CD002290. doi: 10.1002/14651858.CD002290.pub4.

Rysz, J., Franczyk, B., Ciałkowska-Rysz, A., and Gluba-Brzózka, A. 2017. The Effect of Diet on the Survival of Patients with Chronic Kidney Disease. Retrieved August 07, 2017, from https://www.ncbi.nlm.nih.gov/pubmed/28505087.

CHAPTER 9

# CARING FOR CHILDREN WITH ENDOCRINE AND METABOLIC CONDITIONS

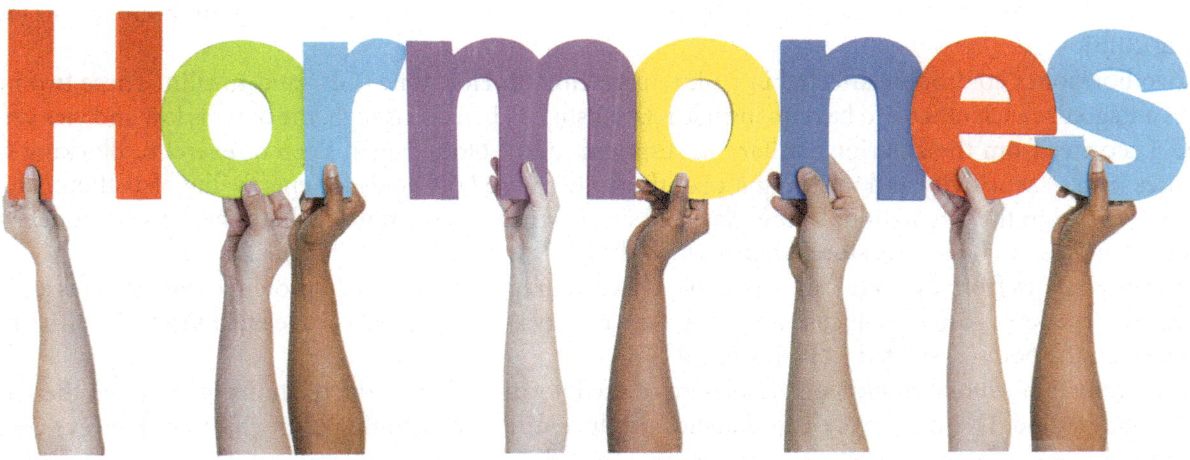


© Rawpixel.com/Shutterstock.com

## LEARNING OUTCOMES

1. Describe hormones and their part in a hormonal cascade.
2. Utilize the nursing process to provide safe, comprehensive health care to children with endocrine and metabolic conditions.
3. Recognize the functions of GH, IGF-1, and insulin.
4. Synthesize data from vital signs and a physical assessment to create a focused assessment.
5. Plan nursing interventions and evaluate outcomes that are developmentally appropriate for infants, toddlers, preschoolers, school-age children, and adolescents with Growth hormone deficiencies.
6. Plan nursing interventions and evaluate outcomes that are developmentally appropriate for infants, toddlers, preschoolers, school-age children, and adolescents with insulin deficiencies.
7. Teaching/learning principles in providing anticipatory guidance in the prevention and treatment of children with endocrine or metabolic conditions.

## KEY TERMS

American diabetes association diet
Anterior pituitary gland
Beta cells
Bone maturation
Diabetic ketoacidosis (DKA)
Epiphyseal closure
Glucometer
Glycosylated hemoglobin (HbA1c)
Hormonal cascades
Growth hormone releasing hormone (GHRH)
Hormones
Hypopituitarism
Insulin resistance
Ketones
Ketogenic, low-fat diet
Kussmaul respirations
Lipohypertrophy
Low-fat vegan diet
Plasma insulin-like growth factor-1 (IGF-1)
Oliguria
Plant-based diet
Polydipsia
Polyphagia
Polyuria
Potassium replacement therapy
Somatotropin

**Hormones** are chemical messengers that communicate messages between the cells and the organs. Hormones regulate metabolism, heart rate, appetite, mood, sexual function, reproduction, labor and birth, growth and development, sleep cycles, and immune function. When hormones are working the body flourishes optimally, when levels are inadequate or excessive, they require medical intervention. Hormones do not function in isolation; they work in **hormonal cascades**, each signaling each other to maintain homeostasis (ATI Testing 2016).

Two hormones commonly affected in children are Growth Hormone (GH) and Insulin. These two hormones antagonize each other and have an inverse relationship. When one is high, the other is low and vice versa.

GH secretes from the anterior pituitary in response to low blood sugar, sleep or exercise. Blocking GH increases insulin sensitivity and releasing it cues the body to use fatty acids for energy, but also allows blood sugar to remain in the circulation. In this way, GH creates **insulin resistance**, where the cells do not absorb insulin when it is available. GH stores energy when the body is hungry (ATI Testing 2016).

Insulin secretes from the **beta cells** of the pancreas and regulates the use of protein carbohydrates and fat through the uptake of glucose. Glucose is used to store energy as fat, liver cells or skeletal muscle. Insulin stores energy when the body is well fed (ATI Testing 2016).

Any study of hormones requires the isolation of each hormone before the relationship between them can best be understood. GH deficiency and diabetes produce different pathologies in children. However, once these hormones are known, the relationship between the two becomes more apparent. Hormone research has not provided all of the answers about hormones. It is a branch of the endocrine system that requires further research (ATI Testing 2016).

## GROWTH HORMONE DEFICIENCY

The hormone human growth hormone (GH), **somatotropin**, is secreted by the **anterior pituitary gland** (see Fig 9-1 and 9-2). GH regulates normal growth, development, and cellular metabolism. Children without adequate levels of GH grow more slowly than their peers. GH is part of a hormonal cascade with adrenocorticotropic hormone (ACTH), thyroid-stimulating hormone (TSH), follicle-stimulating hormone (FSH) and luteinizing hormone (LH) to control metabolism and homeostasis. **Hypopituitarism** is the inadequate secretion of pituitary hormones, primarily GH, but it could originate from the hypothalamus (ATI Testing 2016).

The presentation of the condition corresponds to the severity of the deficiency. Risk factors include injury to the anterior pituitary gland such as tumors, structural defects or surgery. Other hormones that signal GH such as **growth hormone releasing hormone (GHRH)**, or other hormonal deficiencies such as TSH or ACTH can result in deficient levels of GH. Most cases of hypopituitarism are idiopathic. Hypopituitarism should not be confused with short stature. Hypopituitarism is a functional problem, children with short stature have no associated medical condition (ATI Testing 2016).

If a child with GH deficiency does not receive hormone replacement is short with slowed **epiphyseal closure**, delayed bone age, late sexual development, and premature aging later in life (ATI Testing 2016).

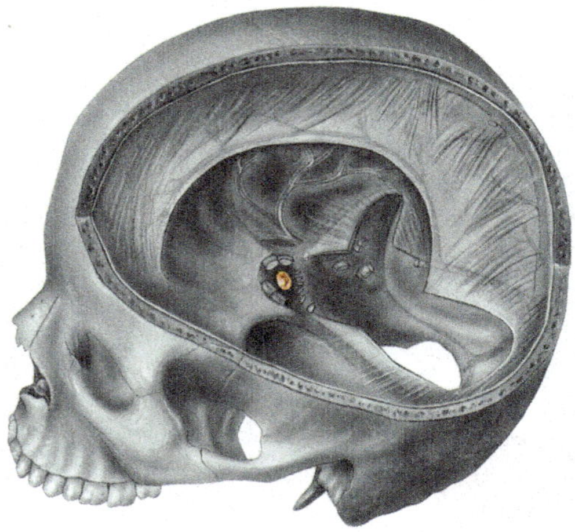



**Fig 9-1** The pituitary gland

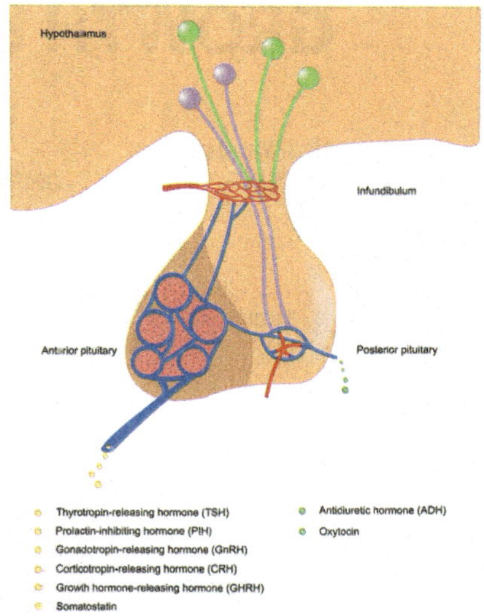




**Fig 9-2** Hormones secreted from the pituitary

## Assessment

Children are shorter than their peers but are proportional regarding height and weight. They have increased insulin sensitivity, delayed dentition, an underdeveloped jaw, and delayed sexual development (ATI Testing 2016).

## Diagnosis

**Plasma insulin-like growth factor-1(IGF-1)** works with GH to grow bones and muscle (see Fig 9-4). It can be normal or decreased in hypopituitarism. IGF binding protein-3 (IGFBP-3) levels confirm GH deficiency, even with a normal IGF-1. The nurse prepares the child and family for the test to make sure they keep the child NPO the night before the test, and to limit the child's activity (ATI Testing 2016).

## Interventions

The nurse evaluates and offers appropriate support for the child and family regarding psychosocial concerns altered body image, bullying, and depression. The nurse also maintains realistic goals for growth based on the child's diagnosis (ATI Testing 2016).

### GH Stimulation Test (see Fig 9-3)

Children who are short for their age, and have a low level of IGF-1 and IGFBP-3 undergo a GH stimulation test (ATI Testing 2016).

The nurse collects baseline blood samples between 0600 and 0800. Then the child receives arginine or GH-releasing hormone to trigger the release of GH, and the nurse takes repeat samples every 30 min for a 3-hr period (ATI Testing 2016).

### Radiologic Assessments

The provider compares the child's long bones and epiphyseal centers to age-appropriate standards. Children under 3 years of age have a general skeletal survey, where older children have X-rays of the wrists and hands. The provider measures bone growth and determines if the epiphyseal plates are active (ATI Testing 2016).

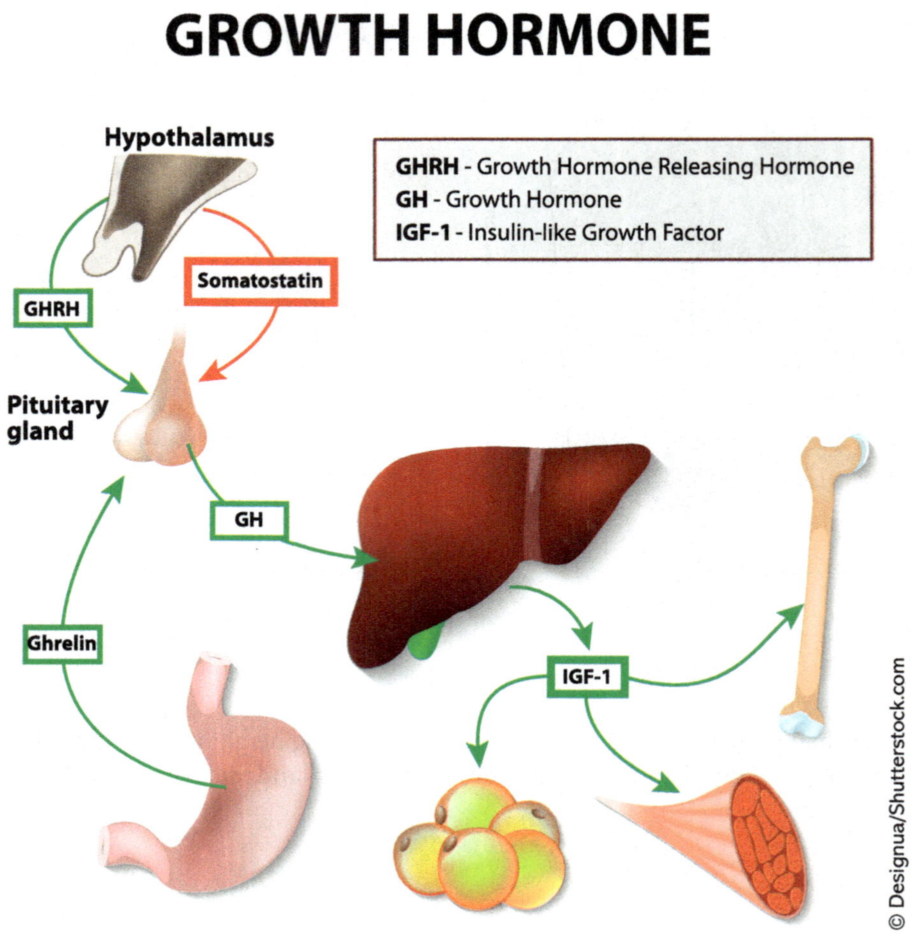


**Fig 9-3** The relationship between the hypothalamus and GH

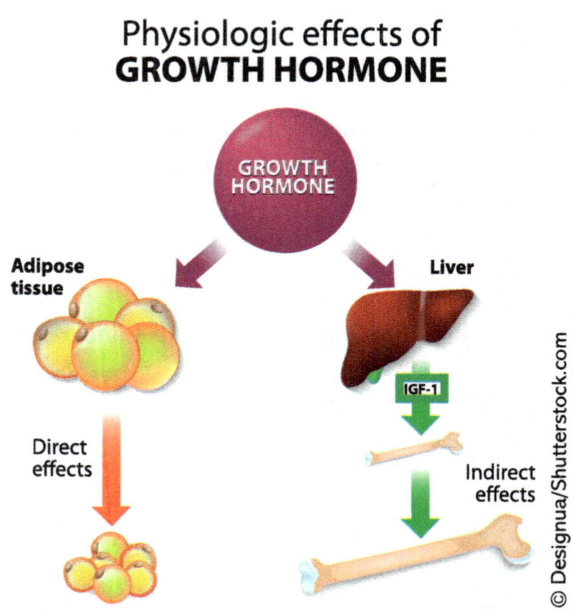


**Fig 9-4** The relationship between GH and GHRH and IGF-1

The nurse positions and possibly sedates the child appropriately for any of the ordered images including Computed Tomographic scanning (CT scan), Magnetic Resonance Imaging (MRI), and skull x-rays to identify tumors or other structural defects. The provider evaluates the child's height and weight increases based on a standardized growth curve. Bone age correlates to height age. Providers monitor children under 3 years of age at least every 6 months and children over 3 years of age every year (ATI Testing 2016).

## Medications

The nurse administers other hormone replacements (thyroid hormone) as ordered.

Somatotropin injections are human growth hormone injections that take replace growth hormone in the body (see Fig 9-5). The endocrinologist should use insulin cautiously as high levels of insulin inhibit fatty acid metabolism and induce insulin resistance (ATI Testing 2016). Growth hormone is shown to increase the height of children approximately 3.7 to 7.5 cm, but children will remain shorter than their counterparts (Bryant, J., Baxter, L., Cave, C.B., and Milne, R. 2007).

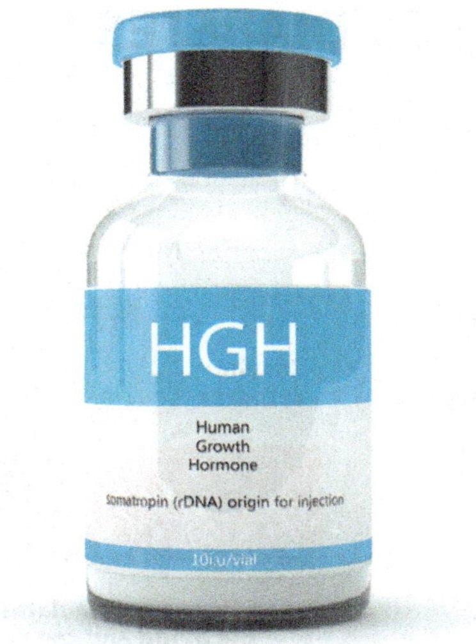




**Fig** 9-5 Injectable somatotropin

## Teaching

The child and parents must learn how to administer medication by subcutaneous injection 6–7 days per week for home use (see Fig 9-6). These injections continue until radiologic evidence reveals **bone maturation** has taken place (14 years of age or older for girls, and 16 years of age or older for boys). The child may continue therapy into early adulthood if ordered (ATI Testing 2016).

# DIABETES MELLITUS

Diabetes Mellitus (DM) presents as a partial or complete metabolic deficiency of insulin. In type 1 DM pancreatic beta cells are destroyed (see Fig 9-7). In type 2 DM, the body fails to use insulin appropriately and develops insulin resistance (see Fig 9-8) (ATI Testing 2016).

The main complication of DM is **Diabetic Ketoacidosis (DKA)**. Long-term complications of DM include the development of cardiovascular disease, hypertension, renal failure, blindness, and stroke. DKA is an acute, life-threatening condition with symptoms that include hyperglycemia (more than 330 mg/dL), glycosuria, ketonuria, ketonemia, and acidosis (pH 7.30 and bicarbonate 15 mmol/L). DKA results in the use of body fat for energy and an accumulation of **ketones** in the blood, urine, and lungs. The onset is quick, and it has a high

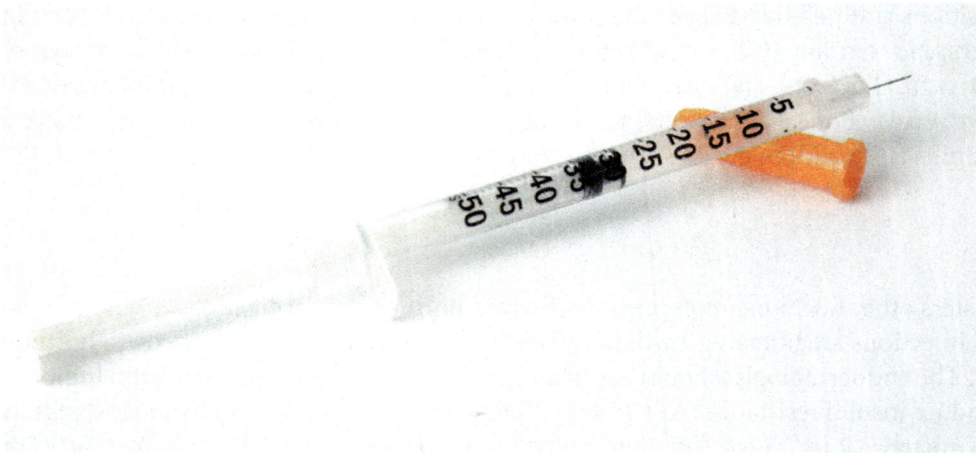



**Fig 9-6** Somatotropin is given subcutaneously

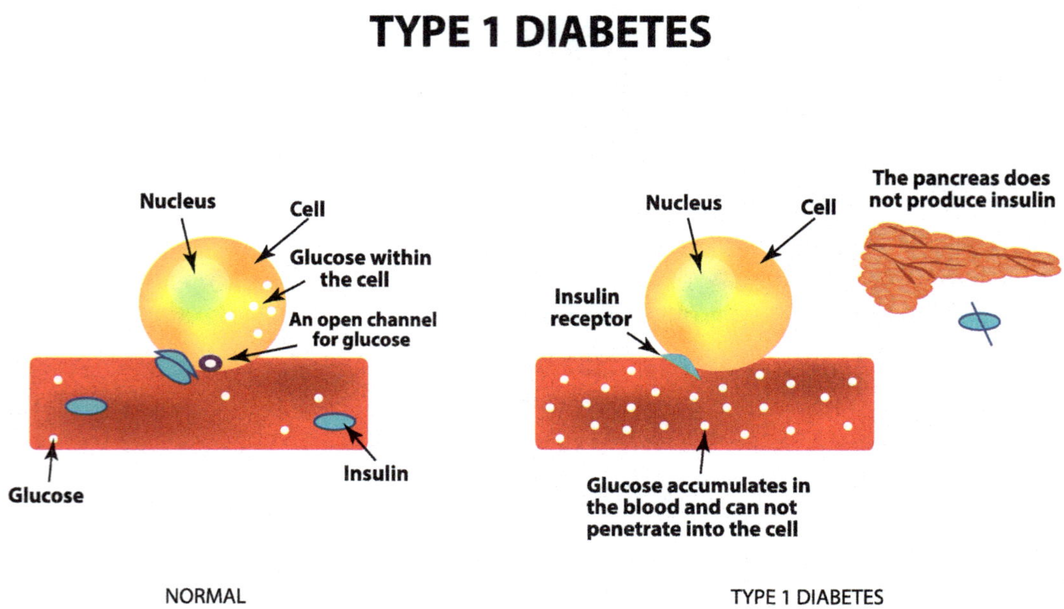




**Fig 9-7** Type I Diabetes mellitus

mortality rate. The causes of DKA include hypoinsulinemia, acute stress, and dehydration related to an acute illness (ATI Testing 2016).

There is a genetic component of type 1 and type 2 diabetes mellitus. DM type one results in an autoimmune response to toxins and viruses that destroy beta cells. Obesity, environmental factors, physical inactivity, high triglycerides (greater than 250 mg/dL), and hypertension can promote insulin resistance and type 2 diabetes mellitus (ATI Testing 2016).

## Assessment

Children with DM fluctuate between high (over 250 mg/dl) and low levels of glucose in the blood (less than 60 mg/dl) (ATI Testing 2016).

Signs and symptoms of hypoglycemia include chronic hunger (**polyphagia**), thirst (**polydipsia**), and **polyuria** (excess urine, early sign) or **oliguria** (minimal urine, late sign). Children may have lightheadedness, shakiness, headache, anxiety and irritability, and pale, cool skin. Other symptoms may include diaphoresis, normal or shallow respirations, tachycardia, and palpitations (ATI Testing 2016).

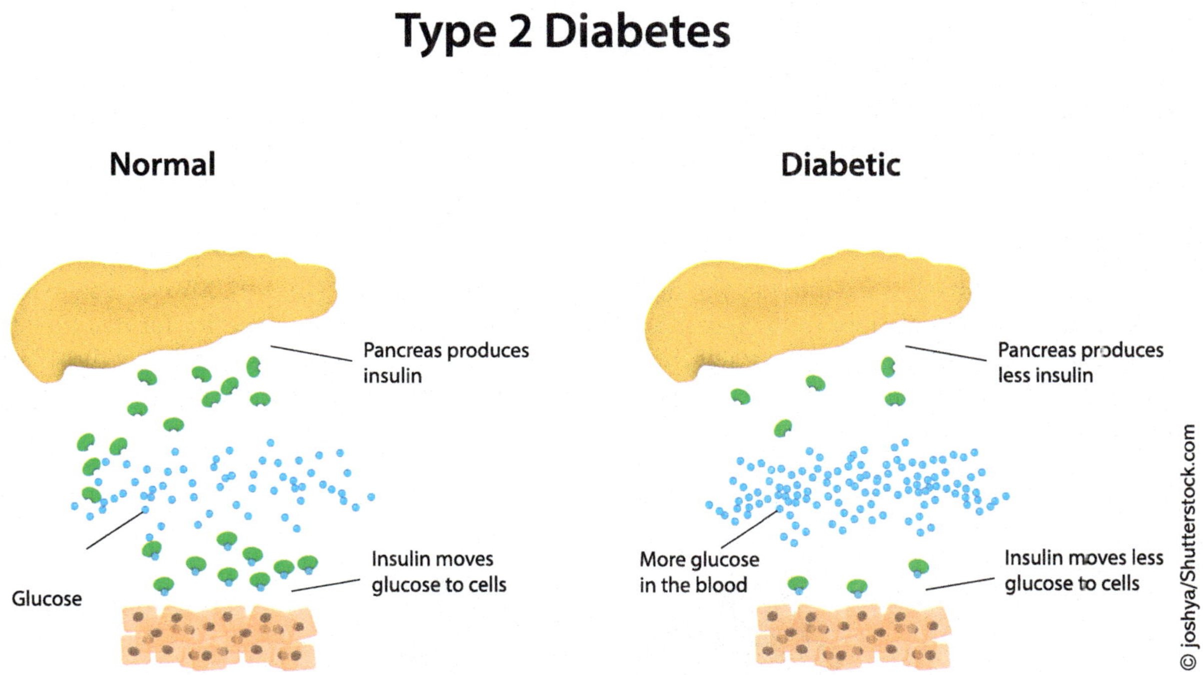


**Fig 9-8** Type 2 Diabetes mellitis

Symptoms of hyperglycemia and include polydipsia, polyuria (early), oliguria (late), nausea, vomiting, and abdominal pain. The child has skin that is warm, dry, and flushed with poor turgor, dry mucous membranes, and a weak pulse. Neurological symptoms include confusion, weakness, lethargy, weak pulse, and diminished reflexes. Acid–base balance is disturbed due to the accumulation of ketones, and rapid, and deep respirations with acetone/fruity odor (**Kussmaul respirations**) (ATI Testing 2016).

As the pathology progresses towards DKA, the child develops ketones in the blood and urine, dyspnea, difficulty in thinking and an inability to concentrate, and mental confusion, and a change in emotional behavior. They also have nausea, vomiting and dehydration, and weight loss. Children can develop slurred speech, blurred vision, and a decreased level of consciousness. Children with advanced DKA have cerebral edema and seizures that lead to coma (ATI Testing 2016).

The nurse takes vital signs including weight, obtains blood glucose levels, I&Os, and evaluates electrolytes, BUN, ABG, and the CBC. A focused assessment evaluates skin integrity and the healing status of any wounds, sensory alterations (tingling and numbness), visual changes, the presence of recurrent infections, the child's diet, and exercise routine, and the child and family's ability to document accurate blood sugars and medicate appropriately (ATI Testing 2016).

## Diagnosis

A child with a random blood glucose of 200 mg/dL or more exhibiting polyuria, polydipsia, and polyphagia or in a 2-hour oral glucose tolerance test a level of 200 mg/dL or more, requires a follow up 8-hour fasting blood glucose test. If levels exceed 126 mg/dL or more, then a diagnosis of Diabetes Mellitis is made (ATI Testing 2016). The nurse administers the 2-hour test by administering a specified amount of glucose. Blood glucose levels are drawn every 30 minutes for 2 hours. The nurse monitors the child for hypoglycemia throughout the procedure.

For a fasting glucose test, the nurse ensures that the child has fasted for 8 hours and that the nurse postpones any medications before the blood draw. The child and family ensure the child eats a high-quality diet for 3 days before the test. The nurse instructs the child to fast for 8 hours before the test. This fasting blood glucose level is an accurate blood sugar unaffected by food (ATI Testing 2016).

### *Glycosylated hemoglobin (HbA1c)*

**Glycosylated hemoglobin (HbA1c)** measures the average glucose levels over a 2-3-month period. The expected reference range is 4%–5.9%, but a realistic target for children who have diabetes can be 6.5%–8%, with a total target goal of less than 7% (ATI Testing 2016).

## Interventions

Blood glucose monitoring is essential to the management of diabetes (see Fig 9-9). Measurements should be assessed at a minimum before meals and at bedtime. The nurse follows agency policy for nail care. Some protocols allow for trimming toenails straight across with clippers and filing edges with a nail file. If a child has severe diabetes, the nurse does not use clippers or scissors; the child should file the nails straight across to minimize skin integrity issues (ATI Testing 2016).

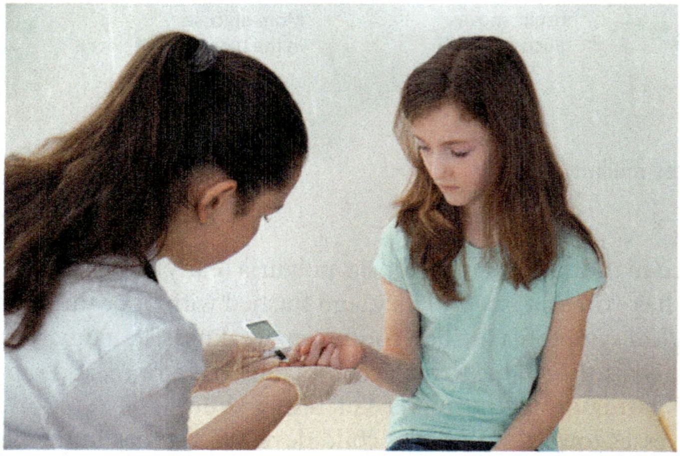

© Andrey_Popov/Shutterstock.com

**Fig 9-9** A nurse taking a blood glucose level

### *Interventions for DKA*

The nurse admits the child to an ICU. The nurse initiates cardiac monitoring and IV access. The nurse begins oxygen therapy to cyanotic children (if arterial oxygen level is less than 80%). The nurse also provides isotonic fluid (0.9% sodium chloride) replacement to support perfusion to vital organs. Large quantities are often required to replace losses. As fluid volume replacement occurs, the nurse looks for evidence of fluid volume excess and cerebral edema. After filling the vascular compartment, the fluid changes to 0.45NS, a hypotonic fluid that pulls fluid from the vascular compartment into the dehydrated cells (ATI Testing 2016).

As serum glucose levels approach 250 mg/dL, the nurse adds glucose to IV fluids to stabilize blood sugars between 120 and 240 mg/dL. The nurse titrates regular insulin continuously through an IV infusion at 0.1unit/kg/hr. The nurse takes a blood glucose level hourly to maintain steady levels of glucose (ATI Testing 2016).

The nurse pays particular attention to serum potassium levels. Potassium levels will initially be elevated. However, as insulin therapy progresses, potassium will shift into cells, and the child is at risk for hypokalemia. The nurse provides **potassium replacement therapy** as indicated by the child's lab values, and ensures adequate urinary output before administering potassium (ATI Testing 2016).

**Table 9-1** Types of Insulin

| Insulin | Type | Onset | Peak | Duration |
|---|---|---|---|---|
| Rapid Acting | Insulin lispro | 15-30 min | 30min-2.5 hrs | 3-6 hrs |
| Short Acting | Regular insulin | 30min-1 hr | 1-5 hr | 6-10 hrs |
| Intermediate Acting | NPH | 1-2 hr | 6-14 hrs | 16-24 hrs |
| Long Acting | Insulin glaring | 70 min | None | 24 hrs |

The nurse gives sodium bicarbonate by slow IV infusion for severe acidosis (pH less than 7.0). The infusion is slow to minimize the rapid migration of potassium into the cells. The nurse tracks potassium levels and the level of consciousness because a correction of acidosis that occurs too quickly can lead to hypokalemia and neurologic sequelae (ATI Testing 2016).

## Medications

Injectable insulin is used to manage DM. The rate of onset, peak, and duration of action varies for each injectable type of insulin (see Table 9-1). Insulin delivery can occur through injections or an insulin pump. Insulin injections are self-administered two or more times per day. Drawing up injections with a needle allows the mixing of rapid-and intermediate-acting insulins. Insulin glargine does not mix with other insulins. When mixing a rapid- or short-acting insulin with a longer-acting insulin, the nurse draws up the shorter-acting insulin into the insulin syringe first and then draws up the longer-acting insulin. This technique minimizes the risk of introducing the longer-acting insulin into the vial of the shorter-acting insulin, contaminating the vial of short acting insulin (ATI Testing 2016).

Insulin injections are painful, and needle length is variable. Research supports a short needle length 4–6 mm to reduce pain and leaking in children (Soo Ting LIM, J., Pei Kwee, L., Yuen Ching HUI, A., Wen Li SEE, W., and Yen, C. 2015). Children who have adverse reactions to injections may benefit from an insulin pump (ATI Testing 2016).

An insulin pump contains regular insulin that delivers a basal amount of insulin, but can also administer a bolus amount of insulin for meals. It can also cover the child during exercise without having to eat carbohydrates. However, the pump needs monitoring by the nurse or the family to ensure the catheter does not come out of place. If the catheter becomes dislodged, the child may go into DKA (ATI Testing 2016).

For either delivery system, the nurse must reinforce instructions, observe return demonstrations, and offer suggestions as needed. Children and/or families must become proficient in medication administration techniques including using a 90° injection angle, and the rotation of sites to prevent **lipohypertrophy** (ATI Testing 2016).

## Teaching

The child and family should familiarize themselves with the **glucometer**, strips, and control test. The nurse checks the accuracy of the glucometer strips by using the control solution (ATI Testing 2016).

The child and family should create a log while they are inpatient that includes the time, date, serum glucose level, food intake, insulin dosage, and environmental or external factors, such as illness or activity level. Children and parents work together to continue the log when they return home (ATI Testing 2016).

Children with diabetes should focus on wellness activities such as infection control strategies, personal hygiene, and foot care. The nurse teaches the child to clean any cuts with warm water and mild soap and applies a dry dressing. The nurse instructs the child and parents to monitor healing and seek intervention promptly.

The child needs to see a doctor or nurse practitioner for regular wellness visits to troubleshoot problems that occur and maintain a healthy lifestyle. Children need yearly eye exams and dental exams twice a year (ATI Testing 2016).

The family should plan meals to coordinate food intake, to activity, onset, and the peak of insulin. The child's caloric needs and food composition should be consistent each day; the child should learn to count carbohydrates (1 carbohydrate exchange = 15 g of carbohydrate). Children should eat at regular intervals and not skip meals. The child and family need support to minimize or eliminate high-fat and high-sugar/high-carbohydrate food items from the family diet (ATI Testing 2016).

## Clinical Pearl

Many children with diabetes live their lives replacing sugar-laden foods for sugar-free laden foods.

The child and family should avoid artificial sweeteners as they induce insulin resistance (Suez, J. et al. 2014). Artificial sweeteners are known to induce insulin resistance and should be contraindicated to the care of a patient with diabetes.

A low-fat, **plant-based diet** containing little to no meat, may help prevent and treat diabetes, by improving insulin sensitivity and decreasing insulin resistance (Tuso, P. J., Ismail, M. H., Ha, B. P., and Bartolotto, C. 2013). In addition, subjects in a randomized, clinical trial on a **low-fat vegan diet**, reduced their HbA1C levels by 1.23 points, compared with 0.38 points for the people on the **American Diabetes Association diet** (Barnard N. D., Cohen J., Jenkins D. J., Turner-McGrievy G., Gloede L., Jaster B., Seidl K., Green A. A., and Talpers. 2006). Similarly, a **ketogenic**, **low fat diet** showed similar results with a reduction of 1.4 A1C points (George, M. M. and Copeland, K. C. 2013). The nurse should support small stepwise goals towards this optimal diet (ATI Testing 2016).

## QSEN Application

Quality Improvement is the "Use data to monitor the outcomes of care processes and use improvement methods to design and test changes to continuously improve the quality and safety of health care systems". Nursing should take the lead to promote lifestyle changes necessary to treat endocrine imbalances effectively. Nurses should "Use a variety of sources of information to review outcomes of care and identify potential areas for improvement. Propose appropriate aims for quality improvement efforts. Assert leadership in shaping the dialogue about and providing leadership for the introduction of best practices."

From Quality and Safety Education for Nurses http://qsen.org/competencies/graduate-ksas/#teamwork_collaboration

The nurse should also help the child to create activity periods for exercise. Children who play competitive sports require a snack 30 minutes before the activity, and snacks every 45–60 min (ATI Testing 2016).

The nurse teaches the child and the family illness management guidelines. Upon the first signs of illness, children should begin to monitor blood glucose levels and urinary ketone levels every three hours, to prevent an episode of DKA. Children should still take insulin or oral diabetic medications and have caffeine free, unsweetened drinks to prevent dehydration (ATI Testing 2016).

Parents and the child should know when there is an emergency. The family should notify the provider if the blood glucose greater than 240 mg/dL, there are positive ketones in the urine, the child is disoriented or confused, tachypnea, episodes of vomiting, or if liquids are not tolerated by the child (ATI Testing 2016).

The child and family should learn the signs if the child is hypoglycemic or hyperglycemic. Hypoglycemic signs include shakiness, diaphoresis, anxiety, nervousness, chills, headache, confusion, labile, difficulty focusing, hunger, dizziness, pallor, and palpitations. The child needs 10–15 g simple carbohydrate (1 tbsp sugar). Some other equivalent glucose sources are 4 oz orange juice, 8 oz. milk, 3–4 glucose tablets, or 4 oz. regular soft drink followed by a complex carbohydrate food (ATI Testing 2016).

If the child loses consciousness or is unable to swallow, the nurse administers glucagon SC or IM and notify the provider. Administer simple carbohydrate as soon as tolerated. The nurse observes for vomiting and takes precautions against aspiration (ATI Testing 2016).

Hyperglycemia causes lethargy, confusion, thirst, nausea, vomiting, abdominal pain, signs of dehydration, rapid respirations, and fruity breath. The parents should encourage oral fluids, administer insulin, and test for ketones (ATI Testing 2016).

Children who have diabetes mellitis type 1 lead full lives if they manage their health on a daily basis. Children who have diabetes mellitis type 2 can not only manage their disease, but also, they can reverse it (ATI Testing 2016).

Both GH and insulin are both hormones in relationship to each other through the endocrine system. Special considerations must be made for deficiencies in GH or insulin and their inverse effects. Children with GH deficiency develop insulin resistance, and children with insulin deficiency have growth deficiencies. Nurses must incorporate these findings into a holistic nursing care plan for children with these hormonal imbalances and realize that all hormones work in relationship to each other (ATI Testing 2016).

## CHAPTER HIGHLIGHTS

- The anterior pituitary gland controls many functions in the body including growth hormone.
- Children with hypopituitarism have a deficiency of endogenous growth hormone (GH).
- Diabetes type 1 is an autoimmune disease where the pancreas does not secrete insulin.
- Ineffective care that results in hypoglycemia includes inaccurate insulin calculation, excessive exercise or illness.
- Diabetes type 2 is a result of insulin resistance that causes the body to produce less insulin.
- DKA treatment seeks to correct dehydration of the body cells and the associated acidosis through fluid resuscitation and correction of electrolyte imbalances.

## REFERENCES

ATI Testing. 2016. Nursing Care of Children. Retrieved from http://www.atitesting.com/ati_next_gen/DisplayResources.aspx?Name=rm_rn_ncc_2016_ebook_20170417.pdf.

Barnard N. D., Cohen J., Jenkins D. J., Turner-McGrievy G., Gloede L., Jaster B., Seidl K., Green A. A., and Talpers. 2006. *Diabetes Care. 2006 Aug*, 29(8), 1777–83.

Bryant J., Baxter L., Cave C. B., and Milne R. 2007. "Recombinant growth hormone for idiopathic short stature in children and adolescents." *Cochrane Database of Systematic Reviews*, Issue 3. Art. No.: CD004440. doi: 10.1002/14651858.CD004440.pub2.

George, M. M. and Copeland, K. C. 2013. "Current Treatment Options for Type 2 Diabetes Mellitus in Youth: Today's Realities and Lessons from the TODAY Study." *Current Diabetes Reports*, 13(1), 72–80. http://doi.org/10.1007/s11892-012-0334-z.

Soo Ting LIM, J., Pei Kwee, L., Yuen Ching HUI, A., Wen Li SEE, W., and Yen, C. 2015. "Can the use of short insulin needles achieve better patient outcomes in adults and children? A systematic review." *Singapore Nursing Journal*, 42(1), 29–38.

Suez, J., Korem, T., Zeevi, D., Zilberman-Schapira, G., Thaiss, C., Maza, O., Elinav, E. et al. 2014. "Artificial sweeteners induce glucose intolerance by altering the gut microbiota." *Nature*, 514(7521), 181–186+.

Tuso, P. J., Ismail, M. H., Ha, B. P., and Bartolotto, C. 2013. "Nutritional Update for Physicians: Plant-Based Diets." *The Permanente Journal*, 17(2), 61–6. http://doi.org/10.7812/TPP/12-085.

# CHAPTER 10

# CARING FOR CHILDREN WITH HEMATOLOGIC CONDITIONS

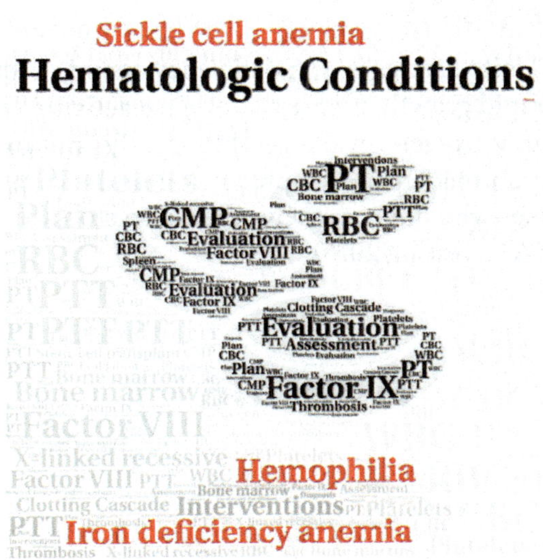


Modified from Shutterstock. © Bay_Design/Shutterstock.com

## LEARNING OUTCOMES

1. Describe the pathophysiology and clinical presentation of iron deficiency anemia.
2. Utilize the nursing process to provide safe, comprehensive health care to children with hematologic conditions.
3. Differentiate between heme and non-heme iron sources, and how they are absorbed.
4. Develop a comprehensive "family-centered" teaching plan for a child with sickle cell anemia.
5. Differentiate between Hemophilia A and B.
6. Develop a comprehensive "family-centered" teaching plan for a child with hemophilia.
7. Teaching/learning principles in providing anticipatory guidance in the prevention and treatment of children with hematologic conditions.

## KEY TERMS

Acute chest syndrome
Aplastic crisis
Cryoprecipitate
Factor VIII
Factor IX
Hemarthrosis
Heme iron
Hip avascular necrosis
Hypochromic RBCS
Microcytic RBCS
Non-heme iron
Prolonged partial thromboplastin time
RICE
Spleen sequestration
Z-track method

## HEMATOLOGIC DISORDERS

Blood nourishes all of the organs in the body with oxygen. Oxygen-rich blood is healthy blood. There are several ways to build and maintain healthy blood. To make healthy blood children must be active, as exercise stimulates erythropoietin, and eat a high quality diet high in minerals particularly iron. Some blood disorders that manifest in children include iron deficiency anemia, sickle cell anemia, and hemophilia.

### Iron Deficiency Anemia (IDA)

The most common anemia in the United States is iron deficiency anemia. Adolescent girls are especially vulnerable, due to a diet low in iron, rapid growth, menses, strenuous activities, and obesity (ATI Testing 2016).

Iron builds hemoglobin to carry oxygen on the red blood cells and oxygenate the body's organs (see Fig 10-1). IDA usually results from an inadequate supply of iron in the diet. It is preventable and reversible. Risk factors include premature babies who did not receive their iron stores from their mothers, cow milk, and a diet low in iron or loss of blood (ATI Testing 2016).

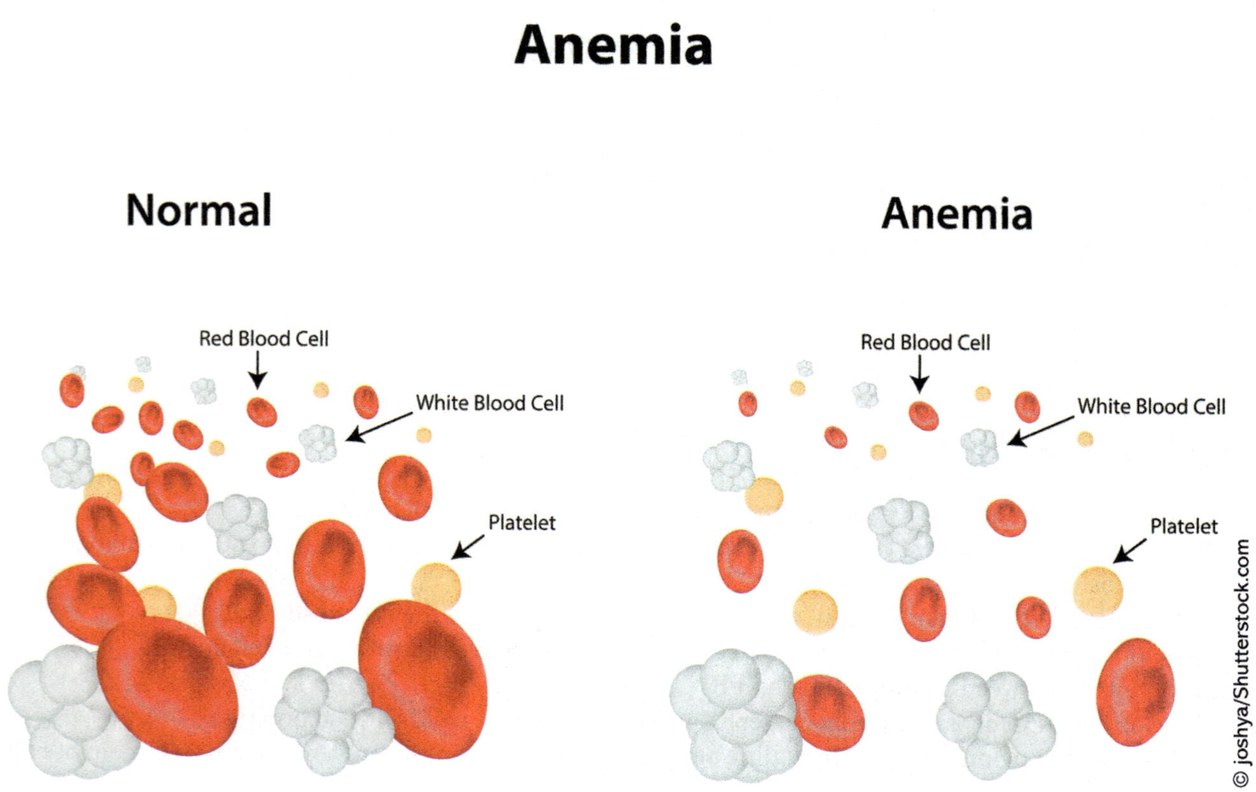


**Fig 10-1** Anemia is a condition of too few red blood cells

Iron comes in two forms animal protein has **heme iron** and **non-heme iron**, and plants contain non-heme iron. Non-heme iron has been easily overlooked as a viable source of iron because it is less absorbable. However, new research may broaden the understanding of iron absorption. Iron absorption turns on in response to the amount of iron already in the body; the body absorbs more iron when iron stores are low. Since the body has no mechanism for iron excretion, absorption is regulated. Vegetarians and vegan have lower iron stores than their meat-eating counterparts but do not have increased rates of IDA (Messina, V. and Mangels, A. 2001).

It is arguable that non-heme iron sources are higher quality sources of nutrition. However, a balance of both can easily meet the iron needs of a child.

As the infant begins solids, non-heme iron sources, such as vegetables, grains, and legumes may promote absorption of iron by dispersing it throughout the day. Non-heme iron is best absorbed with Vitamin C foods found in tomatoes, kale, broccoli, and red peppers. Heme iron sources although highly absorbable may increase the risk for GI cancers as more iron may not be beneficial. Heme iron catalyzes N-nitroso compounds, which are known carcinogens and increases the risk for coronary heart disease (Ward, M. H., Cross, A. J., Abnet, C. C., Sinha, R., Markin, R. S., and Weisenburger, D. D., 2012; Yang, W., Li, B., Dong, X., Zhang, X., Zeng, Y., Zhou, J., and . . . Xu, J. 2014).

Ideally, an infant increases iron stores through delayed cord clamping at birth, breastfeeds from a mother with adequate iron intake, and begins iron-rich foods at 6 months of age when the infant uses up its maternal iron stores (Wang, M. 2016).

Iron-rich foods are preferable to supplementation as foods are better tolerated than supplements without side effects (Wang, M. 2016). Breastfed babies may need supplementation of ferrous sulfate, if there are alterations at any point in the process. Ferrous sulfate can cause GI upset, constipation and diarrhea. The nurse can administer the drops with a vitamin C rich food to promote absorption. Formula fed babies receive iron supplementation through their formula. However, they are subject to the complications of supplementation, such as constipation and dark stools. The complications of iron deficiency early in life include neurological complications and developmental delay (ATI Testing 2016).

## Assessment

A child with IDA presents with tachycardia, pallor, brittle, spoon-shaped fingernails, fatigue, irritability, and muscle weakness, and possibly, a systolic heart murmur (ATI Testing 2016).

Lab tests indicate low RBC with **microcytic** (small RBCs) and **hypochromic** (low hemoglobin) RBCs with decreased Hgb or Hct. The child has a low mean corpuscular volume, a low mean corpuscular hemoglobin concentration (ATI Testing 2016).

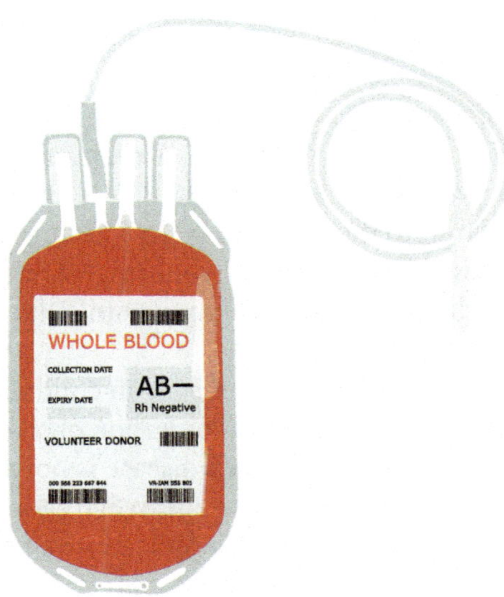

### Interventions

Interventions include iron supplements for preterm and low-birth-weight infants by the age of 2 months and iron supplements to full term infants who are not eating vegetables by the age of 4–6 months. The infant's diet should advance to include foods high in iron and vitamin C.

Formula fed babies should have no more than 32 oz. (960 ml) per day, so that they can intake other high-quality foods. Children should be allowed rest periods as needed. A blood transfusion may occur, if hemoglobin is critically low (ATI Testing 2016).

The nurse checks for the informed consent documentation and checks the blood for safety with another RN. The blood is run with normal saline and is used to prime the tubing. The blood is run very slowly for the first fifteen minutes to look for transfusion reactions and then increases to the ordered rate. The nurse charts vital every fifteen minutes for the first hour. The nurse monitors the effects of the transfusion via laboratory values (ATI Testing 2016).

### Medications

#### *Iron Supplements*

The child receives iron supplements 1 hour before or 2 hours after milk or antacid to prevent decreased absorption. The child can absorb supplements most efficiently on an empty stomach, but the common GI upset may not allow for this. Gastrointestinal (GI) upset (diarrhea, constipation, nausea) occurs at the start of therapy but can decrease over time. The child takes a reduced dose of the iron supplements with meals and gradually increases the dose as tolerated. Supplements given with vitamin C increase the absorption of iron. The use of a straw prevents staining of the teeth for older children (ATI Testing 2016).

If the child does not tolerate oral supplements, an injection can deliver the needed iron. The nurse uses a **Z-track method** (inset like a dart and slowly inject medication, and wait for 10 seconds before removal) to inject the thick fluid into the muscle, with no massage to the injection site (ATI Testing 2016).

### Teaching

The child and family should understand that the stools will change to a tarry-green color if the dose is correct. The parents should reinforce the practice of rinsing the mouth to prevent tooth staining. The stools can be loose to diarrhea to constipation and nausea may present as a side effect but should be self-limited. Fluids and fiber help, if constipation occurs. Children can overdose on iron, so no more than a month's supply with a child-proofed cap, which can protect the child. Follow up lab tests are necessary to monitor the iron level (ATI Testing 2016).

## Sickle Cell Anemia

Sickle cell disease (SCD) is an autosomal, recessive genetic disorder that substitutes hemoglobin S for normal hemoglobin (Hgb A) and disproportionately affects African-Americans. Other forms of SCD can affect individuals of Mediterranean, Indian, or Middle Eastern descent. Children who have the sickle cell trait do not manifest the disease, but can pass the trait to their offspring (ATI Testing 2016).

SCD is a group of genetic diseases characterized by abnormal sickle hemoglobin S (HbS) that replace normal adult hemoglobin (Hgb A) in the circulation. Children with sickle cell disease (SCD) have two copies of the gene that makes hemoglobin-S (ATI Testing 2016).

Sickle cell anemia (SCA) is the most common form of SCD in children.

The sickling of the RBCs causes complications, such as occlusion of blood vessels that causes tissue hypoxia and ischemia (see Fig 10-2). The presentation of sickle cell disease is not always apparent at birth. Once fetal hemoglobin is replaced by adult hemoglobin, symptoms appear. Symptoms can escalate into sickle cell crisis as ischemia and hypoxia manifest as pain for the child. Complications include **acute chest syndrome** (a lung infection that causes more sickling) and cerebral vascular accident (CVA) (ATI Testing 2016).

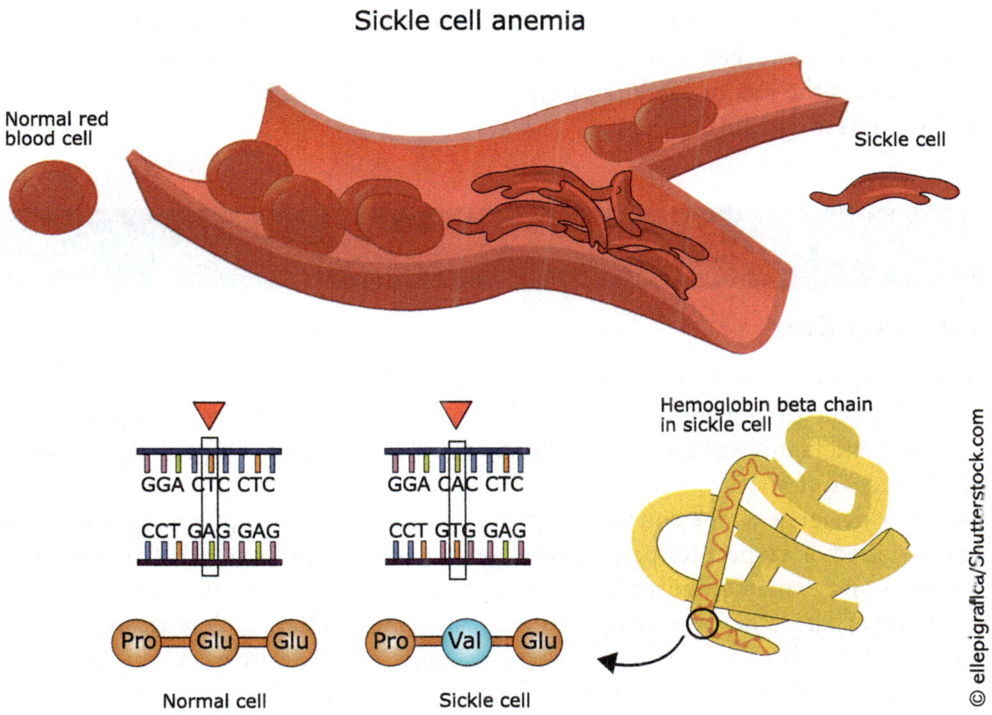


**Fig 10-2** HgbS occludes circulation

## Assessment

A child with sickle cell anemia has a family history of sickle cell disease. They present in a vaso-occlusive crisis (a sickle cell crisis) with complaints of severe pain, shortness of breath, headache, dizziness, pallor, pale mucous membranes, and jaundice. This episode lasts 4–6 days (ATI Testing 2016).

In the acute stage, the child has severe pain and swelling, usually in bones, joints of the hands and feet, and abdomen. The child may have hematuria, obstructive jaundice, or visual disturbances.

Chronic manifestations include a susceptibility to respiratory infection, systolic murmurs, retinal detachment and blindness, enuresis and renal failure, liver cirrhosis and hepatomegaly, seizures, skeletal deformities; shoulder or **hip avascular necrosis** and osteomyelitis (ATI Testing 2016),

**Spleen sequestration**, or the excessive pooling of blood in the spleen (splenomegaly), and/or in the liver (hepatomegaly) is also a complication of SCD. Sequestration decreases the circulating volume and can result in hypovolemia and hypovolemic shock (ATI Testing 2016).

Signs of hypovolemic shock include irritability, tachycardia, pallor, decreased urinary output, tachypnea, cool extremities, thready pulse, and hypotension (ATI Testing 2016).

Children with SCD may experience an **aplastic crisis** or an extreme anemia, jaundice, and/or reticulocytosis caused by decreased RBC production. A viral infection can trigger an aplastic crisis.

Children may also develop acute chest syndrome from a lung infection. Acute chest syndrome which is life threatening. Assessment findings for acute chest syndrome include chest, back, or abdominal pain, a fever of 38.5° C (101.3° F) or higher, cough, retractions, tachypnea, dyspnea, and decreased oxygen saturations. Treatment would include an exchange transfusion and antibiotics (ATI Testing 2016).

## Diagnosis

There is mandatory screening in most states to detect sickle cell anemia using a sickle-turbidity screening tool. The screening can determine sickled cells but cannot distinguish carriers from those with the disease. Hemoglobin electrophoresis separates and identifies the various forms of hemoglobin (Hgb) and diagnoses sickle cell anemia. A CBC determines anemia in the blood (ATI Testing 2016).

A child in a crisis presents with decreased Hgb, an elevated WBC, elevated bilirubin and reticulocyte levels, and a peripheral blood smear reveals sickled cells. A transcranial Doppler (TCD) test determines intracranial vascular flow and detects the risk of cerebro-vascular accident (CVA). Children 2–16 years of age receive an annual TCD test (ATI Testing 2016).

## QSEN Application

### Patient centered Care

Nurses should consider children with chronic diseases, like Sickle cell anemia or hemophilia, to be experts on their disease. Learning to create a rapport, and gain trust helps the nurse elicit personal preferences that make the child and family feel cared for by the medical team. Nurses should develop skills to facilitate this through the recognition of

"the patient or designee as the source of control and full partner in providing compassionate and coordinated care based on respect for patient's preferences, values, and needs", Nurses can"[e]licit patient values, preferences and expressed needs as part of clinical interview, diagnosis, implementation of care plan and evaluation of care". They may also[c]ommunicate patient values, preferences and expressed needs to other members of health-care team, and[p]rovide patient-centered care with sensitivity, empathy, and respect for the diversity of human experience". Finally, nurses can "[a]ssess and treat pain and suffering in light of patient values, preferences, and expressed needs."

Nurses that take time to incorporate patient-centered care provide a better patient experience.

From Quality and Safety Education for Nurses http://qsen.org/competencies/pre-licensure-ksas/

## Interventions

The nurse administers oxygen, if hypoxia is present, and delivers fluid and electrolyte infusions to correct imbalances. The child takes oral fluids when tolerated. The child also may need a blood transfusion to introduce healthy RBCs in the circulation. The nurse monitors intake and output values and promotes rest to decrease oxygen consumption (ATI Testing, 2016).

The nurse will prevent infection through hand washing and administering vaccinations (pneumococcal conjugate vaccine, meningococcal vaccine, and Haemophilus influenza type B vaccine). If the child has an underlying infection, antibiotics may be necessary (ATI Testing 2016).

Pain management requires an interprofessional approach. The child with sickle cell anemia with mild to moderate pain receives acetaminophen or ibuprofen; severe pain requires opioid analgesics (codeine, morphine sulfate, oxycodone, hydromorphone, and methadone). Pain medications are given on a schedule to prevent pain (ATI Testing 2016).

Nonpharmacological pain interventions are done using warm packs on painful joints and using child life for distraction (ATI Testing 2016).

## Teaching

Children with SCD need opiate therapy and blood transfusions for the rest of his or her life. If a child shows negative characteristics associated with opiate use, such as decreased concentration, itching, sleepiness, insomnia, itchiness, depression, and a reduced respiratory rate, these are not signs of drug abuse; these are expected findings based on a lifetime of opiate use. The child will also receive blood transfusions every 3–4 weeks to prevent CVA's. The nurse should offer referrals for emotional and psychological support for the child and family. Fluids are essential to the prevention of a sickle cell crisis. Therefore, the child and family should understand fluid intake as a number of bottles or glasses instead of ounces to consume. (ATI Testing 2016).

The family should understand the disease process, signs of a crisis or infection, and the need for genetic counseling for before child rearing. The child and family should take steps to include rest periods as well as high quality nutrition throughout the day (ATI Testing 2016).

Infection control strategies, including hand-washing, and vaccination maintenance are also necessary to prevent infections that could trigger a crisis. The child should wear a medical identification wristband or medical identification tags (ATI Testing 2016).

## Hemophilia

Hemophilia is a group of bleeding disorders. Children are unable to by control bleeding due to an inability to form a blood clot. Both hemophilia A and B is an X-linked recessive disease; therefore, boys are more likely to have the disease (see Fig 10-3). Bleeding can manifest externally or internally. Hemophilia may reveal itself after a circumcision for boys. Hemophilia varies in severity in relation to the amount of clotting factor that the child makes (ATI Testing 2016).

Hemophilia A is a deficiency of **factor VIII** and is the most common form of hemophilia. Hemophilia B is a deficiency of **factor IX** and is also called Christmas disease. Complications of hemophilia include uncontrolled bleeding, intracranial hemorrhage, and airway obstruction from bleeding in the mouth, neck, or chest (ATI Testing 2016).

### Assessment

Children with hemophilia have episodes of bleeding, reports of joint pain and stiffness, impaired mobility, easy bruising, and activity intolerance. Children can present with active bleeding (bleeding gums, epistaxis, hematuria, and/or tarry stools), hematomas and/or bruising, even with minor injuries (ATI Testing 2016).

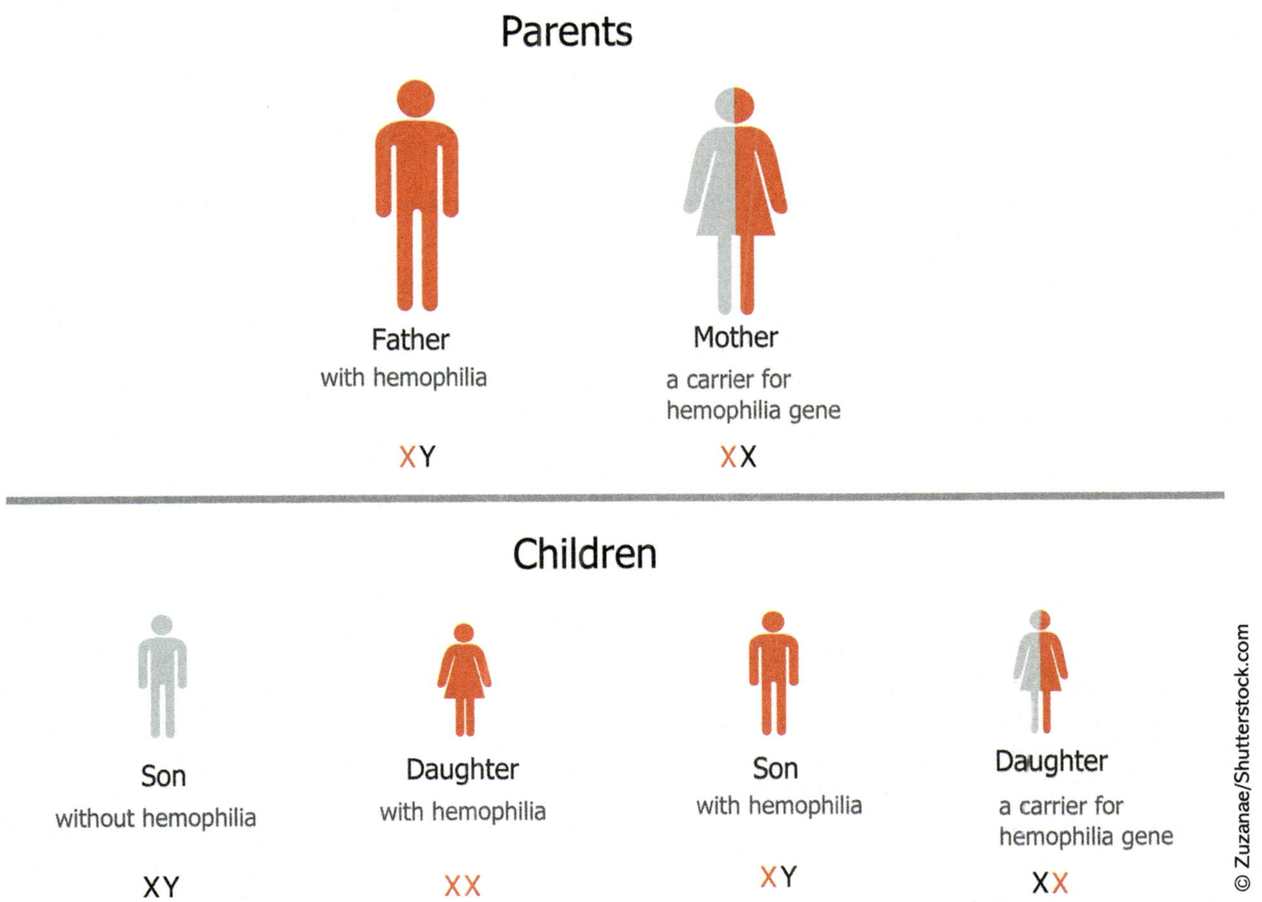


**Fig 10-3** The inheritance of Hemophilia

**Hemarthrosis** (bleeding into a joint) is often the cause of joint pain as evidenced by joint stiffness, swelling, warmth, redness, loss of range of motion, and deformities (see Fig 10-4). A headache, slurred speech, and a decreased level of consciousness occur once the bleeding has become significant. The nurse assesses urine, stool, and nasogastric fluid for occult blood (ATI Testing 2016).

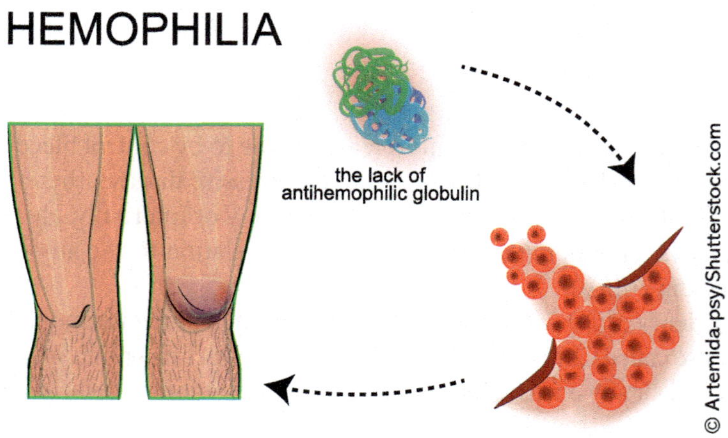


**Fig 10-4** Concealed bleeding in hemophilia

## Diagnosis

A child with hemophilia will have a **Prolonged partial thromboplastin time** (PPTT: the length of time for blood to clot), accompanied by normal platelet levels and a normal prothrombin time (PT: the length of time for plasma to clot). The time for whole blood to clot is also normal. Factor-specific tests determine the type of factor deficiency, and DNA testing detects hemophilia genes in female patients (ATI Testing 2016).

## Interventions

Needle punctures cause bleeding; therefore, the nurse uses the subcutaneous route for injections and venipunctures instead of finger or heel sticks. Children avoid aspirin because of its blood thinning properties; acetaminophen can treat pain in children with hemophilia (ATI Testing 2016).

The child receives IV factor replacement, and the nurse observes for transfusion reaction, flushing, headache, low sodium, and alterations in heart rate and blood pressure. In addition, a blood transfusion can control bleeding, but **cryoprecipitate** (plasma plus clotting factors) provides a high enough concentration of factors to prevent bleeding temporarily. Nonpharmacological interventions for pain include resting, immobilizing, and icing and elevating affected joints (ATI Testing 2016).

## Medications

1-deamino-8-d-arginine vasopressin (DDAVP)

DDAVP is the synthetic version of vasopressin that increases plasma factor VIII (antihemophilic factor). It is useful for children with mild hemophilia, but not for children with hemophilia B (they need factor VIII). A child can receive DDAVP prophylactically for dental or surgical procedures (ATI Testing 2016).

Factor VIII, products that contain factor VIII, recombinant products, and pooled plasma are given intravenously to prevent and treat hemorrhage. This treatment requires several doses, and consistent administration can prevent bleeding complications (ATI Testing 2016).

Corticosteroids treat hematuria and acute episodes of hemarthrosis, and chronic synovitis (inflammation of the synovial membrane). Corticosteroids decrease immune function. Therefore, the nurse and family monitor the child for infection. Nonsteroidal anti-inflammatory agents (NSAID) treat chronic synovitis who but can inhibit platelet function (ATI Testing 2016).

## Clinical Pearl

Children who receive many blood transfusions can develop an allergy to the donor's blood by creating inhibitors. Inhibitors can inactivate the clotting factors infused into the child's blood stream. An immune tolerance induction removes inhibitors. Researchers confirms the induction makes the child not recognize the factor, it would otherwise reject, leading to tolerance of the factor and allows the child to use the clotting factor (Athale, A. H., Marcucci, M, and Iorio, A.2014).

### Teaching

Parents must provide a safe home and play environment. The prevention of bleeding prevents injury to the child. The child should wear an identification bracelet. A disease like hemophilia can prompt parents to be over-protective. However, children still need exercise. Possibly through low-contact sports, such as bowling, fishing, swimming, and golf, and using helmets and padding for potentially hazardous activities. Bleeding episodes require nonpharmacological pain interventions (**RICE**; rest, ice, compression, and elevation). Regular exercise and physical therapy occur once bleeding subsides. Children should use a soft-bristled toothbrush. The family and child should learn the signs of internal bleeding, shock, and hemarthrosis. The child and family should seek psychosocial support through support groups to help them maintain wellness. Children should maintain a healthy weight to minimize stress on joints through a high-quality diet and exercise (ATI Testing 2016).

## CHAPTER HIGHLIGHTS

- Iron deficiency anemia is preventable with a high quality diet. Once deficient, supplementation is necessary until a high quality diet resumes.
- Sickle cell anemia is a genetic disease that causes the red blood cell to become sticky, and take on a sickle shaped that occludes blood vessels.
- Children with sickle cell anemia can develop complications, such as vaso-occlusive crisis, splenic sequestration, and aplastic crisis.
- Children with sickle cell anemia can develop fatal complications, like stroke, acute chest syndrome, and retinopathy.
- Hemophilia is an X-linked genetic disease. There are two forms. Hemophilia A is most common and is a deficiency of Factor VIII.
- Hemophilia B is a deficiency of Factor IX and is less common.
- Children with hemophilia cannot clot their blood in response to injury.
- The treatment goals for hemophilia are to control the bleeding and pain, minimize activity, and support for the child and family who manage a chronic disease.

## REFERENCES

Athale, A. H., Marcucci, M., and Iorio, A. 2014. "Immune tolerance induction for treating inhibitors in people with congenital haemophilia A or B." *Cochrane Database of Systematic Reviews 2014*, Issue4. Art. No.: CD010561. doi: 10.1002/14651858.CD010561.pub2.

ATI Testing. 2016. Nursing Care of Children. Retrieved from http://www.atitesting.com/ati_next_gen/DisplayResources.aspx?Name=rm_rn_ncc_2016_ebook_20170417.pdf.

Messina, V. and Mangels, A. 2001. "Considerations in planning vegan diets: children." *Journal of the American Dietetic Association*, 101(6), 661–9.

Ward, M. H., Cross, A. J., Abnet, C. C., Sinha, R., Markin, R. S., and Weisenburger, D. D. 2012. Heme iron from meat and risk of adenocarcinoma of the esophagus and stomach. Retrieved August 13, 2017, from https://www.ncbi.nlm.nih.gov/pubmed/22044848.

Wang, M. 2016. "Iron Deficiency and Other Types of Anemia in Infants and Children." *American Family Physician*, 93(4), 270.

Yang, W., Li, B., Dong, X., Zhang, X., Zeng, Y., Zhou, J., and ... Xu, J. 2014. "Is heme iron intake associated with risk of coronary heart disease? A meta-analysis of prospective studies." *European Journal of Nutrition*, 53(2), 395–400. doi: 10.1007/s00394-013-0535-5.

CHAPTER 11

# CARING FOR CHILDREN WITH MUSCULOSKELETAL CONDITIONS

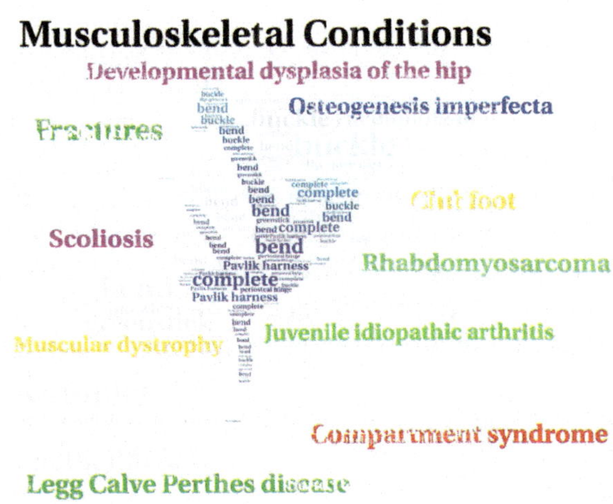


Modified from Shutterstock. © Ahsan Alvi/Shutterstock.com

## LEARNING OUTCOMES

1. Describe the differences between pediatric and adult bone structures.
2. Describe the different types of fractures.
3. Create a nursing care plan for a child in a cast.
4. Utilize the nursing process to provide safe, comprehensive health care to children with hematologic conditions
5. Recognize the assessment findings of compartment syndrome (5Ps) and know when to report to the provider.
6. Synthesize data from vital signs and a physical assessment to create a focused assessment of musculoskeletal conditions.
7. Plan nursing interventions and evaluate outcomes that are developmentally appropriate for infants, toddlers, preschoolers, school-age children, and adolescents in traction.
8. Plan nursing interventions and evaluate outcomes that are developmentally appropriate for infants, toddlers, preschoolers, school-age children, and adolescents with neuromuscular conditions.
9. Teaching/learning principles in providing anticipatory guidance in the prevention and treatment of children with musculoskeletal conditions.

# KEY TERMS

5 Ps
Acetabular dysplasia
Barlow test
Buckle fracture
Bryant traction
Comminuted fracture
Compartment syndrome
Complete bone fractures
Complicated fracture
Dislocation
Greenstick fracture
Halo traction
Heel cord tenotomy
Hip spica cast
Incomplete fracture
Oblique fracture
Ortolani test
Osteoblasts
Osteocyte
Osteogenesis
Osteogenic cells
Pavlik harness
Physeal fracture
Plastic deformation
Range of motion
Spiral break
Stress fracture
Subluxation
Surgical reduction
Talipes calcaneus
Talipes equinovarus
Talipes equinus
Talipes valgus
Talipes varus
Transverse fracture
Trendelenburg sign
Volkmann compression

A child's skeleton is very different than an adult skeleton. **Osteogenesis**, or the formation of bone, begins with cartilage and is then replaced by bone (ossification) (see Fig 11-1). **Osteogenic cells** are the only bone cells that divide. They divide and then differentiate into **osteoblasts**. A bone begins as a cartilage framework. As calcification with calcium and phosphorus occurs and covers the cartilage and cartilage cells die. This process makes the bones porous, and blood vessels fill in these spaces and bring osteoblasts to the bone. Osteoblasts secrete collagen into a mesh matrix and draw calcium into the structure. This process takes the osteoblast into a mature bone cell, the **osteocyte**. This process occurs over childhood with full calcification not occurring until adulthood. Children's bones grow until the epiphyseal plate is no longer active, known as epiphyseal closure. Therefore, child injuries respond differently based on, when they occur during bone development (Gilbert, S. F. 2000).

Children also have congenital musculoskeletal conditions, such as club foot or hip dysplasia. Children respond to casting due to the flexibility of the bones.

A child may also have alterations in the neuromuscular interface causing muscular dystrophy. The lack of muscle tension creates decreased bone mineral density and puts children with muscular dystrophy at risk for fractures (Morgenroth, V. H., Hache, L. P., and Clemens, P. R. 2012). Muscles act on bones to keep them strong (see Fig 11-2). Bones are the framework muscles need to remain strong.

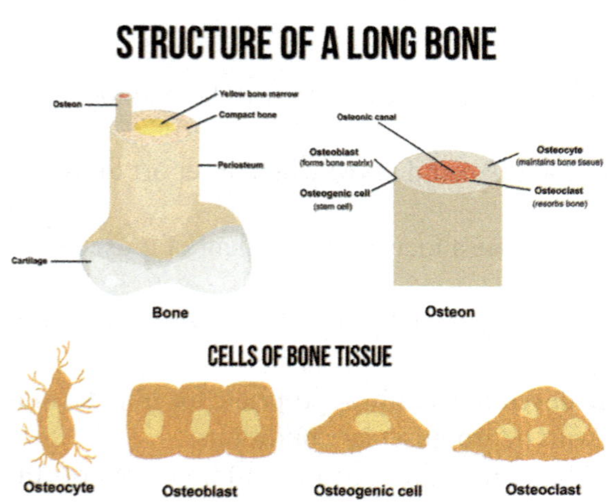



**Fig 11-1** Anatomy of a long bone: cell types

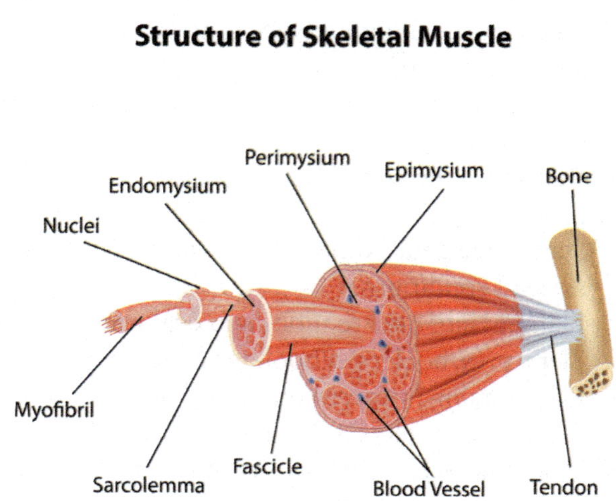



**Fig 11-2** Anatomy of a muscle

# FRACTURES

Fractures are the medical term for a broken bone. Children's bones are different than adults and break in various ways. Bone healing and remodeling occurs faster in children than in adults, as a result of a thicker periosteum and adequate blood supply. Because children still have active epiphyseal plates, injuries can result in altered bone growth. Practitioners can visualize breaks through radiographic evidence that identifies past and present fractures. Such proof can diagnose physical abuse or osteogenesis imperfecta. Risk factors for fractures include poor nutrition, obesity, and risky play activities. Complications include **compartment syndrome**, **Volkmann compression**, or osteomyelitis (ATI Testing 2016).

## Assessment

Children present with pain, edema, ecchymosis, warmth or redness, deformity, and the decreased use of affected area (ATI Testing 2016).

There are different types of fractures (see Fig 11-3). A **plastic deformation** (bend) occurs when the bone is bent, not broken. This break happens due to the high percentage of cartilage in children's bones. A **buckle (torus) fracture** is a compression of the bone that results in a bulge or raised area at the fracture site. A **greenstick fracture** is an **incomplete fracture** of the bone due to the soft nature of children's bones. A **transverse fracture** appears straight across the bone. An **oblique fracture** occurs diagonally across the bone. A **spiral break** twists around the bone and often indicates nonaccidental injury. A **physeal fracture** (break through the growth plate) break goes through the epiphyseal plate of a long bone. A **stress fracture** develops through repeated muscle contractions and causes a crack in the bone. **Complete bone fractures** break away from the bone and are in separate pieces, and **incomplete fractures** are bone fragments that are still attached. A closed or simple fracture does not pierce the skin. An open or compound fracture presents with broken skin with the bone protruding. A **complicated fracture** is a fracture that results in injury to other organs and tissues. A **comminuted fracture** includes small fragments of bone that embed into surrounding tissue (ATI Testing 2016) (see Fig 11-3).

The nurse assesses the affected area for sensation (numbness or tingling), color, movement, temperature, capillary refill, and pulses. The provider makes a diagnosis of the fracture and the fracture type through radiographic imaging (ATI Testing 2016).

## Interventions

Children may need emergency care at the point of the fracture.

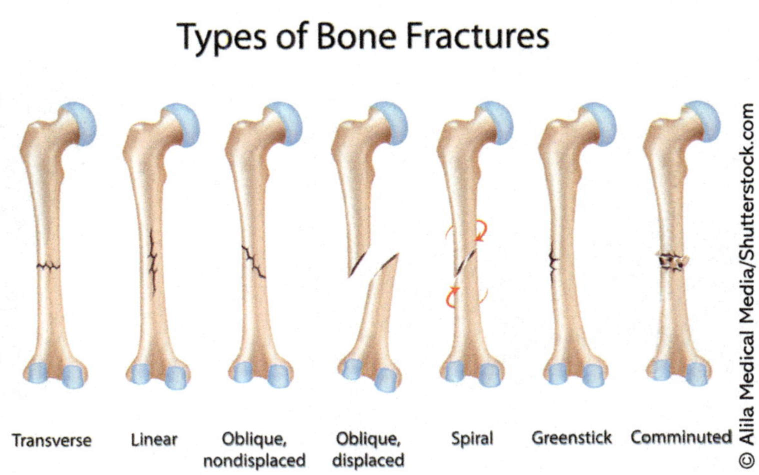


**Fig 11-3** Types of fractures in children

Vitals, pain and a neurovascular status begin the assessment. The nurse administers pain medication and positions the child. The affected limb is elevated, and ice packs (on and off every 20 minutes) are applied. For injuries to the distal arm, pelvis, and lower extremities, the child should be in a supine position. For injuries that occur in the shoulder or upper arm, the nurse places the child in a sitting position. If the nurse suspects a pelvic fracture, urine output becomes a priority assessment to identify hypovolemic shock (ATI Testing 2016).

The nurse administers pain medication using an age-appropriate pain tool and nonpharmacological interventions (ATI Testing 2016).

Opioid administration requires a continuous assessment for respiratory depression and constipation. The nurse, family, and child should assess the affected extremity every hour and perform **range of motion** (ROM) exercises of fingers, toes, and unaffected extremities (ATI Testing 2016).

If the child develops symptoms of compartment syndrome (the 5 Ps), the nurse should notify the provider, loosen the dressing or open and bivalve the cast, and prepare the child for a fasciotomy (ATI Testing 2016).

The nurse will also complete dressing changes or maintain negative pressure wound therapy. The nurse should instruct the child or family to report pain that is not relieved by analgesics, pain that continues to increase in intensity, numbness or tingling, or a change in color of the extremity (ATI Testing 2016).

The nurse encourages adequate hydration and nutrition and administers stool softeners related to immobility (ATI Testing 2016).

## Orthopedic Casting

There are several types of casts, but the nursing interventions for the cast care are the same for each cast type. Cast types include long-leg, short-leg, bilateral long-leg, long-arm, short-arm, shoulder spica, 1½ spica, full spica, and single spica.

The provider decides what material best suits the child. Plaster of Paris is the traditional material (see Fig 11-6). However, plaster of Paris casts are heavy, not water-resistant, and can take 10 to 72 hr. to dry. Synthetic fiberglass casts are light, water-resistant, and dry quickly (5–20 minutes) (see Fig 11-5) (ATI Testing 2016).

## Cast Care

The nurse can help the child by using atraumatic care principles before cast application by demonstrating the procedure using a doll, toy or showing a picture as is appropriate for the age of the child (see Fig 11-8). The child should understand the cast will feel warm when applied but will not cause any harm. One fingerbreadth space should fit between the skin and the cast. The nurse elevates the cast above the level of the heart in a sling during the first 24–48 hours to encourage venous drainage and reduce swelling (see Fig 11-4 and 11-7). Ice decreases the swelling for the first 24 hours. Instruct the child to avoid placing any objects inside the cast to prevent trauma to the skin.

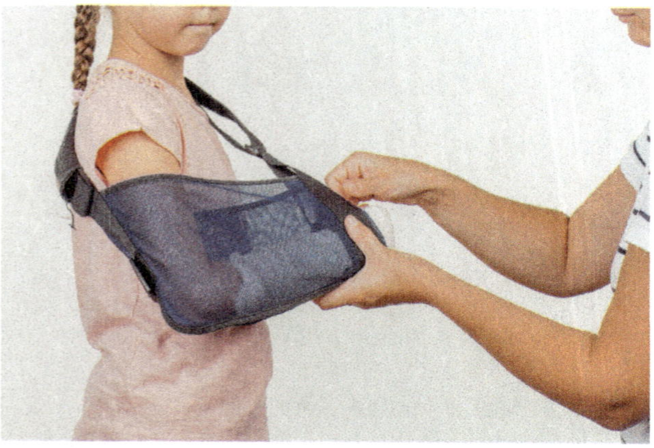


**Fig 11-4** A sling keeps arm at heart level

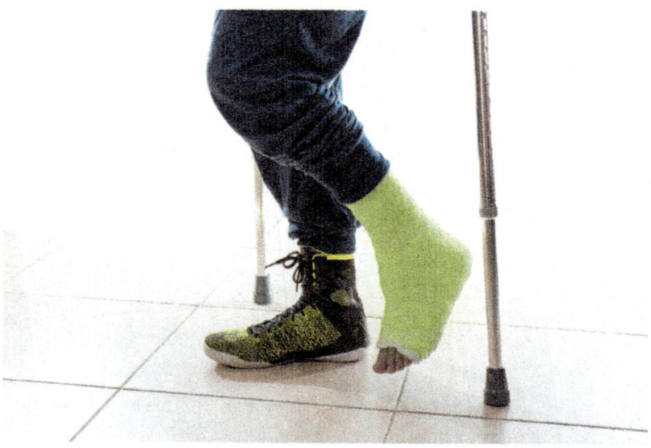


**Fig 11-5** A fiberglass cast

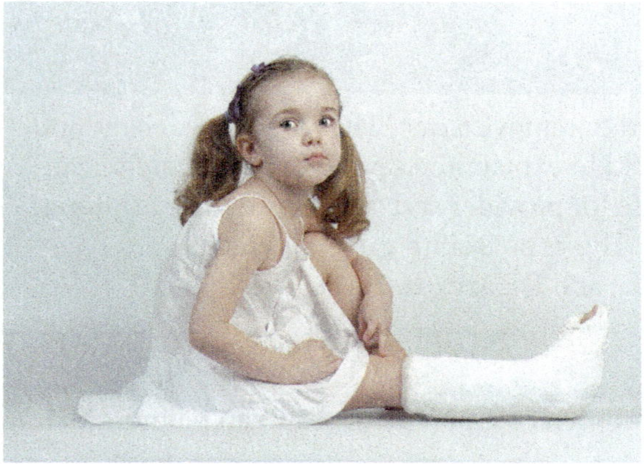


**Fig 11-6** A girl in a plaster of Paris cast

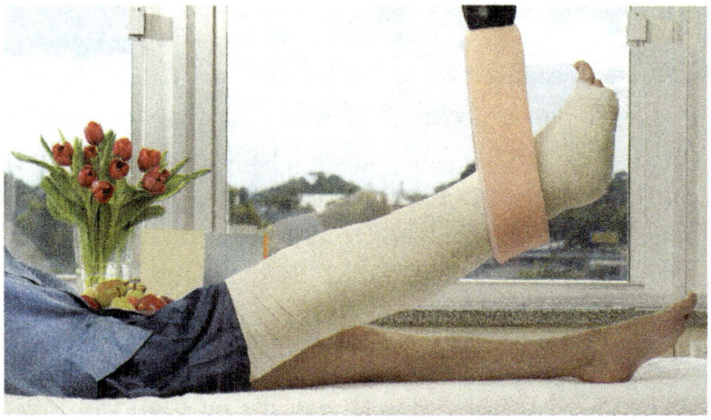


**Fig 11-7** The child feels less pain when the injury is above the level of the heart

The nurse assesses the cast for increased warmth or hot spots on the cast surface, which could signify an infection. The nurse assesses the drainage amount and quality on the cast with a marker and the skin around the cast (ATI Testing 2016).

The nurse makes sure the child turns every 2 hours while supporting all extremities and joints. Turning allows for air to circulate around the cast for faster drying.

Air circulation prevents pressure from changing the shape of the cast. The use of heat lamps or warm hair dryers impairs the proper drying of the cast. For plaster casts, expose the cast to air to promote drying, and use of the palms of hands to prevent denting. The nurse may use moleskin over any spots that apply friction. Plastic protects the cast from urine and feces and allows for showering. The nurse and child maintain skin integrity through routine skin care and perineal care (ATI Testing 2016).

The assessment findings of Compartment syndrome include the compression of nerves and blood vessels inside of the muscle that results in neuromuscular ischemia (ATI Testing 2016).

The symptoms are commonly known as the **5 Ps** and include: pain that is unrelieved with elevation or analgesics; that increases with passive movement; paresthesia or numbness (early finding); pulselessness distal to the fracture (late finding); paralysis or an inability to move digits (nerve damage); and pale, cold skin and cyanosis to nail beds. Compartment syndrome frequently occurs in tibia and forearm fractures (ATI Testing 2016).

A child may also develop a Volkmann contracture or a permanent contracture of the forearm and hand from the ischemia caused by Compartment syndrome (ATI Testing 2016).

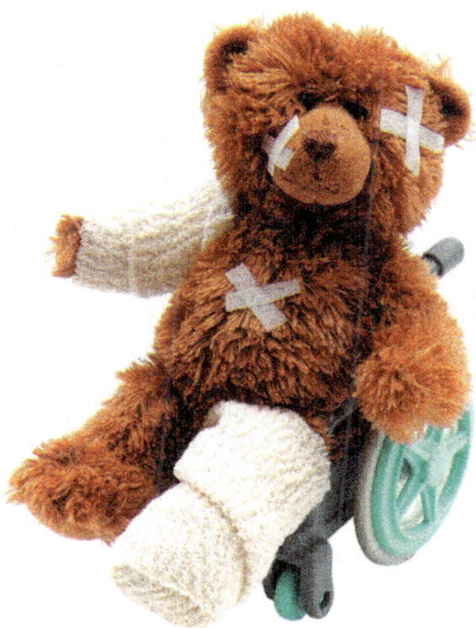


**Fig 11-8** Showing younger children how they will look after surgery with a teddy bear

**Clinical Pearl**

Pediatric patients experience anxiety from the cast saw used to remove a cast. The blade moves back and forth very quickly and makes a lot of noise. It helps the child to explain the saw and then use noise canceling headphones for child and provider. This reduces noise for provider and child. In addition, children benefit from distraction from a personal electronic device. This is an example of atraumatic care (Mahan, S. T., Harris, M. S., Lierhaus, A.M., Miller, P. E., and DiFazio, R. 2017). (see Fig 11-9)

The cast is removed with a cast saw. Children need psychosocial support as the saw can be intimidating and loud.

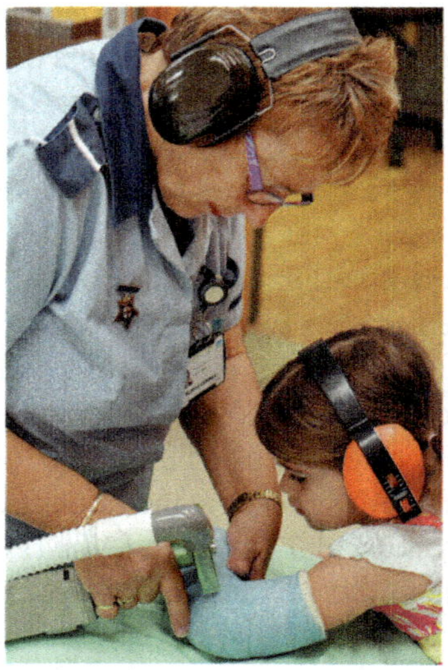


**Fig 11-9**

# OSTEOMYELITIS

Osteomyelitis occurs when a bacterial infection develops secondarily to an open fracture (endogenous source) or from a blood-borne bacterial source (hematogenous source) (see Fig 11-10). A child with osteomyelitis presents with irritability, fever, tachycardia, edema, constant pain increases with movement, decreased movement of the affected extremity, and a localized spot that is tender, swollen, and warm to touch (ATI Testing 2016).

The nurse confirms the complication through the skin, blood, and bone cultures gives IV and oral antibiotics; and monitors super-infections (candidiasis, C. difficile infection).

The child needs monitoring through a course of long-term antibiotic therapy, and adverse effects can develop, such as ototoxicity. The nurse, the family and possibly a Child Life specialist develop diversional activities consistent with the client's level of development (ATI Testing 2016).

The nurse also stresses the relationship between a diet rich in vitamin D, vitamin K, calcium, and high-quality protein help bones to heal (ATI Testing 2016).

## Traction Care

Traction involves the use of a pulling force to reduce a fracture, maintain alignment and provide muscle rest (see Fig 11-11). The priority actions of the nurse are to maintain the traction, performs skin care, provide pain

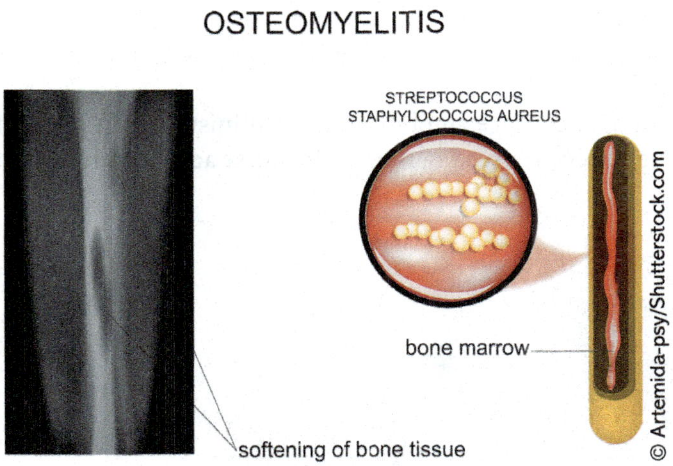


**Fig 11-10** Osteomyelitis is an infection of the bone

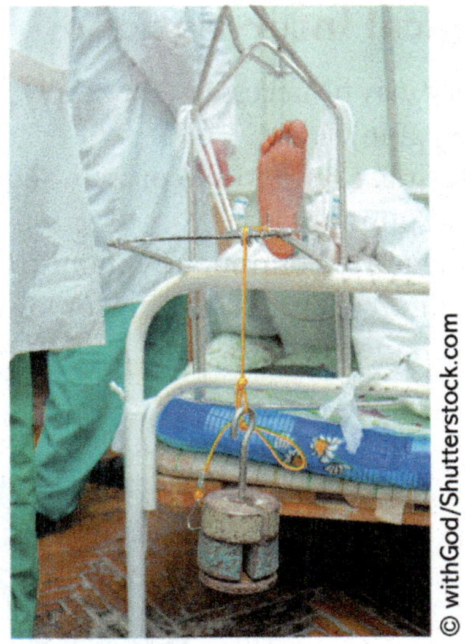


**Fig 11-11** Traction where a weight keeps the bone aligned

management and delivers range of motion exercises as tolerated. The type of traction used depends on the fracture, age of the client, and associated injuries. There are different types of traction. Skin traction reduces pain and maintains the length of the extremity. Skin traction uses a pulling force applied by weights that are attached by a rope to the extremity (Buck, Russell, and Bryant traction) (ATI Testing 2016).

Skeletal traction uses a continuous pulling force that is applied directly to the skeletal structure and/or specific bone. Skeletal traction is appropriate when the pulling force needed is more than skin traction can withstand. A surgeon inserts a pin or rod through or into the bone and attaches weights to the limb with a rope. The nurse never removes the weights. There are different types of traction. **Halo traction** (cervical traction) uses a halo-type bar that screws into the head. The child's halo attaches to either bed traction or rods secured to a vest worn by the child (ATI Testing 2016).

The nurse's priority intervention is to maintain the traction. A child in traction needs proper body alignment, both nonpharmacological and pharmacological interventions for pain and muscle spasms. The nurse continuously monitors for compartment syndrome skin integrity, and pin care. The pin sites should be free of pain, redness, swelling, drainage, or odor. Ensure that all the hardware is tight and that the bed is in the correct position, making sure the weights hang freely, and the knots do not contact the pulley. Weights are not touched unless prescribed and supervised by the provider. Similarly, the nurse should consult with the provider for an over-bed trapeze to assist the child to move in bed.

The nurse provides range of motion and promotes mobility in nonimmobilized extremities to prevent contractures, and promotes frequent position changing within restrictions of traction. The child should take deep breaths and use incentive spirometry to prevent respiratory infections and atelectasis. Frequent position changes prevent skin integrity issues. The nurse should remove the bed sheets from the head of the bed to the foot of the bed, and remade that way as well (ATI Testing 2016).

## Halo Device

The nurse places the wrench within easy access to the health-care team if CPR necessitates the removal of the rods. The child moves as a unit without applying pressure to the rods to prevent loosening of the pins and pain.

The child and family should know how to provide pin site care, identify signs of infection and compartment syndrome, and to avoid powder under the halo vest (ATI Testing 2016).

## Surgical Interventions

Surgery may be necessary, especially for supracondylar fractures and fractures of the humerus and femur (ATI Testing 2016).

**Surgical reduction** corrects alignment through a closed (no incision) or open (with incision) with or without pinning.

The nurse continuously monitors for infection, encourages mobilization, administers pain medications, and reinforces crutch training for lower-extremity fractures (see Fig 11-12). The nurse administers antipruritic and pain medications.

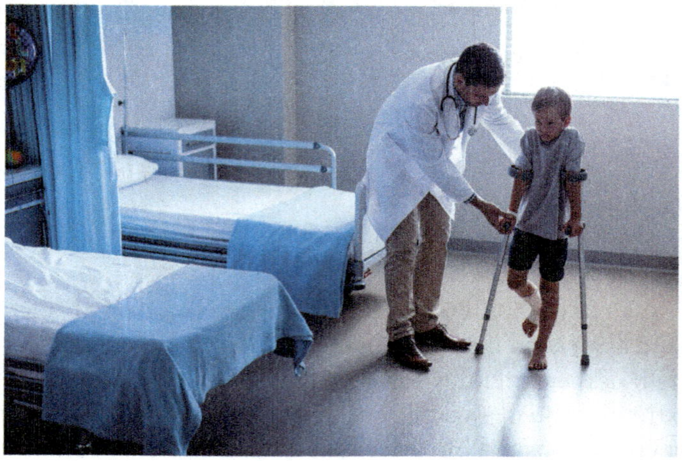

© wavebreakmedia/Shutterstock.com

**Fig 11-12** A boy learns to walk on crutches

The nurse prepares the child and family for surgery, including NPO status. The health-care team enlists an orthopedic specialist for fracture care in children. The nurse may contact a social service worker if nonaccidental accident is suspected (ATI Testing 2016).

The family must understand proper cast or pin care, perform a neurovascular check, and knows indications to call the provider (ATI Testing 2016).

## Teaching

The nurse assists the child with proper crutch use. The nurse also teaches the parents about pain medications, neurovascular checks, and when to contact the provider. Severe pain that is not relieved 1 hour after the administration of pain medication may indicate the loss of circulation to the limb. As the bone heals, the nurse teaches the family and child about cast removal and the use of a cast cutter (ATI Testing 2016).

Once the child's bone is healed and the cast removed, the extremity should soak in warm water. Once dried, a moisturizing lotion hydrates the skin (ATI Testing 2016).

# CONGENITAL MUSCULOSKELETAL DISORDERS

Musculoskeletal congenital disorders for children are identified at birth or might not be present until later in infancy, childhood, or adolescence.

These disorders include clubfoot, Legg-Calve-Perthes disease, Developmental dysplasia of the hip (DDH), osteogenesis imperfecta, scoliosis, Juvenile Idiopathic Arthritis (JIA), and Muscular dystrophy. The nurse manages musculoskeletal conditions and promotes the child's growth, development, and mobility (ATI Testing 2016).

## QSEN Application

**Safety**

QSEN defines safety as something that

"[m]inimizes risk of harm to patients and providers through both system effectiveness and individual performance".

Nurses "[p]articipate as team members to design, promote and model through, [the] effective use of technology and standardized practices that support safety and quality", Nurses commit to use "national patient safety resources for own professional development and to focus attention on safety in care settings". The nurse should also "[c]ommunicate observations or concerns related to hazards and errors to patients, families and the health-care team, and identify and correct system failures and hazards in care". In addition, nurses [d]esign and implement micro-system changes in response to identified hazards and errors. The nursing focus should be to "engage in systems focus rather than blaming individuals when errors or near misses occur". Desirable outcomes originate from nurses who "[r]eport errors and support members of the health-care team to be forthcoming about errors and near misses, and [who] participate appropriately in analyzing errors and designing, implementing and evaluating system improvements".

Nurses develop and support a culture of safety to protect patients by implementing these QSEN practices.

From Quality and Safety Education for Nurses http://qsen.org/competencies/pre-licensure-ksas/

## Clubfoot

Club foot is an inherited complex deformity of the ankle and foot (see Fig 11-13). Clubfoot originates from three places. A positional clubfoot occurs from intrauterine crowding, syndromic club foot often occurs in children with Cerebral palsy or spina bifida, and congenital clubfoot is idiopathic (ATI Testing, 2016).

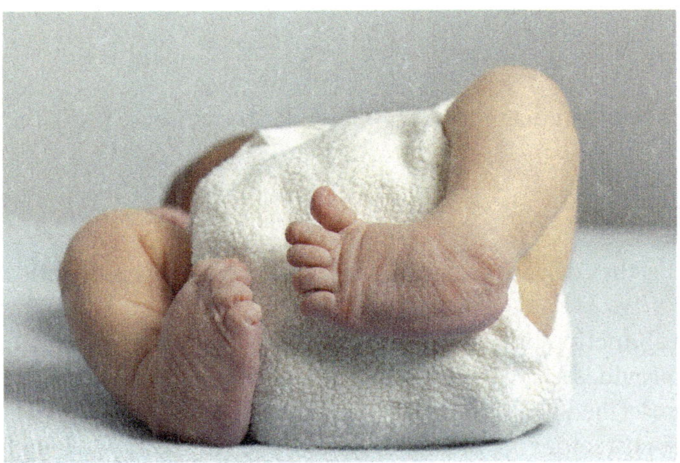


**Fig 11-13** A baby with clubfeet

## Assessment

There are five variations of club foot. **Talipes varus** refers to the inversion (bending inward) of the foot. **Talipes valgus** is eversion (bending outward) of the foot. **Talipes calcaneus** occurs when the toes are higher than the heels (dorsiflexion). **Talipes equinus** occurs when toes are lower than the heels (plantar flexion). In **talipes equinovarus** toes are facing inward and lower than the heel (ATI Testing 2016).

## Diagnostic

A series of ultrasounds verifies the malformation (ATI Testing, 2016).

## Interventions

### Castings

A series of castings that start shortly after birth, and continue until maximum correction occurs. The child needs weekly manipulation of the foot to stretch the muscles with subsequent placement of a new cast.

After the casting, a **heel cord tenotomy** procedure is performed to release the tendon and is followed by a long leg cast for 3 weeks. A Denis Browne bar that connects specialized shoes can be applied to maintain the correction and prevent recurrence.

The nurse continuously monitors the neurovascular status of the child and performs cast care. The nurse also monitors growth and development while being immobile. The nurse also provides basic skin care and monitors for signs of breakdown (ATI Testing 2016).

## Legg-Calve-Perthes Disease

Legg-Calve-Perthes disease is the aseptic necrosis of the femoral head can be unilateral or bilateral. Risk factors include children 2–12 years of age, but it is most common between ages 4 and 8 years of age, and are more common in boys. Any trauma that causes inflammation also predisposes a child to Legg-Calve-Perthes disease (ATI Testing 2016).

## Assessment

Children with Legg-Calve-Perthes disease presents with an intermittent painless limp, hip stiffness, limited ROM, hip, thigh, and knee pain, shortening of the affected leg, and muscle wasting (ATI Testing 2016).

## Diagnosis

Radiograph of the hip and pelvis can diagnose Legg-Calve-Perthes disease (ATI Testing 2016).

## Interventions and Teaching

Treatment for Legg-Calve-Perthes disease varies with the child's age and the functionality of the femoral head (ATI Testing 2016).

The provider places an abduction brace. The nurse administers NSAIDs as prescribed, promotes rest and limits weight bearing, and provides cast care. Traction can help with range of motion and promotes advancement to active motion as prescribed (ATI Testing 2016).

The surgeon performs an osteotomy of the hip or femur. The family should help the child adhere to weight bearing limitations and learn developmentally appropriate strategies as prescribed (ATI Testing 2016).

## Developmental Dysplasia of the Hip (DDH)

Developmental dysplasia of the hip (DDH) includes a variety of disorders resulting in abnormal development of the hip (ATI Testing 2016).

DDH manifests in three disorders that can occur. **Acetabular dysplasia** creates a delay in acetabular development creating an acetabular roof is shallow and oblique. **Subluxation** is incomplete dislocation of the hip, and **dislocation** occurs when the femoral head does not have contact with the acetabulum.

Risk factors include birth order (firstborn), female gender, family history, breech intrauterine position, delivery type, and joint stability issues. Complications are related to postoperative complications and the effects of immobilization and casting (ATI Testing 2016).

Postoperative complications include atelectasis, ileus, and infection. The effects of immobilization include decreased muscle strength, bone demineralization, and altered bowel motility. The effects of casting include skin breakdown, neurovascular alterations, and infection (usually *Staphylococcus aureus* (ATI Testing 2016)).

### Assessment

Infants present with asymmetry of gluteal and thigh folds, limited hip abduction, the shortening of the femur, a widened perineum, a positive **Ortolani test** (hip reduces by abduction) (see Fig 11-14) and a positive **Barlow test** (hip dislocates by adduction) (see Fig 11-15) (ATI Testing 2016).

A child presents with one leg shorter than the other, a positive **Trendelenburg sign** (while bearing weight on the affected side and the pelvis tilts downward), walking on toes on one foot, and walking with a limp (ATI Testing 2016).

### Diagnosis

An ultrasound performed at 2 weeks of age to determine the cartilaginous head of the femur and an x-ray can diagnose DDH in infants older than 4 months of age. Treatment starts as soon as DDH is diagnosed and depends on the child's age and the extent of the dysplasia (ATI Testing 2016).

The nurse promotes bonding by encouraging the parents to hold and cuddle the infant/child and provide for his or her developmental needs of the infant/child (ATI Testing, 2016).

### Intervention and Teaching

Newborns to 6 months of age can use a **Pavlik harness** (see Fig 11-15). The child wears a harness for up to 12 weeks, but the assessment of the straps occurs every 1–2 weeks for adjustment. The nurse educates each the

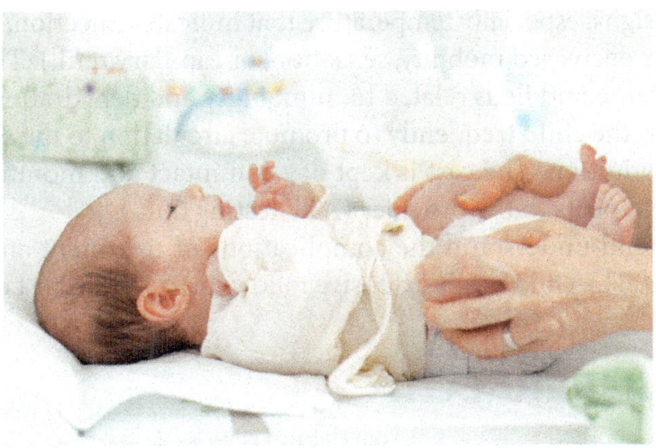



**Fig 11-14** The Ortolani test

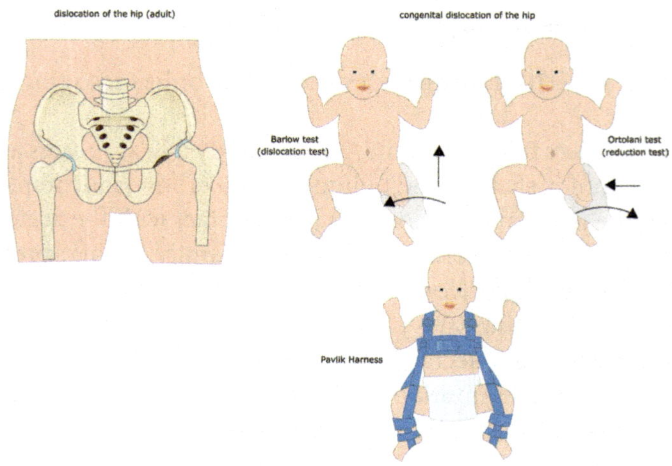




**Fig 11-15** The Barlow test and Pavlik harness

family member not to adjust the straps. The nurse monitors neurovascular and skin integrity checks. Skin care includes wearing an undershirt and knee socks, performing gentle massage of the skin under straps, not using lotions and powders, and placing diaper under the straps (ATI Testing 2016).

When adduction contractures are present **Bryant traction** is applied. Bryant traction is a type of skin traction that uses a **hip spica cast**. The nurse must maintain the child's hips flexed at a 90° angle, with the buttocks raised off of the bed (ATI Testing 2016).

The nurse also monitors neurovascular checks, maintains traction (ropes, boots, pulleys, and weights), performs skin care, and ensures the child maintains alignment. The nurse performs cast care for a child in the hip spica cast. The nurse reinforces teaching regarding positioning, turning, neurovascular assessments, and care of the cast. The cast can rest on pillows, as long as the child's bottom is suspended.

The nurse gives sponge baths to avoid wetting the cast and uses a waterproof barrier around the genital opening of the spica cast to prevent soiling with urine or feces.

The family will understand using appropriate equipment, such as a stroller, wagon, and car seat for maintaining mobility (ATI Testing 2016).

If the child is 6 months of age up until 2 years of age, then a surgery is necessary. The child receives a closed surgical reduction with the placement of a hip spica cast. The nurse prepares the family and child for surgery and teaches the child and family about spica cast and home care management.

Older children also undergo surgical reduction with presurgical traction. The child may need a femoral osteotomy (removal of the bone of the femoral head), reconstruction, and tenotomy (cutting of adductor tendon) (ATI Testing 2016).

The nurse monitors vital signs, especially temperature that indicates infection, and changes in neurovascular status (numbness, tingling, decreased mobility, sensation, or capillary refill). The child's bowel and urinary system are subject to constipation and ileus related to immobility and dehydration (ATI Testing 2016).

The nurse also repositions the child frequently to promote circulation to the skin, and maintain a high-fiber diet and with adequate hydration. The cast is kept dry and intact and monitored for any foul odor from cast or urine which the nurse reports to the provider (ATI Testing 2016).

The child and family should understand the complications of treatment and the procedure and know when to report to the provider. The child needs extensive follow up to get the best outcome (ATI Testing 2016).

## OSTEOGENESIS IMPERFECTA

Osteogenesis imperfecta (OI) is a rare genetic condition that impairs collagen and results in brittle bones that grow slowly, easily fracture and cause deformities (see Fig 11-16). Complications for OI include disuse osteoporosis, hearing loss, and permanent deformities (ATI Testing 2016).

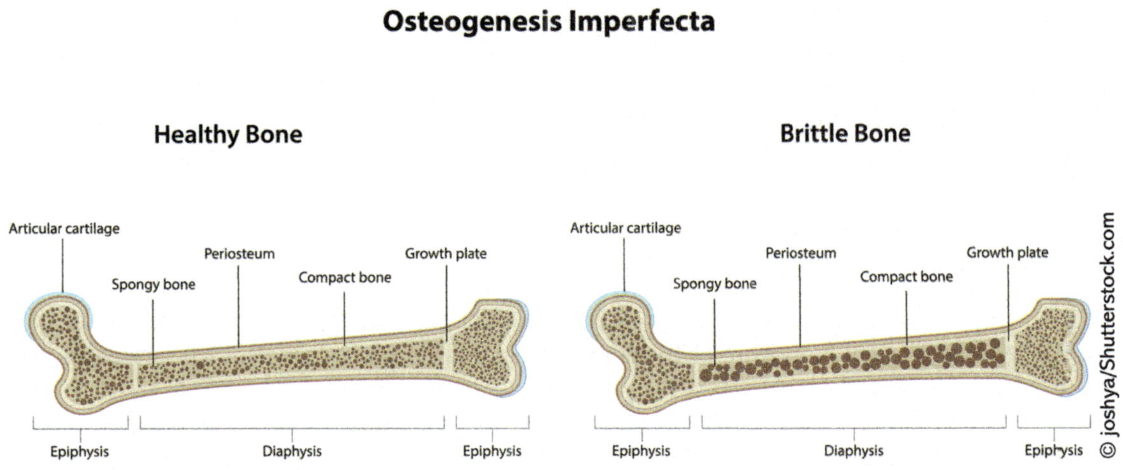


**Fig 11-16** The brittle bones of a child with OI

## Assessment

Children with OI experience multiple bone fractures from minor trauma, but they may occur before birth with severe cases. Children have a blue sclera, early hearing loss, and small, discolored teeth (ATI Testing 2016).

## Diagnosis

The provider makes a diagnosis through a bone biopsy. The nurse prepares the child and family for the procedure and helps position the child (ATI Testing 2016).

## Interventions

Children with OI receive supportive care as OI is a genetic disease that affects every bone cell in the body. Treatment focuses on prevention and medication administration (ATI Testing 2016).

## Medications

### Pamidronate

Pamidronate is a bisphosphonate that increases bone density. The nurse starts an IV and administers pamidronate, and observes for adverse effects (hypokalemia, hypomagnesemia, hypocalcemia, hypophosphatemia, thrombocytopenia, neutropenia, dysrhythmias, kidney failure, general malaise).

For children with severe cases of OI correction of bone deformities and the placement of rods may help (ATI Testing 2016).

## Teaching

The child and family must understand the need for a high-quality diet, the necessity of using low-impact exercise, and the prophylactic administration of antibiotics for dental work (ATI Testing 2016).

In addition, the child and family must understand adverse effects and when to call the provider.

The child needs physical therapy and braces or splints as prescribed. The child needs a proactive family able to help the child meet developmental milestones (ATI Testing 2016).

OI is a difficult pathology to manage, especially in childhood. The child with OI is often mistaken as a child suffering from abuse. It is the health-care team's responsibility to use good assessment skills and not jump to conclusions. The last thing the health-care team needs to do is cause undue stress for a family working to manage a challenging chronic disease. The family and child need support groups to help manage this disease (ATI Testing 2016).

## SCOLIOSIS

Scoliosis is a complex malformation of the spine that also affects the ribs and posture (see Fig 11-17 and Fig 11-18). Scoliosis is a lateral curvature of the spine and spinal rotation that results in rib asymmetry (ATI Testing 2016).

Scoliosis can present as idiopathic, but structural scoliosis is the most common presentation. Risk factors for a child with scoliosis include a family history, being a girl child between 8 and 15 years of age. Complications include breathing difficulties (with severe curvatures), spine or nerve damage, infection and lowered self-esteem (ATI Testing 2016).

### Assessment

Children present with asymmetry in scapula, ribs, flanks, shoulders, and hips. Children may have ill-fitting clothing (one leg shorter than the other) (ATI Testing, 2016).

### Diagnosis

A scoliosis screening during preadolescence for boys and girls can identify the curvature. A scoliometer measures truncal rotation, the Cobb technique measures the degree of curvature, and the Risser scale indicates skeletal development. Radiography helps identify any impact on respiratory and cardiac organs (ATI Testing 2016).

### Interventions

Treatment directly relates to the degree, location, and type of curvature.

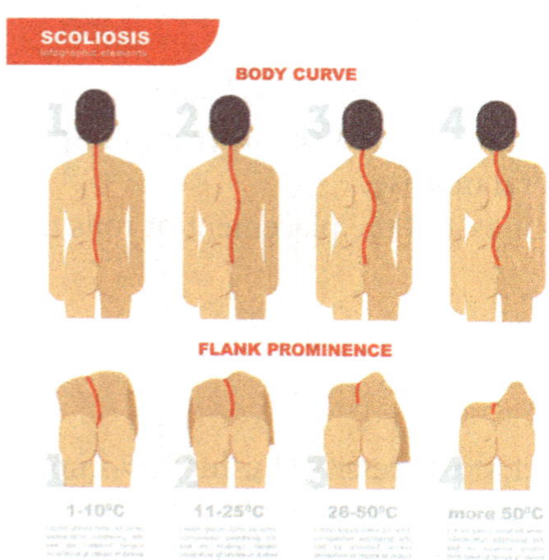




**Fig 11-17** Presentation of scoliosis

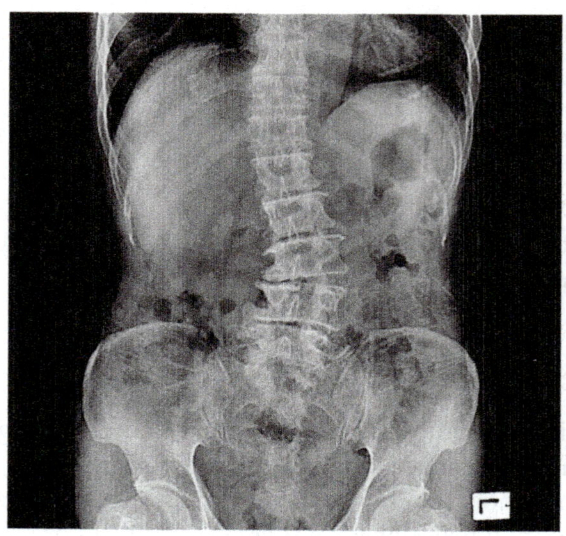



**Fig 11-18** X-ray of a spine with scoliosis

## Bracing

Bracing uses customized braces to slow the progression of the curve (see Fig 11-19).

The nurse assists with fitting the client with a brace, provides a medical assessment focused on the skin, and supports a positive self-image of the child. The nurse teaches the child how to wear the brace (ATI Testing 2016).

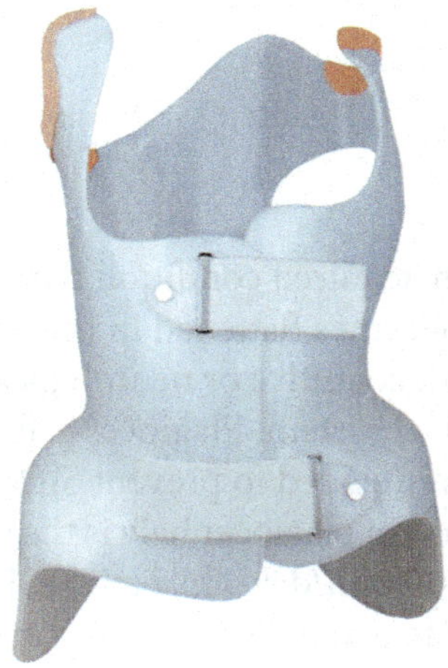

© Popoudina Svetlana/Shutterstock.com

**Fig 11-19** A brace to correct the curvature

## Surgical Interventions

A child with a curvature greater than 45° will undergo spinal fusion with rod placement (ATI Testing 2016).

### *Preoperative Interventions*

The nurse educates the family about autologous (self-donated) blood donations that are necessary for the procedure. The nurse draws blood to obtain laboratory values that include a type and cross-match, if additional units are needed.

The nurse familiarizes the family and child with the Pediatric Intensive Care Unit (PICU) and explains expectations for the post-procedure period. The nurse introduces invasive equipment, such as monitoring equipment, NG tube, chest tubes, indwelling urinary catheters, and self-administering analgesic pumps. The nurse also teaches the use of incentive spirometer, turning, coughing, and deep breathing to prevent complications (ATI Testing 2016).

### *Postoperative Interventions*

The nurse's priority intervention is log rolling to prevent damage to the spinal fusion. The nurse monitors neurovascular and skin status. The child must frequently be turned to prevent skin breakdown, especially if there is a brace. The nurse also monitors pain using an age appropriate tool, and the child uses a patient-controlled analgesic (PCA) pump as prescribed. The child's surgical and drain sites are monitored for infection or hemorrhage as prescribed. The nurse will administer a self-donated blood transfusion as prescribed. The nurse looks for complications, including paralytic ileus, hemorrhage, and infection.

The child should complete ROM on unaffected extremities and ambulate. Encourage mobility as soon as tolerated (ATI Testing 2016).

The family and nurse can engage in age-appropriate activities with the child and find opportunities for the child to visit with friends and family during the hospital stay. The child and family must understand the necessity of physical therapy and proper positioning of the spine. The adolescent with a brace needs encouragement to be independent and engage in social activities (ATI Testing 2016).

## Teaching

The child and family must understand the expected outcomes, the course of treatment and recovery. The family should also promote independence in the adolescent and understand the necessity of follow up care (ATI Testing 2016).

# PLAGIOCEPHALY

Plagiocephaly, or flat-head syndrome, is an acquired condition that occurs from the flattening of the head in infancy (see Fig 11-20). The infant's head becomes flattened in the occipital region. There is no evidence that positional plagiocephaly leads to permanent cognitive or neurological damage is not to be confused with craniosynostosis that can affect the neurological system. Plagiocephaly is caused by only using the supine sleep position. The supine sleep position is recommended to prevent SIDS.

The most important point for prevention of plagiocephaly is the importance of allowing the infant to lie in the prone position ("tummy-time") for 30–60 min/day while awake. Parents and caretakers should also change the infant's head position from side to side to avoid constant pressure on the occiput.

Children with plagiocephaly need physical therapy and wear a customized helmet to reshape the head. Risk factors include too much time in the supine position and torticollis.

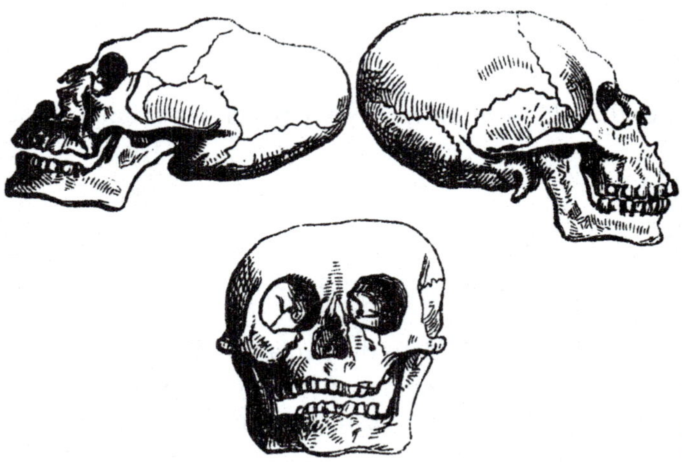



**Fig 11-20** the flattening of the skull in plagiocephaly

## Assessment

Children with plagiocephaly present with an oblique shape of the head, an asymmetrical skull, and facial features, a flattened occiput, frontal and parietal bossing, prominent cheekbones and/or the anterior displacement of an ear. Children who also have torticollis also have a possible decreased range of motion in the neck.

## Interventions and Teaching

The parents can use a cranial molding orthosis helmet to reshape the child's head. The treatment time is approximately 3 months and requires the child to wear it 23 hours a day. There is good evidence that a helmet is more effective than no treatment at all (Slowey, D. 2016). The nurse educates parents about the importance of daily "tummy time" when the infant is awake, and to minimize the time the child spends in a car seat, bouncer, or swing. Parents can alternate the infant's head position during sleep. Parents should understand the infant should still sleep in the supine position.

Torticollis, or tightening of the sternocleidomastoid muscle on one side of the neck, can develop. Physical therapy can successfully treat torticollis within 4–8 weeks by increasing neck ROM.

# JUVENILE IDIOPATHIC ARTHRITIS

Juvenile idiopathic arthritis (JIA) is a chronic autoimmune inflammatory disease affecting joints and surrounding tissues. JIA causes chronic inflammation of the synovium of the joints that result in damage to the articular cartilage. JIA can cause residual joint deformities and altered joint function. JIA is classified depending on the involvement of a rheumatoid factor. Risk factors include immunogenic susceptibility and environmental triggers. Complications include joint deformity, functional disability, and uveitis (ATI Testing, 2016).

## Assessment

Children present with joint swelling, stiffness, redness, and warmth. Symptoms tend to be worse in the morning or after inactivity. Children also have mobility limitations, fever, rash, and delayed growth (ATI Testing 2016).

## Diagnosis

Laboratory results reveal an elevated Erythrocyte sedimentation rate (ESR) and WBCs, especially during exacerbations. Antinuclear antibodies indicate an autoimmune disease and elevation in JIA and mean an increased risk for uveitis. Although rheumatoid factor is rare for children, the lab result can be helpful. Radiographic studies are valuable for baseline comparison. X-rays can show increased synovial fluid in the joint, which causes edema or widening of the joint. As the pathology progresses narrowed, joint spaces may develop. A slit lamp eye examination can diagnose uveitis (see Fig 11-21) (ATI Testing 2016).

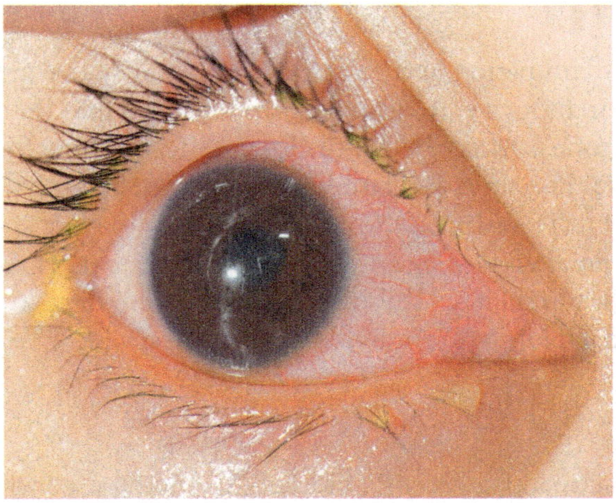



**Fig 11-21** An eye with uveitis

## Interventions and Teaching

Children with JIA receive treatment in an outpatient setting.

The nurse evaluates the child's pain response to prescribed analgesics as well as reinforces relaxation techniques and nonpharmacological pain management (ATI Testing 2016).

The nurse encourages physical therapy program to increase mobility and prevent deformities. The child should engage in activity as tolerated and full ROM exercises. The nurse or parents can use heat or warm moist packs to the child's affected joints before exercise to decrease pain. The nurse can recommend warm baths after a day of exercise (ATI Testing 2016).

Wellness priorities for a child with JIA are a nutrient rich diet and regular eye exams. The nurse can evaluate the child's diet for high nutrient foods and encourage a well-balanced diet with an appropriate fluid intake (ATI Testing 2016).

The nurse should also identify alternate ways for the child to meet developmental needs, especially during periods of exacerbation. The family should expect exacerbations that worsen with illness (ATI Testing 2016).

The child needs regular social contact to promote the child's development, including participation in school and contact with peers and a support group of similarly aged children.

The family will need to work with the school nurse and teachers to meet medication and in-school physical therapy goals (ATI Testing 2016).

## Medications

### NSAIDS

Nonsteroidal anti-inflammatory medications, such as ibuprofen, naproxen, diclofenac, indomethacin, and tolmetin control pain and inflammation.

The child should take NSAIDs with food to minimize gastric irritation. The parents should report changes in stool and GI discomfort or increase in bruising immediately to the provider (ATI Testing 2016).

### Methotrexate

Methotrexate is classified as a cytotoxic disease-modifying antirheumatic drug (DMARD) that delays joint degeneration and progression of rheumatoid arthritis when NSAIDs are ineffective. The health-care team monitors liver function and Complete Blood Count tests. Adolescents should not mix methotrexate with alcohol, and use birth control as methotrexate is a teratogen (ATI Testing 2016).

### Corticosteroids

Prednisone provides relief of inflammation and pain for uveitis and severe arthritis. The child may receive prednisone as an eye solution, orally, or IV. Additionally, an injection into the intra-articular space can provide effective pain relief. Prednisone is prescribed in the lowest effective dose for short-term therapy and then discontinue by tapering the dose. The child and family should understand that weight gain, especially in the face, is a common adverse effect (ATI Testing 2016).

Prednisone can also create an alteration in growth and development. Therefore, the nurse and provider monitor height and weight measurements. Children on prednisone have a depressed immune function. Therefore, infection control and avoiding sick individuals is necessary (ATI Testing 2016).

### Etanercept

Etanercept is a tumor necrosis factor alpha-receptor blocker (DMARD) used when methotrexate is ineffective for immunosuppressive action. Before administration of etanercept, a tuberculin skin test is necessary, and then yearly while taking the medication. Etanercept lowers the immunity making fatal infections easy to contract. Etanercept is administered once or twice each week by subcutaneous injection (ATI Testing 2016).

A child with JIA needs a multidisciplinary team, including a physical therapist, occupational therapist, ophthalmologist, dentist, dietitian, social worker, school nurse (ATI Testing 2016).

# MUSCULAR DYSTROPHY

Muscular dystrophy (MD) is a group of inherited conditions where the muscles degenerate causing progressive muscle weakness and muscle wasting (see Fig 11-22). There are several types of muscular dystrophy. Three of types of muscular dystrophy are Duchenne, Facioscapulohumeral, and Limb-girdle. The onset of the disease, the pace of muscular degeneration, and the muscle group affected depend on the type of MD (ATI Testing 2016).

Duchenne MD affects the most children and is an X-linked recessive trait. Children with Duchenne (pseudohypertrophic) are affected between 3 and 5 years of age. The disease is progressive, with a life expectancy into early adulthood (ATI Testing 2016).

Facioscapulohumeral muscular dystrophy is an autosomal dominant inherited disorder with the age of onset occurring during early adolescence. It affects the muscles of the face, shoulder blades and upper arms. Progression is slow children have a normal life span (ATI Testing 2016).

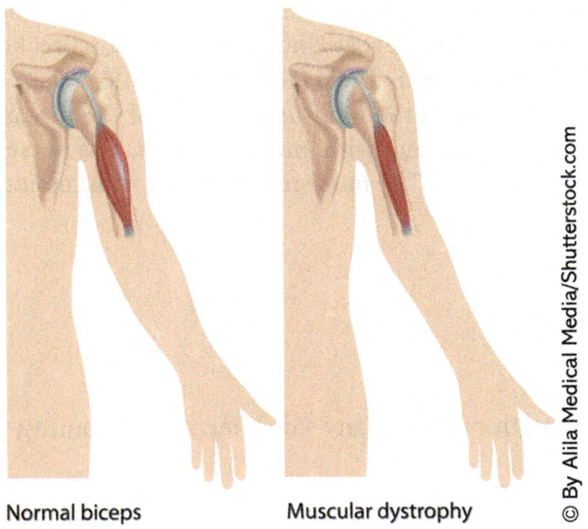


**Fig 11-22** Muscle wasting in MD

Limb-girdle muscular dystrophy is an autosomal dominant and recessive, heterogeneous disorder. It affects shoulders, upper arms, pelvic area, and thighs. It has an onset later in childhood with a slow progression. Complications include a progressive weakening of respiratory muscles that impair a child's ability to ventilate the body. The child with respiratory compromise will receive a tracheostomy, feeding tube and mechanical ventilation (ATI Testing 2016).

## Assessment

Children with MD present with muscle weakness beginning in the lower extremities, an unsteady gait with a waddle, fatigue, and lordosis. Children have delayed motor skill development, frequent falling, difficulty getting out of bed, and difficulty rising from a seated position or climbing stairs. Children with MD may have learning difficulties or mild cognitive delays that do not worsen with disease progression. Children have difficulty walking, or lose the ability to walk, progressive muscle weakness and atrophy that leads to respiratory and cardiac problems as the disease progresses (ATI Testing 2016).

## Diagnosis

A serum polymerase chain reaction is run on the child's DNA to detect the dystrophin gene mutation. The serum creatine may be elevated right before symptoms. A muscle biopsy and an electromyogram (EMG) also give indications (ATI Testing, 2016).

## Interventions

The nurse monitors respiratory function, including depth, rhythm, and rate of respirations during sleep and daytime hours and encourages the use of incentive spirometry. The nurse positions the child in semi-Fowlers to promote the expansion of lungs. The nurse teaches the child, how to use a mechanical cough device and gives oxygen as prescribed. The nurse can administer oxygen and suction the airway for patency. The child may need intermittent positive pressure ventilation and mechanically-assisted cough devices if indicated. The child may need antibiotics related to decreased immune function from the corticosteroids (ATI Testing 2016).

Fluids are encouraged as well as adequate nutritional intake.

The nurse monitors cardiac function, and the ability to perform ADLs. The nurse and parents promote the child's independenceby allowing the child to perform ADL's for as long as possible (ATI Testing, 2016).

Children need appropriate physical activity that includes stretching exercises, strength and muscle training, and breathing exercises. As immobility increases, the nurse maintains the child's body alignment. The child repositions himself or herself, or by the nurse, every 2 hours to avoid skin breakdown. If the child has orthoses and braces the skin is monitored for skin breakdown (ATI Testing 2016).

Children and parents must understand the long-term effects of the disease. The child and family must receive annual physical exams and keep current with immunizations. The nurse identifies the family's support system for coping mechanisms and support. The nurse may facilitate a discussion of end-of-life decisions when appropriate (ATI Testing 2016).

## Medication

### Corticosteroids

Prednisone increases muscle strength but has many side effects on immunity, and growth and development milestones (ATI Testing 2016).

## Surgical Interventions

The child with MD may need surgery to release or repair contractures or the insertion of a gastrostomy tube or tracheostomy (ATI Testing 2016).

A multidisciplinary approach, including a neurologist, genetic counselor, physical, occupational, and respiratory therapists; dietitian, social workers, nurses, and school teachers are all necessary for the best outcome (ATI Testing 2016).

Parents should consider home health nursing, respite care, long-term care, and palliative care to assist him/her, as the child declines. Support for the family is as important as psychosocial support for the child (ATI Testing 2016).

# CHAPTER HIGHLIGHTS

- Children have musculoskeletal conditions as a result of trauma, a congenital condition or a neuromuscular alteration.
- Children commonly experience fractures related to sports injuries, trauma, and nonaccidental injury.
- Talipes equinovarus (clubfoot) is a common congenital condition treated by casting or surgery.

- Children with Legg-Calve-Perthes disease is common in preschool aged boys that causes ischemia and necrosis of the femoral head of the femur.
- Children with mild DDH are treated with a Pavlik harness, more severe cases require surgery.
- Children with osteogenesis imperfecta need careful handling by the family and health-care team to avoid fractures, yet still attempt to meet developmental milestones.
- Children with scoliosis have a lateral curvature of the spine that is corrected with a brace or surgical spinal fusion.
- Children with plagiocephaly have a misshapen head from too much time in the supine position. They do not have neurological deficits as a result.
- Children with JIA is an autoimmune condition that affects the joints that occurs in females more than males.
- Children with muscular dystrophy have an inherited disease characterized by progressive muscle weakening and atrophy.

## REFERENCES

ATI Testing. 2016. Nursing Care of Children. Retrieved from http://www.atitesting.com/ati_next_gen/DisplayResources.aspx?Name=rm_rn_ncc_2016_ebook_20170417.pdf.

Mahan, S. T., Harris, M. S., Lierhaus, A.M., Miller, P. E., and DiFazio, R. 2017. "Noise Reduction to Reduce Patient Anxiety During Cast Removal: Can We Decrease Patient Anxiety With Cast Removal by Wearing Noise Reduction Headphones During Cast Saw Use?" *Orthopaedic Nursing*. 36(4):271–8.

Morgenroth, V. H., Hache, L. P., and Clemens, P. R. 2012. "Insights into bone health in Duchenne muscular dystrophy." *BoneKEy Reports*, 1, 9. http://doi.org/10.1038/bonekey.2012.5.

Gilbert S. F. 2000. *Osteogenesis: The Development of Bones. Developmental Biology*, 6th ed. Sunderland (MA): Sinauer Associates; 2000. Available from: https://www.ncbi.nlm.nih.gov/books/NBK10056/.

Slowey, D. 2016. The Role of Cranial Molding Orthosis (Helmet) Therapy. Retrieved August 19, 2017, from https://www.cns.org/guidelines/guidelines-management-patients-positional-plagiocephaly/Chapter_5.

CHAPTER 12

# CARING FOR CHILDREN WITH CANCER

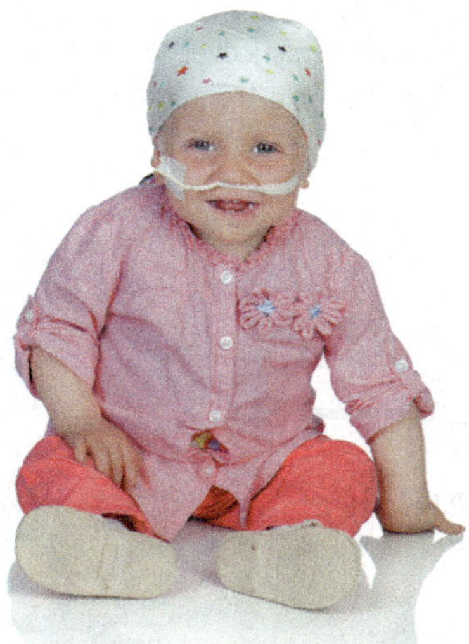



## LEARNING OUTCOMES

1. Describe the pathophysiology and clinical presentation of cancers.
2. Utilize the nursing process to provide safe, comprehensive health care to children with cancer.
3. Create a comprehensive "family-centered" teaching plan for a child with a blastoma tumor.
4. Develop a comprehensive "family-centered" teaching plan for a child undergoing a stem cell transplant.
5. Differentiate among blastomas, blood neoplasms, and bone tumors.
6. Develop a comprehensive "family-centered" teaching plan for a child with leukemia.
7. Create a comprehensive "family-centered" teaching plan for a child with a bone tumor.
8. Teaching/learning principles in providing anticipatory guidance in the prevention and treatment of children with cancer.

## KEY TERMS

Alopecia
Blastoma
Bone marrow aspiration
Inferior venacavogram
Malignant
Metastasize
ONS/ONCC chemotherapy certified nurse
Pancytopenia
PICC line

## ORGAN NEOPLASMS

A **blastoma** is a group of immature, undifferentiated cells are tumors. A cancerous tumor is the result of rapidly dividing **malignant** (cancerous) cells that take over space from the healthy cells of the body (see Fig 12-1). Two types of blastomas common in children are nephroblastoma (Wilm's tumor) and neuroblastoma. Neuroblastoma is a tumor found in nerve cells of the sympathetic nervous system (Dumba, M., Jawad, N., and McHugh, K. 2015).

### Wilm's Tumor and Neuroblastoma

Wilm's tumor (nephroblastoma) (see Fig 12-2) is a malignancy found in the kidneys or abdomen. The tumor is usually unilateral and usually does not metastasize. Most children are diagnosed between 2 and 3 years of age. Wilm's tumor is a tumor that develops in the adrenal gland, kidneys or abdomen. The tumor is usually

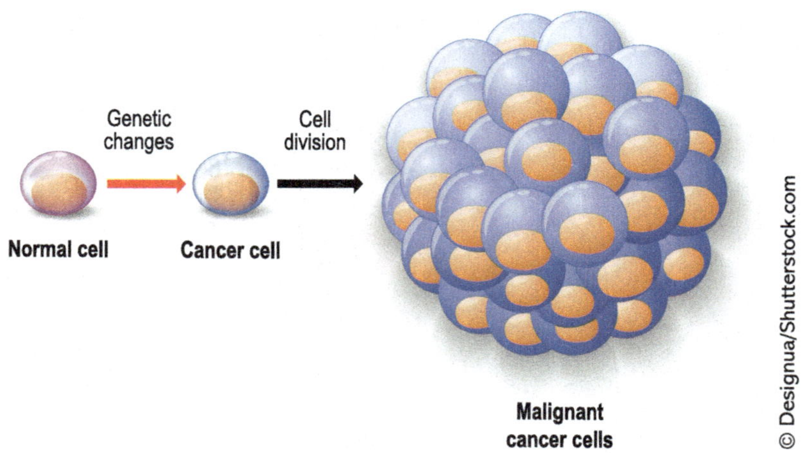


**Fig. 12-1** Rapid division of malignant cells forms a tumor

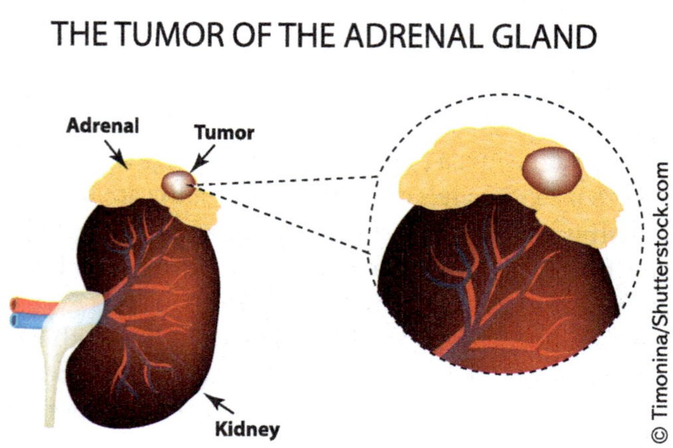


**Fig 12-2** Wilm's tumor is an adrenal tumor

in one adrenal gland (unilateral) with only 10% of the cases presenting bilaterally. Children often present with the tumor before 5 years of the tumor does not usually **metastasize** (spread to other organs) (ATI Testing 2016).

Neuroblastoma causes a tumor that also can appear in the adrenal gland. It can also present in the sympathetic chain of the retroperitoneal area, head, neck, pelvis, or chest. It is a malignancy of primordial neural cells that are found in the sympathetic nervous system. Children are usually affected in their toddler years, with 95% of cases before age 10. Neuroblastoma affects males more than females. Neuroblastoma metastasizes quickly with half of all cases presenting with metastasis. Treatments option any combination of surgery, chemotherapy, and radiation (ATI Testing 2016).

## Assessment

### Wilm's Tumor

A child with Wilm's tumor presents with a painless, firm, nontender abdominal swelling or mass, fatigue, malaise, weight loss, fever, hematuria, and/or hypertension. A child with metastasis has dyspnea, cough, shortness of breath, and chest pain as additional symptoms. The nurse assesses the child and family for coping mechanisms. The nurse also tracks any delays in the child's development, height or weight that is related to illness (ATI Testing 2016).

### Neuroblastoma

There is a range of responses in children with neuroblastoma depending on the affected area. Children may present with abdominal or pelvic tumors—pain, distention, constipation, urinary retention, or hypertension. Children with thoracic or cervical tumors have a neck mass or swelling, and respiratory distress. Children with metastatic disease may have petechiae, ecchymoses, and pallor due to **pancytopenia** resulting from bone marrow metastases. They may also have periorbital ecchymoses, proptosis (displacement of the eye), bone pain, and irritability (ATI Testing 2016).

Complications include metastasis, kidney failure, pancytopenia, bone marrow depression, anorexia, nausea and vomiting, alteration in bowel elimination, mucositis, dry mouth, and **alopecia** (hair loss) (ATI Testing 2016).

## Diagnosis

### Wilm's Tumor

A Wilms' tumor diagnosis requires an abdominal ultrasound and a biopsy collected during resection of the tumor. Laboratory tests include a CBC that may reveal microcytic anemia and a possible WBC elevation. A Comprehensive Metabolic Panel (CMP) detects elevated BUN and creatinine. Urinalysis may show microscopic hematuria in 25% of the cases (ATI Testing 2016).

Children with Wilm's tumor need an abdominal ultra-sonography and chest computed tomography (CT) scan, an **inferior venacavogram** (to rule out involvement with the vena cava), and bone marrow aspiration to rule out metastasis (ATI Testing 2016).

### Neuroblastoma

A child with neuroblastoma receives a skeletal survey; skull, neck, chest, abdominal, and bone CT scans; in addition a **bone marrow aspiration** can rule out metastasis (ATI Testing 2016).

A metaiodobenzylguanidine (MIBG) (a chemical similar to norepinephrine) scan identifies cancer cells, determines bone mass, bone marrow content, and soft tissue involvement. A biopsy of the tumor is the most diagnostic indication.

A urinalysis identifies catecholamines (vanillylmandelic acid, homovanillic acid, dopamine, and norepinephrine) elevation. CBC and coagulation studies indicate severe disease with bone marrow involvement (ATI Testing 2016).

## QSEN Application

**Patient-centered care**

Nurses should consider children with chronic diseases, like cancer, experts on their disease. Learning to create a rapport, and gain trust helps the nurse elicit personal preferences that make the child and family feel cared for by the medical team. Nurses should develop skills to facilitate this.

The nurse should "[r]ecognize the patient or designee as the source of control and full partner in providing compassionate and coordinated care based on respect for patient's preferences, values, and needs. Elicit patient values, preferences and expressed needs as part of clinical interview, diagnosis, implementation of care plan and evaluation of care. The nurse can also [c]ommunicate patient values, preferences and expressed needs to other members of health care team." Nurses should "[p]rovide patient-centered care with sensitivity, empathy and respect for the diversity of human experience." Furthermore, nurses should "[e]nsure that the systems within which ones practices support patient-centered care for individuals and groups whose values differ from the majority or one's own".

Especially, in a chronic disease like cancer, nurses must [a]ssess and treat pain and suffering in light of patient values, preferences, and expressed needs.

Patient-centered care empowers the child to participate in the healing plan of care.

From Quality and Safety Education for Nurses http://qsen.org/competencies/pre-licensure-ksas/

# Interventions

## Wilm's Tumor

The most significant safety concern for Wilm's tumor is keeping the tumor intact, by refraining from palpating the suspected tumor in the abdominal assessment. The nurse should exercise caution when handling or bathing the child to prevent trauma to the tumor site (ATI Testing 2016).

The nurse provides education and support to the child and family regarding diagnostic testing, treatment plan, ongoing therapy, and prognosis. The nurse administers antibiotics as ordered for infection. The nurse keeps the child's skin clean, dry, and lubricated provides oral hygiene, and keeps the child's lips lubricated (ATI Testing 2016).

The nurse and/or child life should schedule age appropriate diversional activities. The nurse should provide high-quality psychosocial support for the child and family that include avoiding false assurances, listening to the child's concerns, preparing for procedures, allowing time for the grief and loss process (ATI Testing 2016).

The nurse prepares the child and family for the surgical removal of the tumor and kidney soon after diagnosis (ATI Testing 2016).

Then the child begins a regimen of preoperative chemotherapy or radiation. In rare cases where the kidneys are affected, chemotherapy may decrease the size of the tumors and potentially preserve one kidney (ATI Testing 2016).

Children may undergo postoperative radiation and/or chemotherapy for large tumors, metastasis, reoccurrence, and residual disease. Radiation affects rapidly growing cells in the body but can also kill healthy cells with a fast turnover rate. Radiation is dose calculated and delivered in divided treatments over several weeks. Nurses should take steps to protect themselves through the use of lead aprons and becoming an **ONS/ONCC chemotherapy certified nurse** (ATI Testing 2016).

### *Medications and Chemotherapy*

#### Acinomycin D and Vincristine

Children with tumors at more advanced stages, or with an unfavorable histology, or that recur after treatment may receive medications, such as doxorubicin and cyclophosphamide. The nurse administering chemotherapeutic agents gives an antiemetic before administration (ATI Testing 2016).

## Neuroblastoma

A child with neuroblastoma undergoes the surgical removal of the tumor, and chemotherapy and/or radiation for metastasis and residual disease. The child has a long-term central venous access or **PICC line** placed for chemotherapy (ATI Testing 2016) (see Fig 12-3). A PICC line is a central venous access device that delivers fluids and medications. A PICC also allows for blood draws. A PICC line saves the child from multiple needle sticks. However, infection is common and preventable. The nurse and child should wear a mask or have the child turn his or her head away if he or she can adequately follow commands. The nurse assesses the site for infection and removes the dressing towards the insertion site. The nurse assesses the entire site and documents any length of the catheter that appears outside of the body. The nurse changes the dressing using sterile technique, cleans the site and uses an antimicrobial chlorhexidine patch (biopatch) (the blue color faces the sky) and a sutureless securement device as the best way to prevent catheter-related blood stream infection (Ullman, A. J., Cooke, M. L., Mitchell, M., Lin, F., New, K., Long, D. A., Mihala, G., and Rickard, C. M. 2016).

Children might also have an implanted venous port for chemotherapy, fluid, and blood draws. The nurse cleans the site with chlorhexidine. A Huber needle is inserted at a 90-degree angle, until it hits the back of the port. If a brisk blood return occurs, the nurse can flush the port, and use the port. The needle may be used for up to a week depending on the facilities protocol (ATI Testing n.d.).

Peripherally Inserted Central Catheter (PICC)

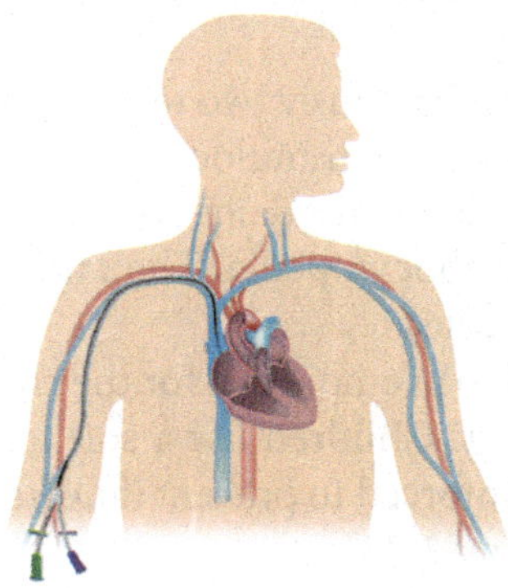

**Fig 12-3** A PICC line is inserted into the basilic or cephalic vein and rests in the superior vena cava above the right atrium

### Clinical Pearl

A breakthrough was made for high-risk neuroblastoma (children have a 50/50 chance of 5-year survival) using monoclonal antibodies that attach to cancer cells and mark them for attack by the immune system. A trial for dinutuximab, a monoclonal antibody, established efficacy and prompted a first line change that includes cytokines and isotretinoin for the treatment of high-risk neuroblastoma. Monoclonal antibodies are a scientific breakthrough that causes less side effects than chemotherapy. However, the administration of monoclonal antibodies requires pre-medication with analgesics, antihistamines and antipyretics (McGinty, L. and Kolesar, J. 2017; Hoy, S. and Hoy, S. M. 2016).

### *Medications and Chemotherapy*

A child with neuroblastoma receives a combination of agents: cyclophosphamide, doxorubicin, cisplatin, etoposide, vincristine, ifosfamide, and carboplatin.

The nurse administers chemotherapeutic agents and an antiemetic before administration and monitors for mucosal ulceration. If ulceration occurs, cool fluids prevent dehydration and soothe raw mucous membranes (ATI Testing 2016).

## Teaching

The nurse educates the child and family about the procedure and side effects of chemotherapy, such as mouth sores, loss of appetite, nausea and vomiting, hair loss, diarrhea or constipation, increased risk of infection, easy bruising or bleeding, and fatigue (ATI Testing 2016).

The family and the child must understand the importance of immunizations and follow-up appointments and good infection control practices (ATI Testing 2016).

### *Complications*

Bone marrow suppression is a serious complication that occurs in both pathologies. A child with bone marrow depression develops further complications, such as anemia, neutropenia, and/or thrombocytopenia. The nurse monitors vital signs and reports temperatures greater than 37.8° C (100° F) and looks for signs of infection, such as lung congestion, redness, swelling and pain around IV sites, and lesions in the mouth. The nurse performs wound care and ensures immunization compliance. The nurse administers antimicrobial, antiviral, and antifungal medications (ATI Testing 2016).

The child may receive epoetin alfa subcutaneously two to three times per week to produce RBCs to resolve anemia. The child may also receive filgrastim, a granulocyte colonystimulating factor that makes WBCs to manage neutropenia. Children take a subcutaneous, daily dose. Finally, oprelvekin subcutaneous daily injections stimulate platelet formation for thrombocytopenia. The nurse looks for signs of a headache, fever, and mild to moderate bone pain (ATI Testing 2016).

All nursing interventions are clustered to promote rest for the child with scheduled rest periods. The nurse handles the child carefully to prevent injury. Children use a soft toothbrush with gentle brushing. Infection control principles and hand hygiene are reinforced to prevent illnesses. Children should avoid people who may be possible sources of infection (ATI Testing 2016).

Children should refrain from fresh fruits and vegetables, and flowers. The nurse also avoids invasive procedures, such as injections, rectal temperatures, and catheters. Any puncture sites receive 5 minutes of constant pressure from the nurse, to stop bleeding. The nurse does not administer aspirin and NSAIDs (ATI Testing 2016).

Complications of chemotherapy include anorexia, nausea, and vomiting. The nurse administers anti-emetics before meals. The nurse can help the child by keeping the environment free of strong smells. Foods eaten during chemotherapy may cause an aversion. Therefore, the child should not just eat his or her favorite foods. Small, frequent, nutrient dense foods are encouraged (ATI Testing 2016).

Children experience diarrhea as a result of radiation to the abdominal area. Some chemotherapeutic agents can cause constipation. The nurse provides skin care and suggests a nutrient rich diet. It may be pureed or liquid and should contain nonacidic foods. The nurse monitors the child for dehydration (ATI Testing 2016).

Children experience mucositis and dry mouth. The nurse keeps the child's lips moist, applies topical anesthetics and analgesics, but refrains from hydrogen peroxide and lemon glycerin swabs due to mucosal drying and irritation on the eroded tissue. The child can use chlorhexidine mouth wash or salt rinses using ½ tsp table salt mixed with 1 tsp baking soda and 1-quart water. A softly brushed toothbrush is gentle on gums, and dental maintenance is essential (ATI Testing 2016).

Children with alopecia related to chemotherapy lose hair for 3–6 months before hair regrows. Children learn scalp care, use gentle shampoos, and use gentle brushing without heat styling. Children should have the option to cut their hair before it falls out, and they may choose to wear a surgical cap as the hair falls out. Children may want to wear a cotton hat or a scarf; adolescents may prefer wigs or turbans. The child needs psychosocial support from the nurse and family (ATI Testing 2016).

## BLOOD NEOPLASMS

Leukemia is a blanket term for a group of malignancies that affect the bone marrow and the lymphatic system. Leukemia refers to the type of WBCs that becomes neoplastic that fall into two categories: acute lymphoid leukemia (ALL) and acute myelogenous or nonlymphoid leukemia (AML) (ATI Testing 2016).

Leukemia causes an increase in the production of immature WBCs, which floods the circulation to organs and tissues (see Fig 12-4). Bone marrow infiltration precipitates crowding of cells that would typically produce RBCs, platelets, and mature WBCs. This causes anemia, neutropenia, and thrombocytopenia. These immature cells can build up in the spleen, liver, and lymph nodes causing tissue fibrosis. Infiltration of the central nervous system causes increased intracranial pressure. Other areas susceptible to build up of immature cells include the testes, prostate, ovaries, gastrointestinal tract, kidneys, and lungs (ATI Testing 2016).

Leukemia is the most prevalent form of childhood cancer, and is the model disease for cancer biology (Freireich, E. J., Wiernik, P. H., and Steensma, D. P. 2014). Risk factors include male gender, European descent, a family history, or a diagnosis of Down syndrome. Children present with leukemia typically between 2 and 5 years of age. Complications include infection and hemorrhage (ATI Testing 2016).

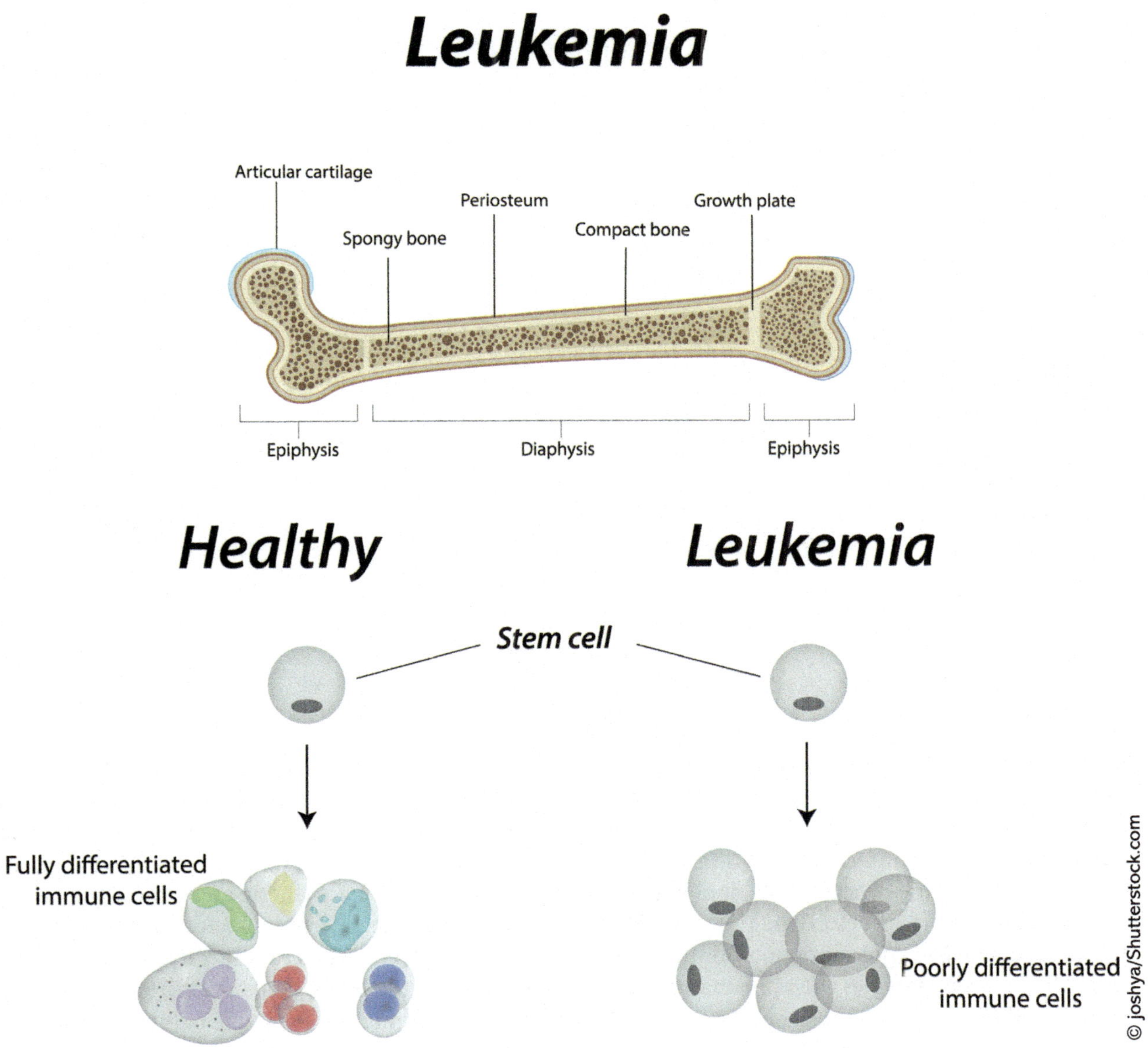


**Fig 12-4** Leukemia produces too many immature blood cells

## Assessment

Children may have chronic complaints of anorexia, headache, and fatigue. The early presentation in the child includes a low-grade fever, pallor, ecchymosis and petechiae, lethargy, hepatomegaly, lymph nodes, and joints, abdominal, leg, and joint pain, constipation, headache, vomiting, anorexia and an unsteady gait. As the disease progresses, children have pain, hematuria, ulcerations in the mouth, enlarged kidneys and testicles, and manifestations of increased intracranial pressure (ATI Testing 2016) (see Fig 12-5).

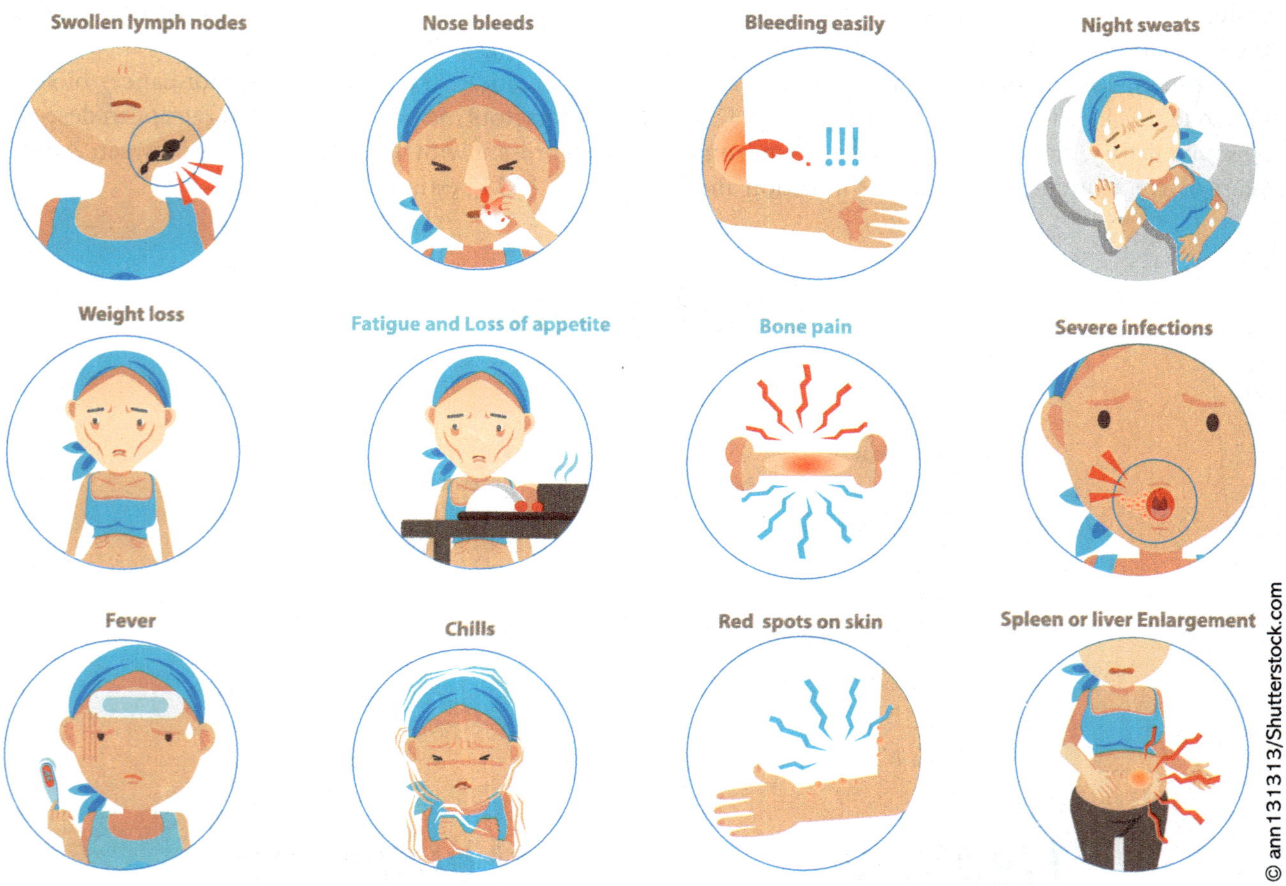


**Fig 12-5** Assessment findings for Leukemia

## Diagnosis

Children undergo a bone marrow aspiration or biopsy analysis as the most definitive diagnostic procedure. Children with leukemia have large amounts of immature leukemic blast cells and protein markers that indicate a particular type of leukemia. Blood work includes a CBC to detect anemia, thrombocytopenia, neutropenia, and leukemic blasts or immature WBCs.

Nurses assist in the procedure by applying a eutectic mixture of local anesthetic cream over the biopsy area 45 minutes to 1 hour before the procedure. The nurse also administers Propofol and helps position the child for access to the posterior or anterior iliac crest or the tibia in infants as it is easier to access and hold the infant. The provider samples the bone marrow. After the procedure, the nurse holds pressure to the site for 5–10 min and then places a pressure dressing on the site. The nurse monitors for stable hemodynamics and signs of infection (ATI Testing 2016).

### Cerebrospinal Fluid (CSF) Analysis

Children also undergo CSF analysis to discover potential CNS effects. The nurse assists with positioning and psychosocial support during the lumbar puncture is assessed to determine CNS involvement. The nurse prepares the child by making sure the child voids and applies a topical anesthetic cream to the puncture site. The child lies down in the side-lying position with the head flexed and knees drawn up towards the chest (ATI Testing 2016).

The nurse may administer sedation as ordered (fentanyl and midazolam). The provider collects three to five test tubes of CSF and takes pressure readings. The nurse maintains a pressure dressing over the puncture site. The nurse and /or child life provide activities that require the child to lie flat for 4–8 hours in a flat position to prevent loss of CSF that causes a spinal headache. This position might not be realistic for an infant, toddler, or preschooler and they may not meet the goal.

The nurse monitors lab values for liver and kidney functions, and any deleterious effects of chemotherapy (ATI Testing 2016).

## Interventions

Use pharmacological and nonpharmacological interventions to provide around-the-clock pain management (ATI Testing 2016).

### Chemotherapy

Chemotherapy agents used are specific to the type of leukemia, age, and whether leukemic cells have collected in the cerebrospinal fluid. Chemotherapy is administered in four phases to treat leukemia: Induction therapy, CNS prophylactic therapy, intensification therapy (consolidation), and maintenance therapy. The goal of induction therapy is complete remission, or less than 5% of leukemic cells in the bone marrow. The goal of CNS prophylactic therapy is to prevent the infiltration of the CNS by leukemic cells. The goal of intensification therapy is to destroy any remaining leukemic cells, then a delayed intensification effect occurs to prevent any resistant leukemic cells from emerging. The goal of maintenance therapy is to prolong the remission phase (ATI Testing 2016).

#### *Side Effects of Treatment*

Chemotherapy side effects are the same as the solid tumor chemotherapy effects and include mucosal ulceration, constipation, anorexia, nausea, vomiting, and alopecia. The child is pretreated for nausea and vomiting with anti-emetics and possibly dexamethasone before treatment. There are further complications, such as foot drop neuropathy, jaw pain, and hemorrhage cystitis. A child with foot drop uses a footboard in bed and needs assistance with ambulation. Children with jaw pain benefit from a soft or liquid diet. A child with hemorrhage cystitis needs fluids and regular voiding. The nurse initiates chemotherapy early in the morning to promote adequate fluid intake and voiding. The nurse administers the medication mensa (a cytoprotective)to protect the bladder from hemorrhagic cystitis. As the disease progresses cardio-myopathy, cognitive and neuropsychological defects develop (ATI Testing 2016).

Children can develop moon face, decreased immune function, skin breakdown, nutritional deficiency, and mood swings from the use of prescribed corticosteroids.

The nurse provides emotional support to the child and parents and promotes peer contact, if possible. Instruct the child and parents about bleeding precautions and the management of active bleeding. Instruct the parents in the proper use of vascular access devices (ATI Testing 2016).

### Hematopoietic Stem Cell Transplant (HCST)

HCST can be indicated for children who have AML during the first remission and for children who have ALL after a second remission. Children undergo an allogeneic transplant (donor blood-forming stem cells). The goal of an HCST is to coordinate administration of high-dose chemotherapy and possible full-body radiation. The nurse infuses donor stem cells via IV infusion (see Fig 12-6). The nurse places the child on protective isolation precautions in a private, positive-pressure room that cycles through at least 12 air exchanges/hour and uses HEPA filtration for incoming air. The nurse wears a respirator mask, gloves, and gowns. The environment is free of bacterial sources, such as dried or fresh or potted plants. The nurse's goal is to keep the child infection free until the transfused stem cells grow. The nurse monitors for complications, such as pulmonary complications, congestive heart failure or graft vs. host disease (ATI Testing 2016). In addition to traditional treatments for HCST music therapy, exercise therapy, art therapy and telecommunication should be available to all school-aged and adolescent bone marrow transplant recipients during the first year following transplant to improve quality of life (Cincinnati Children's Hospital Medical Center 2012).

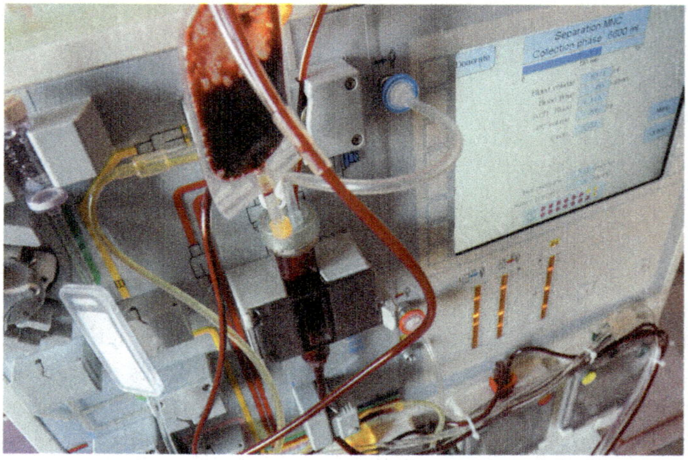



**Fig 12-6** Infusing stem cells for leukemia

### Radiation Therapy to the Brain

The nurse positions the child manages side effects of the radiation promotes a healthy diet and rest, and provides emotional support to the child and family.

A second malignancy and cognitive and neuropsychological defects are indicative of advancing disease (ATI Testing 2016).

## Complications and Teaching

### Infection

Infection is a complication of myelosuppression. The nurse manages infection through the use of a private room, infection control strategies, and hand hygiene. The nurse administers antibiotics for infection found in the blood, stool, urine, and/or nasopharyngeal cultures. The nurse promotes adequate protein and caloric intake (ATI Testing 2016).

The nurse monitors the absolute neutrophil count (ANC). The ANC calculation determines the total percent of neutrophils (the "polys" or "segs" plus the "bands").

Take the product ofthe total WBC count by the percentage of neutrophils to calculatethe ANC. Infections are common when the ANC is very low (ATI Testing 2016).

The child receives vaccinations before treatment according to IDSA Clinical Practice Guideline (Rubin, L., Levin, M., Ljungman, P., Davies, E., Avery, R., Tomblyn, M., Bousvaros, A., Dhanireddy, S., Sung, L., Keyserling, H., andKang, I. 2013). The nurse holds vaccinations if the immune system is severely depressed until the treatment is complete.

### Hemorrhage

Bleeding (thrombocytopenia) is a complication of myelosuppression.

The nurse avoids rectal temperatures, unnecessary skin punctures. The nurse uses surgical aseptic technique when needed and applies pressure for 5 minutes to stop bleeding. If the child has a nose bleeds treatment includes cold therapy and holding pressure. The nurse administers platelets concentrates or platelet rich plasma as ordered, and monitor for petechiae, ecchymoses, hematuria, bleeding gums, hematemesis, and tarry stools. Teach the child and parents the importance of oral care to prevent gingival bleeding through the use of a soft toothbrush. The child should avoid harsh, astringent mouthwashes. The child and family learn methods for preventing and managing epistaxis (ATI Testing 2016).

### Anemia

Anemia is a complication of myelosuppression.

The nurse may administer oxygen, fluids, and blood transfusions as prescribed while promoting rest. A diet high in iron helps stabilize anemia (ATI Testing 2016).

## BONE AND SOFT TISSUE CANCERS

A child with malignant tumors in the bone originates from the osteoid matrix, blood vessels, and/or cartilage (see Fig 12-7). Osteosarcoma usually presents in the metaphysis of long bones, commonly found in the femur. Treatment often includes amputation or a limb salvage procedure of the affected extremity and chemotherapy. Ewing's sarcoma (a primitive neuroectodermal tumor) presents in the shafts of long bones and trunk bones. Treatment options include: surgical biopsy, intensive radiation therapy to the tumor site, and chemotherapy, but does not require amputation. The prognosis depends on the progression of the disease.

Soft tissue malignancies arise from undifferentiated cells in the soft tissues anywhere in the body that includes muscles, tendons, connective or fibrous tissue, and blood or lymph vessels. Rhabdomyosarcoma originates in skeletal muscle but frequently occurs in the head and neck, especially the orbit of the eye. Treatment for tumors consists of surgical biopsy, local radiation therapy, and chemotherapy, in lieu of invasive surgical procedures (ATI Testing 2016).

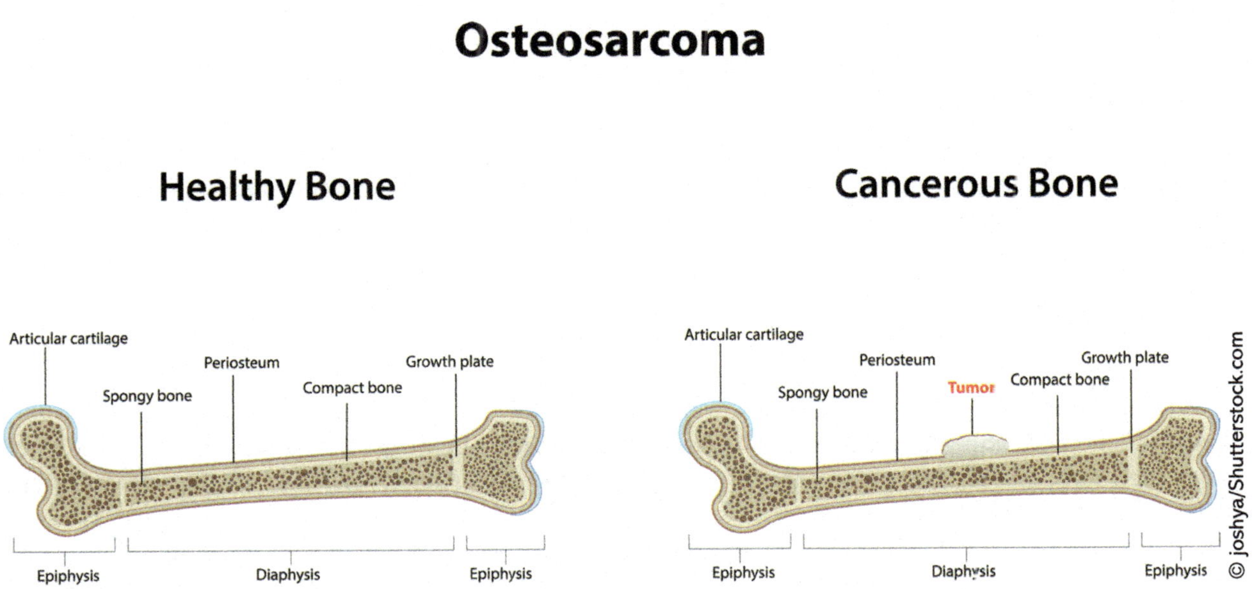


Fig 12-7 Bone tumors deform the bone

Children may also undergo irradiation for malignancies if the malignancy presents in or near the pelvic area child can develop secondary cancers and lose fertility. Risk factors for osteosarcoma include the male sex and children experiencing rapid growth in the teen years. Ewing's sarcoma presents in people under 30 years of age and of European descent. Complications are similar to other cancers discussed, including myelosuppression. Children may also develop skin desquamation (ATI Testing 2016).

# BONE TUMORS

## Assessment

Adolescents complain of nonspecific bone pain that parents and providers may mistake for injury or rapid growth spurts.

The child experiences temporary relief of pain with flexion of the extremity. The child presents with weakness, swelling, or decreased movement of the extremity (see Fig 12-8), palpable lymph nodes near the tumor, anemia, the inability to hold a heavy object, generalized infection, and/or unexplained weight loss (ATI Testing 2016).

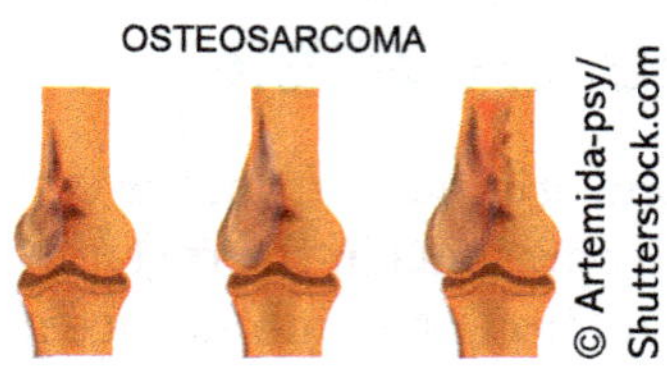


**Fig 12-8** Most cases of osteosarcoma affect the knee

## Diagnosis

### Ewing's Sarcoma

A child with Ewing's sarcoma receives x-rays, computed tomography (CT) scans, or magnetic resonance imaging (MRI) of the primary site, a bone marrow biopsy, and CT of the chest and bone scans to evaluate the progression of the disease.

A CBC helps rule out infection, iron deficiency anemia, and other possible causes of findings (ATI Testing 2016).

## Interventions

The nurse administers medication and offers psychosocial support, including the reinforcement of a realistic clinical picture. The child and family need several days to prepare for surgery and chemotherapy. The child may also undergo radiation treatment (ATI Testing 2016).

## Medications

Chemotherapy

Osteosarcoma

Several chemotherapy agents are used singly or in combination before and/ or after surgery. These agents include high-dose methotrexate with citrovorum factor rescue, doxorubicin, cisplatin, ifosfamide, and etoposide (ATI Testing 2016).

Chemotherapy agents for Ewing's sarcoma include vincristine, doxorubicin, and cyclophosphamide that alternate with ifosfamide and etoposide. The nurse premedicates the child with anti-emetics before treatment (ATI Testing 2016).

### Amitriptyline

Amitriptyline is a tricyclic antidepressant to treat neuropathic pain or phantom pain in adolescents who have had an amputation. Side effects and adverse effects include drowsiness, orthostatic hypotension, anti-cholinergic effects, seizures, mania, and cardiac dysfunction (ATI Testing 2016).

## Surgical Interventions

### Surgical Biopsy

The child's tumor is biopsied under anesthesia to determine the type of cancer and progression of the disease. The nurse performs routine preoperative and postoperative care (ATI Testing 2016).

### Limb Salvage Procedure for Bone Cancers

Limb salvage procedure for bone cancers includes chemotherapy to reduce the tumor, bone and joint replacement after the tumor resection. The nurse supports the family through the fitting and wearing of a temporary prosthesis (ATI Testing 2016).

## Teaching

The nurse educates the child and family about preoperative, postoperative care, and chemotherapy. Limb amputation may require chemotherapy preoperatively and postoperatively. The nurse teaches the child and family about stump care and phantom limb pain. The nurse explores coping mechanisms for the child and family to handle questions about the prosthesis. The nurse offers emotional support to the child and family and provides resources for support groups in the community for cancer patients with amputations and mental health wellness. The child will also receive physical and occupational therapy referrals that begin inpatients and continue after discharge (ATI Testing 2016).

## Complications

Interventions for myelosuppression are the same as other cancers discussed and include infection control and hemorrhage. Skin desquamation presents with dry or moist skin with permanent hyperpigmentation and possible injury to deep tissues underneath. The nurse dresses the child in loose fitting clothes and avoids direct sunlight or high temperatures in hopes of maintaining the skin integrity. The nurse looks for signs of infection (ATI Testing 2016).

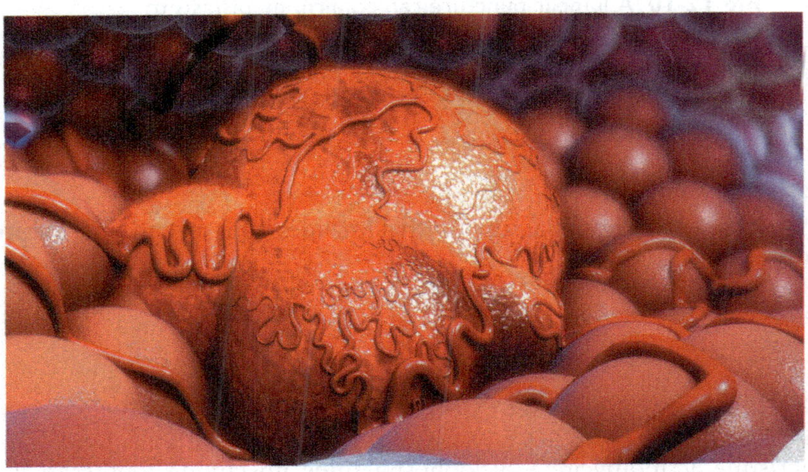



**Fig 12-9** A tumor produces its own blood supply and is highly vascular

# RHABDOMYOSARCOMA

Rhabdomyosarcoma originates in skeletal muscle creating tumors that impair muscle function. Risk factors include children under 5 years of age and European descent (ATI Testing 2016).

## Assessment

The child with rhabdomyosarcoma presents with, either pain related to the compression of soft tissue from the tumors or no pain from the complete obstruction of blood flow (ATI Testing 2016).

The assessment varies based on the location of the tumors. Children may present with headaches, diplopia, vomiting, unilateral proptosis, ecchymosis of the conjunctiva, and strabismus. They may complain of a stuffy nose, pain, nasal obstruction, and epistaxis. Children may have palpable neck nodes and a visible mass in the advanced stages of the disease. Other symptoms include nasal obstruction, pain, discharge, sinusitis, swelling, chronic otitis media, pain, sanguinopurulent discharge from the nose, and facial paralysis. Gastrointestinal assessment findings include an abdominal mass, and pain or obstruction. Genitourinary findings include obstruction and a visible superficial mass on the perineum. Children may complain of extremity pain, a palpable fixed mass, and lymph node enlargement (ATI Testing 2016).

The child undergoes a CT or MRI of the primary site. Then the provider takes a biopsy of the tumor. A lumbar puncture confirms any metastasis (ATI Testing 2016) (see Fig 12-10).

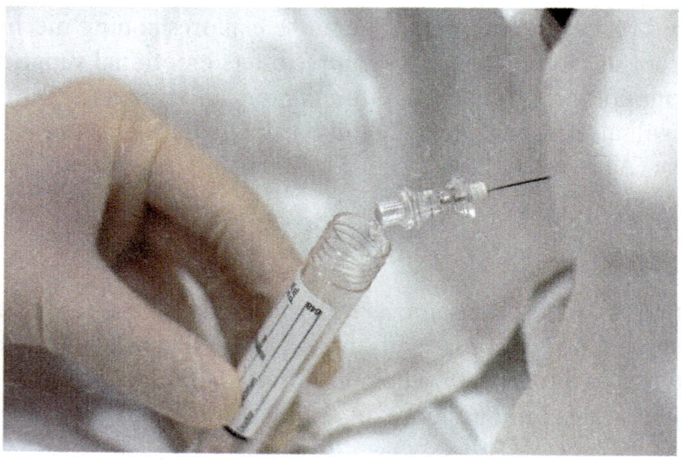



**Fig 12-10** A lumbar puncture can confirm metastasis to the CNS Diagnosis

## Interventions

The nurse provides high-quality psychosocial support that includes honesty and time for processing this family event (ATI Testing 2016).

## Medications

### Chemotherapy

The child receives vincristine, actinomycin D, cyclophosphamide, ifosfamide, topotecan, irinotecan, and doxorubicin for about 1 year. The nurse pre-medicated with anti-emetics before treatment (ATI Testing 2016).

### Localized Radiation Therapy

Radiation therapy, in combination with chemotherapy and surgery, is standard treatment. The nurse administers chemotherapy and assists with radiation treatments (ATI Testing 2016).

## Surgical Interventions

### Surgical Biopsy

A surgical biopsy of the tumor is biopsied under anesthesia to identify the type of cancer and the progression of the disease. The nurse performs preoperative and postoperative care and initiates physical and occupational therapy referrals that begin as an inpatient and continue after discharge (ATI Testing 2016).

The family and child need high-quality psychosocial support that includes preparation for pre-and post-procedure care. They will also need referrals to support groups for the child and the family. Older children need a developmentally appropriate support group with kids their own age. Mental health wellness support is essential to encourage the child to resume regular activities. Physical and occupational therapy referrals to start while in the hospital and to continue after discharge (ATI Testing 2016).

## Interventions for Complications

Interventions for skin desquamation and myelosuppression are the same as for other cancers discussed (ATI Testing 2016).

# CHAPTER HIGHLIGHTS

- Cancer has a genetic, environmental, infectious origin.
- Cancer treatments include surgery, chemotherapy, radiation, immunotherapy and stem cell transplantation.
- Common assessment findings for children with cancer include pain, anemia, infection, bruising, bleeding, and a mass.
- Nursing interventions for children with cancer include medication and chemotherapy administration, pain management, infection control, hydration and ways to preemptively manage side effects of chemotherapy.
- Wilm's tumor is found in the adrenal gland and should not be palpated.
- Neuroblastoma is cancer that responds to immunotherapy.
- Leukemia is a common childhood cancer caused by an overcrowding of immature blood cells.
- Bone cancers, such as osteosarcoma and Ewing sarcoma, are common in adolescents.

# REFERENCES

ATI Testing. 2016. Nursing Care of Children. Retrieved from http://www.atitesting.com/ati_next_gen/DisplayResources.aspx?Name=rm_rn_ncc_2016_ebook_20170417.pdf.

ATI Testing. n.d. Retrieved from http://www.atitesting.com/ati_next_gen/skillsmodules/content/cvad/viewing/CVAD_dressing_change.html.

ATI Testing. n.d. Retrieved from http://www.atitesting.com/ati_next_gen/skillsmodules/content/cvad/viewing/accss_imp_prt.html.

Cincinnati Children's Hospital Medical Center: BESt Evidence Statement—School-aged and Adolescent Bone Marrow Transplant (BMT) Recipients: Quality of Life Interventions, http://www.cincinnatichildrens.org/svc/alpha/h/health-policy/best.htm, BESt 128, 1–7, May 30, 2012.

Dumba, M., Jawad, N., and McHugh, K. 2015. Neuroblastoma and nephroblastoma: a radiological review. Cancer Imaging: The Official Publication of the International Cancer Imaging Society, 155. doi: 10.1186/s40644-015-0040-6.

Freireich, E. J., Wiernik, P. H., and Steensma, D. P. 2014. "The leukemias: a half-century of discovery." *Journal of Clinical Oncology: Official Journal of the American Society of Clinical Oncology*, 32(31), 3463–9. doi: 10.1200/JCO.2014.57.1034.

Hoy, S. and Hoy, S. M. 2016. Dinutuximab: A Review in High-Risk Neuroblastoma. Targeted Oncology, 11(2), 247–253. doi: 10.1007/s11523-016-0420-2.

McGinty, L. and Kolesar, J. 2017. Dinutuximab for maintenance therapy in pediatric neuroblastoma. American Journal of Health-System Pharmacy, 74(8), 563–7. doi: 10.2146/ajhp160228.

Rubin, L., Levin, M., Ljungman, P., Davies, E., Avery, R., Tomblyn, M., Bousvaros, A., Dhanireddy, S., Sung, L., Keyserling, H. and Kang, I. 2013. "IDSA Clinical Practice Guideline for Vaccination of the Immunocompromised Host." *Clinical Infectious Diseases*, 58(3), 309–18.

Ullman A. J., Cooke M. L., Mitchell M., Lin F., New K., Long D. A., Mihala G., and Rickard C. M. 2016. "Dressings and securement devices for central venous catheters (CVC)." *Cochrane Database of Systematic Reviews 2015*, Issue 9. Art. No.: CD010367. doi: 10.1002/14651858.CD010367.pub2.

CPSIA information can be obtained
at www.ICGtesting.com
Printed in the USA
LVOW05s2159270118
564060LV00003B/32/P